SCRIBE PUBLICATIONS
Punishing The Patient

Richard Gosden, PhD, was born in Sydney, Australia in 1945. He was originally trained in advertising, but has since travelled extensively and worked in numerous occupations. Most recently he has been an environmental campaigner and a university lecturer. He is currently employed as a research officer working on disability issues at the University of Wollongong.

Dr Gosden's doctoral thesis was a study of psychiatric controversies over the cause of the symptoms of schizophrenia. He is the author of a number of articles on environmental issues, early treatment of schizophrenia, psychiatry and human rights, and the use of psychiatry in social control. *Punishing the Patient* is his first book.

To life beyond Normal

Punishing The Patient

How Psychiatrists Misunderstand and Mistreat Schizophrenia

Richard Gosden, PhD

Scribe Publications
Melbourne

Scribe Publications Pty Ltd
PO Box 287
Carlton North, Victoria 3054, Australia
Email: scribe@bigpond.net.au

First published by Scribe Publications Pty Ltd 2001

Copyright © Richard Gosden 2001

All rights reserved. Without limiting the rights under copyright reserved above, no part of this publication may be reproduced, stored in or introduced into a retrieval system, or transmitted, in any form or by any means (electronic, mechanical, photocopying, recording or otherwise) without the prior written permission of both the copyright owner and the above publisher of this book.

Cover design by Pauline McClenahan, Captured Concepts
Typeset in Sabon by the publisher

Printed and bound in Australia
by Griffin Press, Netley, South Australia

National Library of Australia
Cataloguing-in-Publication data

Gosden, Richard.
  Punishing the patient: how psychiatrists misunderstand and mistreat schizophrenia.

  Includes index.
  ISBN 0 908011 52 0.

  1. Schizophrenia. 2. Schizophrenia - Diagnosis. 3. Schizophrenia - Treatment. I. Title.

616.898206

www.scribepub.com.au

Contents

Abbreviations		vi
Preface		vii
Acknowledgements		ix
	Introduction	1
1	Human Rights and the Medical Containment of Deviance	7
2	The Medical Model: schizophrenia as a disease	28
3	Theories Galore: the quest for a cause	53
4	Behind the Medical Model: interest groups and human rights	90
5	Non Medical Models: schizophrenia as a spiritual/mystical emergency	112
6	Shrinking Free Thought: human rights and mystical experience	151
7	Mental as Anything: schizophrenic symptoms as manufactured artefacts	165
8	Punishing the Patient: human rights and psychiatric coercion	197
9	Early Psychosis: expanding the market for preventive medicine	224
	Conclusion	248
Endnotes		265
Bibliography		285
Index		307

Abbreviations

APA American Psychiatric Association
DSM-II *Diagnostic and Statistical Manual of Mental Disorders* (2nd edn.)
DSM-III *Diagnostic and Statistical Manual of Mental Disorders* (3rd edn.)
DSM-IV *Diagnostic and Statistical Manual of Mental Disorders* (4th edn.)
EPPIC Early Psychosis Prevention and Intervention Centre
EPSE extrapyramidal side effect
ICCPR International Covenant on Civil and Political Rights
ICD-10 International Classification of Diseases (10th edn.)
ICESCR International Covenant on Economic, Social and Cultural Rights
NAMI National Alliance for the Mentally Ill
NEPP National Early Psychosis Project
PACE Personal Assistance and Crisis Evaluation
UN United Nations

Preface

I have been researching theories of schizophrenia—and about the rights of schizophrenics—for many years. Initially I undertook the research for a PhD thesis on controversies over the cause of schizophrenia. Later, it was to write this book, which is largely derived from the doctoral research.

Most books on schizophrenia are written by people who have had some kind of direct involvement with the condition as therapists, carers, or victims. At the professional level, these books range from the party line of mainstream psychiatry to the cry-in-the-dark of dissident psychiatrists who know that something is wrong with the attitudes of their mainstream colleagues, but can't say what it is. At the personal level, these books include first-hand accounts of the tribulations of caring for a child with schizophrenia, and descriptions of what it is like to be branded a schizophrenic, and to suffer the torment of living with drug treatment. All of these types of book are necessarily limited to the personal experience of the author. However, I am not a psychiatrist, or a sufferer of schizophrenia; nor am I a parent of a schizophrenic child. This book has been written from a perspective that is quite different from the usual books on schizophrenia.

My academic training is as an analyst of science and medicine. I come from that school of thought which looks upon scientific 'truths' as knowledge that has been constructed through social negotiation, like any other kind of knowledge. This background has given me some useful tools with which to deconstruct psychiatric claims and to take what I hope is an informed, fresh look at medical notions about the nature of schizophrenia.

But it was not academic work that first interested me in psychiatry and schizophrenia. I have come to academic research relatively late in life. Most of my adult life has been spent as a wanderer, and much of my knowledge about the problems of schizophrenics comes from a passage through the school of hard knocks. My dedication to human rights was cultivated by a long sojourn as a draft dodger and peace activist, and I have had abundant personal experience of social alienation and ostracism as a result of being, at different times, an unemployed person and an environmental activist. I have travelled extensively and worked in various occupations. I have also made an extended comparative study of world mystical traditions, and I have lived for several months in a Tibetan Buddhist community in which mystical practices were taught.

Throughout my years on the social margins, schizophrenia was a frequent topic of conversation amongst people I encountered. So was the threat of forced psychiatry. Being labelled with schizophrenia is considered something of an occupational hazard for people who march to the beat of a different drum, and my sincere hope is that this book might play some small part in reducing that risk.

Acknowledgements

I would like to thank Sharon Beder for her constant support throughout the many years of this project. Without her willingness to discuss ideas, read drafts, and offer advice and encouragement I could never have completed it. I would also like to thank Brian Martin, my PhD supervisor from the Science, Technology and Society Program at the University of Wollongong, for his guidance and many suggestions during the preparation of my doctoral thesis. I also want to thank David Cohen, Professor of Social Work at the Florida International University, for the sound advice he gave after reading my PhD thesis.

I am also greatly in debt to many members of the Support Coalition, World Network of (Ex-)Users and Survivors of Psychiatry, and MadNation email discussion groups. My research has benefited immeasurably from the privilege of interacting on a daily basis with these extraordinary international networks of psychiatric survivors. In this regard I want to particularly thank the co-ordinators of these organisations—David Oaks, Sylvia Caras and Vicki Fox Wieselthier—for their tireless work in bringing these vibrant electronic communities into existence.

I would also like to thank Chris Bowker for sharing her experience as a human rights advocate in the mental health field; Heather Nolan for her wonderfully descriptive letters and poignant arguments against the injustice of psychiatric coercion; and Don Weitz, for allowing me to reproduce parts of his passionately written personal story of psychiatric abuse.

I'd like to express my appreciation to my editors, Caroline Williamson and Gillian Fulcher. I'm also in debt to my courageous publisher, Henry Rosenbloom, for his willingness to take a chance, for his many hours of tireless editing, and for his many intelligent and insightful suggestions for improving the manuscript.

The diagnostic criteria for schizophrenia taken from the *Diagnostic and Statistical Manual of Mental Disorders,* fourth edition, are reprinted here with the permission of the copyright holders, the American Psychiatric Association (© 1994).

Introduction

In the mid-1990s an anxious mother began a letter-writing campaign to persuade legislators of the need to amend the Mental Health Act in the Australian state of New South Wales. Describing herself as a medical doctor with experience in psychiatry, she wrote to newspapers and politicians about her twenty-year-old son who was behaving strangely. She said that he was suffering from psychosis but was refusing to be treated. Her problem was that the mental health laws then in force in New South Wales would not allow for his involuntary treatment. To be eligible for forced treatment, her son was required to be at risk of causing serious physical harm to himself or to other people. Being a peaceful sort of young man, he didn't fit either of these criteria, and so he was allowed to remain free.

Out of frustration, she began lobbying to have the law changed. She wanted the criteria for dangerousness removed from the legislation, so that peaceful people such as her son could be forced into treatment if they were unwilling to go voluntarily. Her local member of state parliament, Dr Peter Macdonald, was a medical doctor himself, and he joined her campaign. In an effort to persuade his political colleagues to change the legislation, he read one of her letters into the parliamentary record:

> Our twenty-year-old son developed a psychosis about three years ago. He was a top student at his school, a promising musician, well liked and respected by his peers. Our relationship with him was good, and we had hopes that he would be a well-adjusted adult, able to take his place in society. Today he is wandering the

beaches and streets of Manly, to all intents and purposes a 'homeless youth'.

His psychosis (diagnosed as schizo-affective disorder) takes the form that he believes he has to convert all to Christianity because all are doomed to go to hell. He cannot explain why he believes this and he seems to think that the world is going to end soon. He gives away all his belongings and money to people he believes God is directing him to save, e.g. he gave away $2000 at Christmas. This was his entire savings.

For a while he was bringing home vagrants and they would spend the night in his bed while he wandered the streets looking for more people to save. We lost various possessions to these people, some of whom were also obviously suffering from psychosis themselves. He deprives himself of sleep as he believes he has to be 'working' i.e. evangelising.

He has lost all his friends and his relationship with us is under great strain as he puts his 'work' before all other considerations. But he is not a danger to himself or to others so he cannot be taken to hospital under the present Mental Health Act.

The doctors involved say he would probably benefit from medication for his psychosis and they want to put him on the clozapine programme but their hands are tied until such time as he deteriorates further and does something to actively harm himself or others. Meanwhile his family suffers, his relationships with all his mates are lost, he loses all his money, he smells, he neglects all that he formerly held dear when he was well.

I think it is a disgrace that our society can let this happen, and I know it is not just my son to whom this is happening. It involves many other youths who are also wandering the streets in the grip of mental illness.[1]

In 1997 the New South Wales Mental Health Act was in fact amended so that people who have unusual but peaceful habits can be forced into treatment. This change, however, was not entirely due to one person's efforts. It was part of a widespread trend all over the world to weaken civil liberties protections, in order to make it easier to force involuntary psychiatric treatment on people diagnosed as being 'psychotic'.

Psychosis, the term used to describe the young man's condition, is psychiatric language for a state of altered consciousness. To observers, psychotic people appear to have lost the ability to control their own minds and behaviour.

In psychiatric classification systems, schizophrenia is the most serious sub-type of a spectrum of psychotic disorders. The principal symptoms of schizophrenia are mental activity such as hallucinations, delusions, and disordered thinking. The hallucinations are usually in the form of inner voices that sometimes pass judgement on the person experiencing them. The inner voices also frequently supply the person with esoteric knowledge about religious and political affairs, and reveal secret meanings behind everyday events that are hidden from normal people. Unusual beliefs are formed from these internal experiences, and disordered thinking accompanies attempts to communicate the beliefs to other people.

As well as these so-called 'positive' symptoms, psychiatrists also use an alternative range of 'negative' symptoms to indicate schizophrenia. These are the opposite of the positive symptoms, in that a lack of self-expression is taken to indicate a similar lack of inner mental activity. On top of these, degrees of social and occupational dysfunction are also used as diagnostic tools. There are no laboratory tests to verify the presence of schizophrenia, and identification of the condition relies on the subjective opinions of those making the diagnosis.

Despite all this apparent certainty about the condition, and after almost one hundred years of recognition as a valid and distinct mental illness by mainstream psychiatry, schizophrenia still remains controversial in many ways. There is controversy about the psychiatric classification system that identifies a diverse range of signs as symptoms of a distinct mental disorder; there is controversy over diagnosis for the condition; there is controversy over treatments, particularly when the treatment is given without informed consent; and there is controversy over the causes.

It is the linked issues of diagnosis, treatment and causes that are together the main focus of this book. On the one hand, I believe that the diagnostic criteria for schizophrenia are so broad that people are included who clearly do not have medical problems. There are some people, for instance, who are diagnosed when they are undergoing a spiritual/mystical emergency, and others who are only diagnosed for having problems of living arising from social or occupational dysfunctions. Many others are misdiagnosed with schizophrenia when they actually have drug- or substance-related disorders that have other diagnoses.

On the other hand, schizophrenia is almost always treated with drugs upon a diagnosis being made, whether the patient consents or not. In fact, more than half of all people treated for schizophrenia are involuntary patients. Unlike voluntary patients, people who have psychiatric treatment forced on them are not 'consumers'; instead, their forced treatment is justified with what I think are often cynical interpretations of 'the right to treatment' and 'informed consent'.

The drugs used to treat schizophrenia manage but do not cure the condition. They are also dangerous, and have a wide range of debilitating side effects. Even so, there are now insistent demands being made by mental health professionals and support groups for patients' relatives that drug treatment be given at the earliest signs of schizophrenic symptoms. These demands are supported by an international lobbying campaign sponsored by drug companies to alter mental health legislation to make it easier for psychiatrists to force treatment on unwilling patients.

For all the above reasons, I have developed serious concerns about the human rights of people who receive psychiatric treatment for schizophrenia, whether voluntarily or involuntarily. My greatest concern is that when psychiatrists force treatment on people they bypass the normal doctor/patient contractual arrangements, and other human rights come into play that are not normally associated with medicine. People who are forced into treatment when they are undergoing a mystical experience, for instance, are entitled to feel that their 'right to the freedom of thought and belief' is being violated. This is a fundamental human right guaranteed in United Nations' covenants and declarations.

Similarly, people who are incarcerated and forcibly treated for only having social or occupational problems can complain legitimately that their rights to 'liberty' and to protection against 'torture, or cruel, inhuman or degrading treatment or punishment' are being violated. These rights are also guaranteed by international law.

As things stand, psychiatrists deflect complaints such as these by claiming that all people who are diagnosed with schizophrenia are, by definition, mentally ill and therefore have a 'right to treatment'. According to this way of thinking, forcing treatment on patients is merely a way of respecting this right. Any claims to the contrary by patients are simply further signs of their mental illness. To put it mildly, I disagree. The central objective of this book is to show that there are serious problems of truth and justice arising from these psychiatric beliefs and attitudes. I hope this book demonstrates that spiritual/mystical emergencies and social alienation are not medical problems, and that when people undergoing these experiences are diagnosed and forcibly treated for schizophrenia they clearly have valid complaints that their human rights are being violated.

The description of the young man above, who was the subject of his mother's letter-writing and political campaign, raises many of the uncertainties that surround the mental disorder which psychiatrists call psychosis. Did he have a problem with his mind, or was his problem primarily one of social adjustment? If he had a mental problem, was it caused by an imbalance in his brain chemistry (which should have been rectified with medication) or was he undergoing a religious/spiritual emergency (which forced drug treatment would have suppressed but left unresolved)?

His mother's opinion—that he was in desperate need of medical attention—wasn't just that of an anxious parent. She was a medical doctor with experience in psychiatric problems. She had to be taken seriously. When she said her son was suffering from psychosis, she presumably knew what she was talking about. But can we be certain that she did? Ordinary lay people wouldn't necessarily read signs, such as his apparent selfless generosity, as indications of mental illness. To some people, he might have been showing signs of a virtuous spirit. Some might even argue that he appeared to be acting under the influence of a perfectly legitimate religious inspiration. If he believed that he was acting under God's direction, and he was doing more good than harm by helping homeless people, was it right for his mother and her psychiatric consultants to intervene? At twenty years of age, after all, he was a grown man.

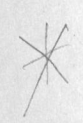

Other people might see this particular young man as having been under the influence of something far less dramatic than either madness or sainthood. Like so many young people before him, perhaps he was simply rebelling against the middle-class values of his parents. But his mother didn't think so. And, as she said, there are a great many young people like her son wandering around. The question is this: are differently minded people like her son in need of forced psychiatric intervention to alter the direction of their lives? If they remain untreated, are they at risk of harm greater than the risks of their treatment, and do they cause social problems that are more serious than the obvious disappointment and distress they bring to their loving parents?

1

Human Rights and the Medical Containment of Deviance

The problems of truth and justice associated with forced psychiatric treatment are not confined to schizophrenia. There is a widespread trend in developed countries to expand the use of psychiatric coercion by medicalising various forms of mental and behavioural deviance that were formerly considered problems of character, intelligence, morals, and discipline. Children and adolescents are particularly targeted in this expansion. A recent report in a leading British newspaper described what has become a growing reliance on psychiatric drugs to control the behaviour of children. The headline, 'Doctors could soon prescribe behaviour-controlling chemicals to pre-teens against their parents' wishes', was an accurate summary of the report:

> More than three-quarters of a million children could be given drugs to control their behaviour—against their wishes and those of their parents. The spectre is raised by legislation planned by the government to give more powers to psychiatrists.
> Mental-health workers are warning that the new legislation is being drawn so widely that doctors will be given the right to drug children just because they have a difficulty with math or spelling.

The concern over the legislation follows alarming evidence that tens of thousands of schoolchildren with mild behaviour problems are being drugged with Ritalin—dubbed the 'chemical cosh' or 'kiddie crack'—simply in order to control them.

In England, the number of prescriptions for the mind-drug Ritalin—which is given to so-called 'hyperactive' children to improve concentration—has shot up from just 3500 in 1993 to 126,500 in 1998.

The UK is rapidly following in the path of the US, where a report last week showed that three million children—one in every 30—are now being given Ritalin. Children as young as two are being given mood-altering drugs, including anti-depressants.

The new legislation will give far greater powers to psychiatrists to give compulsory treatment in the community to both adults and children.[1]

Surveys have demonstrated the need for the expansion of psychiatric powers by uncovering mental illness in epidemic proportions in a number of countries. A recent survey in the Australian state of South Australia found that more than one-quarter of the adults it studied were in need of psychiatric attention: the researchers claimed that 26.4 per cent of 1,009 ordinary rural adults had mental illnesses, and that 11 per cent had two or more disorders. A similar study in Christchurch, New Zealand found that 20.6 per cent of the general population had mental illnesses, and two studies in the United States found rates of 20 per cent and 29 per cent.[1]

The South Australian study found that only 4.2 per cent of the people with mental illnesses had seen a psychiatrist or psychologist in the previous twelve months; it agreed with US researchers that 'most community residents are not treated for their psychiatric problems'. The blame for this was aimed at general practitioners, who were thought to be under-diagnosing mental illness.

But the findings can be interpreted in an entirely different way. Of 1,009 people in South Australia, eleven acknowledged that they had mental problems and had sought specialist treatment for them.

A further 255 people were 'diagnosed' by the researchers with mental illnesses but were not receiving treatment. From the medical point of view, these 255 people should have been receiving treatment. But the people themselves apparently disagreed, and seemed prepared to cope with life in their untreated state. Experience tells us that if they were not coping without treatment it is likely that they would have already come into contact with psychiatry as either voluntary or involuntary patients.

By finding more than one-quarter of the population to be mentally ill, when these same people were willing to carry on with life as they were, the South Australian researchers raised an interesting question. Are we living in a society that is quite literally part mad, in which a quarter of the population are unaware that they have already developed mental illnesses, and the rest of us appear unwilling to acknowledge that soon it might be our turn? Or is there something wrong with the diagnostic techniques used by the researchers? Is there something about the way psychiatry is practised that predisposes psychiatrists to find mental pathology where ordinary non-medical people might find foolishness, stupidity, aggression, laziness, drunkenness, boorishness, unhappiness, self-doubt, and numerous other character flaws—faults that affect most people at some time or another, making us unpleasant company, but which do not really distinguish us as having diseased minds?

This non-medical approach is sometimes referred to as the 'moral model' to distinguish it from the medical or psychiatric approach. In a discussion about the differences between the moral and the medical models, Ronald Leifer has observed:

> When the moral model is used to explain human behaviour, it is assumed the person has the capacity for free choice and is responsible and accountable for his or her actions. The medical model, on the other hand, is deterministic and explains human actions in terms of antecedent causes. These causes may be biochemical, social, psychological or historical.[3]

The South Australian survey shows the huge gap that exists between the medical view of the community's state of mental well-being and the community's own view of itself. This confirms sociological research which has found that 'lay beliefs are often quite distinctive in form and content' to clinical medicine.[4]

The DSM Diagnostic System

Here we come to a key document used internationally in the diagnosis of 'mental illness', and one that will be referred to repeatedly in this book. The Australian researchers used a manual devised and published by the American Psychiatric Association (APA) to identify mental disorder in their state of South Australia. The APA is the main professional organisation of psychiatrists in the United States, and its diagnostic manual—the *Diagnostic and Statistical Manual of Mental Disorders* (DSM)—has become one of two international standards for psychiatric diagnosis. (The other is the World Health Organisation's ICD-10, which will be discussed in detail in Chapter 2.) The DSM system is so deeply entrenched in the medical practice of English-speaking countries such as the United States and Australia that codes from the manual are used for making medical claims for psychiatric expenses.

Early versions of the DSM had little pretence of being scientific, and were largely heuristic guide-books that incorporated much of the psychiatric lore derived from Freudian psychoanalytical techniques.[5] But with the third revision in 1980, a 'fateful point in the history of the American psychiatric profession was reached ... The decision of the APA first to develop DSM-III and then to promulgate its use represents a significant reaffirmation on the part of American psychiatry to its medical identity and its commitment to scientific medicine'.[6] Subsequent revisions of the manual have also claimed scientific status.

The recent editions of DSM attempt to classify all deviant personality types so as to provide a universal reference for aspects of human expression and identity that require psychiatric modification. The preparation of the most recent edition of the manual, DSM-IV, was a 'team effort' involving more than one thousand people. In its pages, codes and descriptions are supplied for nearly four hundred separate mental disorders. They range in scope from 'Disorders Usually First Diagnosed in Infancy, Childhood or Adolescence' such as the learning disorders (315.00 Reading Disorder and 315.1 Mathematics Disorder) and the disruptive behaviour disorder (313.81 Oppositional Defiant Disorder) through to a whole range of adult forms of deviancy, including substance abuse of various kinds, sexual dysfunctions, personality disorders, and psychoses. A recent reviewer, prompted by the breadth of its scope, facetiously observed that, 'According to the Diagnostic and Statistical Manual of Mental Disorders, Fourth Edition, human life is a form of mental illness'.[7]

There are obvious dangers to civil liberties arising from the empowerment of medical practitioners to use the DSM system as a template for dividing the general population into a normal 75 per cent and an unfit 25 per cent. But even if the alienation of a quarter of the population were acceptable in terms of civil liberties, why should a conservative American professional organisation be relied upon to specify the types of people that are socially unacceptable in other countries such as Australia? Consider, for instance, some of the features of 301.7 Antisocial Personality Disorder:

> Irresponsible work behaviour may be indicated by significant periods of unemployment ... or by the abandonment of several jobs without a realistic plan for getting another job. There may be a pattern of repeated absences from work ... They may have an inflated and arrogant self-appraisal (for example feel that ordinary work is beneath them or lack a realistic concern about their current problems or their future) and may be excessively opinionated, self-assured or cocky.[8]

This type of person may be unattractive to employers in the United States, and indeed to employers in other parts of the world as well. But do most people really believe that these character traits are manifestations of mental disease? Some Australian psychiatrists have argued against the respect given to the DSM system in Australia, particularly by courts of law, complaining that 'the DSM is no more than a distillate of the prejudices and power plays of a group of aging American academics, of no interest to most Europeans and only passing relevance to some Australasians.'[9]

Apart from the doubtful classification system, which purports to match aspects of personality and self-expression with specific underlying mental diseases, there is also uncertainty about whether diagnosticians are able to consistently identify the forms of deviance that the manual describes. Because the classification system largely deals with manifestations of mind and personality, doctors are obliged to identify and diagnose the mental disorders that the system specifies by making subjective value judgements without the assistance of definitive methods of measurement or laboratory tests.

This means that someone who is 'excessively opinionated, self-assured and cocky' to one diagnostician could easily be 'well-informed, confident and amusing' to another. In fact, when two psychiatrists are required to interview the same patient on admission to a psychiatric hospital, it has been found that the level of agreement between them is often little better than chance. In regard to schizophrenia, for instance, researchers concluded—after assessing six studies conducted in the United States and the United Kingdom—that diagnostic agreement between psychiatrists was 'no better than fair'.[10]

Growth of the Mental Health Industry

Despite the known shortcomings of psychiatric diagnosis, the mental health industry continues to expand. Between 1975 and 1990 the number of psychiatrists in the United States increased from 26,000 to 36,000; clinical psychologists increased from 15,000 to 42,000; and clinical social workers increased from

25,000 to 80,000. The total cost of mental health care rose between 1980 and 1990 from about $20 billion to about $55 billion.[11]

The 'medicalisation of deviance' is becoming particularly apparent in the socialisation of children; in fact, the early detection of supposedly serious psychiatric problems in children is a widely discussed imperative. In New South Wales (NSW), Australia's most populous state, the Schizophrenia Information Centre warns parents to be watchful for early signs of schizophrenia in their children, advising that treatment should be given immediately if any symptoms are observed. One of the signs they advise parents to look for is a child who is observed to 'say or do things most people find socially embarrassing—such as telling someone they're ugly or their nose is a funny shape ... It is as if their brain disorder involves some damage to the internal "filter" which helps people sort out what's appropriate from what's not.'[12]

A recent paper on childhood schizophrenia in the United States gives a number of examples of supposedly psychotic symptoms that have been observed in child patients. The observations include:

> An 8-year-old girl reported hearing multiple voices including the voice of a dead baby brother saying—'I love you sister, sister I'm going to miss you'. An 11-year-old boy heard God's voice saying, 'Sorry D., but I can't come now, I'm helping someone else'. An 8-year-old girl reported an angel saying things like, 'You didn't cry today' and 'You've been a very nice girl today'. An 8-year-old boy stated, 'I can hear the devil talk—God interrupts him and the devil says "shut up God". God and the devil are always fighting'. A boy described monsters calling him 'Stupid F ...' and saying they will hurt him.'[13]

The researcher reports that the mean age of the onset of non-psychotic symptoms in these children was 4.6 years; the mean age of the onset of psychotic symptoms was 6.9 years; and the mean age at diagnosis of schizophrenia was 9.5 years.[14]

It is worth noting that this particular study was conducted in

Los Angeles on 38 children, seventeen of whom were black, sixteen Hispanic, four white, and one Asian. All the children had been screened to ensure that their symptoms met strict DSM criteria for schizophrenia.[15] The DSM description of schizophrenia is normally used to determine abnormality in adults, and it is extraordinary to read a paper such as this, published in a prestigious journal of the United States' National Institute of Mental Health, reporting research that had adapted these diagnostic criteria for use on children without any explanation. The researcher seemed to believe that children should meet the same standards of conformity in their thoughts, beliefs, and expression that are expected of adults.

Perhaps the racial background of the children can help explain why the researcher apparently held such a view. Observers of psychiatric trends in the United States have become concerned about a tendency to fund research into a perceived link between inner-city street crime and an assumed imbalance of brain chemistry in the perpetrators. A part of this line of research involves the development of new psychiatric drugs that, it is hoped, will pacify aggressive people by increasing the availability of serotonin in their brains. Young black males are seen as the prime targets for this type of therapy. The accompanying debate has inspired the headline in at least one black newspaper, 'Plot To Sedate Black Youth'.[16]

Social Control, Youth, and Unemployment

The use of psychiatry as a means of social control is becoming apparent in preventive medicine programmes for various mental illnesses. These programmes are designed to detect children and young people who have divergent thinking and behavioural patterns, and to get them into treatment before their supposed mental illnesses develop. In Australia, as part of the National Mental Health Strategy, programmes have recently been initiated which are aimed at the early detection and treatment of psychosis in young people. Clinical guidelines for best practice in this area describe the risk factors and signs that can be used to identify young people who are in need of prophylactic drug treatment to prevent the development of psychotic conditions such as schizophrenia. (See Chapter 9.)

Unfortunately, even official human rights watchdogs such as the Australian Human Rights and Equal Opportunity Commission seem to be unaware of the harm that might be done by encouraging the early diagnosis and treatment of mental illness. A 1993 report by the Commission on human rights and mental illness claimed that:

> Conduct disorder and other disruptive behaviours are a source of considerable morbidity in child and adolescent mental health with problems occurring in 3.2–6.9 per cent of young people ... Prevention of conduct disorders in childhood and adolescence, or their early and effective treatment, is of special significance given the great personal, social and economic costs produced by antisocial behaviour and other disorders.[17]

Conduct disorder is specifically confined to children and adolescents, and some psychiatrists believe it is a precursor of schizophrenia.[18] According to DSM-IV, 'The essential feature of Conduct Disorder is a repetitive and persistent pattern of behaviour in which the basic rights of others or major age-appropriate societal norms or rules are violated.'[19] Staying out late at night despite parental prohibitions is one of the signs. The textbook recommendation for treating this kind of waywardness is dosing with haloperidol,[20] a high-strength neuroleptic drug used for treating schizophrenia. (Neuroleptic drugs are a subset of mind-altering drugs known as psychotropics. They were previously known as anti-psychotics and major tranquillisers.)

The Commission's report was particularly enthusiastic about the early diagnosis and treatment of schizophrenia:

> Psychiatrists working with general practitioners in an English community have been able to detect the earliest signs of

schizophrenia—and with education, supportive interventions and short-term psychotropic medication—prevent the onset of an episode ... Obviously this research must be repeated and tested in different settings, including Australia, but these early findings are encouraging and warrant urgent attention.[21]

The Commission was implying that it might be useful to screen the general population for 'the earliest signs of schizophrenia'. But if this screening were to be carried out, and people with the 'earliest signs' were coerced into preventive mental health programmes, the effect would be to lower the community's tolerance level for individual differences in thoughts and beliefs. The current tolerance level is only crossed when a person demonstrates the degree of individual difference indicated by the symptoms of psychosis. But in the absence of any laboratory tests for schizophrenia, the 'earliest signs' might simply be minor deviations from expected norms in speech and behaviour. Children and adolescents who are thought to be in need of discipline, and people marginalised through unemployment and homelessness, might be particularly vulnerable.

Unemployment and lower socio-economic status have long been closely linked with schizophrenia. During the Great Depression of the 1930s, researchers in Chicago found that the rate for treated schizophrenia was nearly three times higher in the slum areas than in the most affluent areas. Modern psychiatrists believe that 'it has become so common for schizophrenics to be out of work' that unemployment has become one of the main indicators of the disorder.[22] United States-based dissident psychiatrist Thomas Szasz has argued that youth unemployment is a major risk factor for receiving a diagnosis of schizophrenia.[23]

DSM-IV defines a mental disorder as a condition that 'causes clinically significant distress or impairment in social, occupational, or other important areas of functioning'.[24] This suggests that a psychiatrist charged with making an assessment of an unemployed person might begin with the assumption that the person's 'occupational impairment' indicates the presence of a mental disorder in need of diagnosis. This approach is reinforced by more specific advice on how to identify schizophrenics: 'Many individuals are unable to hold a job for sustained periods of time and are employed at a lower level than their parents (downward drift).'[25]

Another authoritative diagnostic manual, the World Health Organisation's ICD-10, contains a description of schizophrenia that might be even more threatening for unemployed people. The following diagnostic guidelines are given to identify one of the ICD-10 sub-types of schizophrenia called 'simple schizophrenia':

> Simple schizophrenia is a difficult diagnosis to make with any confidence because it depends on establishing the slowly progressive development of the characteristic 'negative' symptoms of residual schizophrenia without any history of hallucinations, delusions, or other manifestations of an earlier psychotic episode, and with significant changes in personal behaviour, manifest as a marked loss of interest, idleness, and social withdrawal over a period of a least one year.[26]

It should be noted that this sub-type of schizophrenia does not require the usual signs of psychosis. It is quite likely that the description of 'simple schizophrenia' would easily fit a great number of people who have been forced to adapt to the experience of long-term unemployment.

Unemployment is now at chronically high levels in most parts of the world and, apart from the link with schizophrenia and other mental diseases, there is also a traditional tendency to view unemployed people as a socially destabilising force, in need of control. Unemployment for 15-19 year olds in Australia, for instance, currently hovers around 20 per cent.[27] This means that at any given time about 20 per cent of the country's youth workforce could be said to suffer from the psychiatric symptom of 'occupational dysfunction'. The assumed link between mental illness and unemployment is now so deeply entrenched in contemporary thinking that the Human Rights Commission's report on mental illness naively repeated claims that 'more than 50% of unemployed young people suffer from depression'.[28]

Expanding Captive Drug Markets

For the past decade, increasingly insistent psychiatric hyperbole has been promising imminent breakthroughs in knowledge and treatments for a number of mental illnesses, particularly schizophrenia. These exaggerated claims have frequently been combined with drug company-funded 'right to treatment' campaigns run by support groups for the relatives of mental patients. The combined force of drug companies, psychiatrists, and relatives' support groups has persuaded both the public and governments that mental health services and budgets should be expanded, and that civil liberties protections should be weakened, so that more people can be forced into treatment.

An example of the type of pressure arising from this situation can be found in the 1995 annual report of the NSW Mental Health Review Tribunal—a quasi-judicial body constituted under the NSW Mental Health Act with designated responsibilities for hearing appeals and reviewing the cases of detained mental patients. Scattered throughout the 1995 report were repeated references to a perception by members of the tribunal that involuntary commitment to mental hospitals was being unnecessarily restricted.

The tribunal claimed that civil liberties protections were being interpreted in a way that was too restrictive of psychiatric practice, and that a much wider net should be cast for coercive use of psychiatry. The tribunal even went so far as to argue that the criteria for involuntary commitment should be expanded to include people with personality disorders 'who would benefit from behavioural modification, rehabilitation, or drug and alcohol programmes'.[29]

Ironically, in the same report, the tribunal also drew attention to the rate at which the numbers of involuntary patients had been steadily increasing under the existing criteria.[30] The total number of involuntary hospital admissions in NSW rose from 5,499 in 1992,[31] to 7,370 in 1995,[32] a 34 per cent increase in three years. (By 1998 this number had risen to 10,078, almost double the 1992 figure.)[33]

This increase had been accompanied by an even more accelerated rise in the numbers of community counselling orders (CCOs) and community treatment orders (CTOs). Both orders are legal devices that facilitate the commitment of people as outpatients, and allow for mobile treatment teams to enter people's homes and forcibly inject them with long-acting drugs. The law provides for arrest and incarceration in a mental hospital for non-compliance. The combined total of CCOs and CTOs issued in NSW had risen from 510 in 1992[34] to 1,901 in 1995[35]—a 270 per cent increase in three years. (The 1998 figure was 2,998, nearly six times the number in 1992.)[36] Strangely, even though the tribunal was calling for a weakening of civil liberties protection, they still made the observation that there was a developing 'trend towards coercive, as opposed to consensual treatment' under the existing criteria.[37]

Outpatients' commitment is currently being introduced in the United States, state by state. This concept introduces a new dimension to mental health arrangements that worries many observers. One of the major concerns is the lack of restriction on the number of people who might eventually be controlled by forced drugging. Before the development of outpatients' commitment, a person had to be incarcerated in a hospital to receive involuntary treatment. This requirement placed finite limits, in terms of the availability of accommodation and funding, on the total number of people who could be subjected to forced treatment at any given time. But outpatients' commitment removes those limitations. It remains to be seen how many people will eventually be diagnosed with mental illnesses such as schizophrenia, and then placed into forced treatment programmes, while still living in their own homes.

There are indications that drug company profits might be a factor in this trend. Involuntary patients are quite literally a captive market for psychiatric drugs. One analyst of the pharmaceutical market recently argued that the $1 billion-a-year US market for schizophrenia drugs could be expanded to $4.5 billion a year if all the people with identifiable symptoms of schizophrenia could be forced into treatment with the newer, more expensive drugs.[38]

On top of the market expansion promised by outpatients' commitment in developed countries, a lot of attention has also been directed towards expanding psychiatric applications in developing countries. In 1997, psychiatric researchers claimed that schizophrenia was afflicting about 24.4 million people in low-income societies. This was said to be a 45 per cent increase since 1985.[39]

This increasing tendency to medicalise deviance in poorer countries might force mainstream human rights groups such as Amnesty International to pay more attention to violations arising from psychiatric practices. To date, human rights activists have under-rated the significance of psychiatric abuse, despite the historical role that psychiatric atrocities have played in developing the concept of human rights.

Human Rights and Psychiatry

The international system for the protection of human rights was developed after the Second World War, largely in response to Nazi atrocities. The Nazis had held a collective belief that the German nation was a living organism, and that its wellbeing was threatened by 'useless eaters' and 'life unworthy of life'.[40] German doctors, 45 per cent of whom belonged to the Nazi Party in the early 1930s, were empowered to tend to the health of the national organism. The psychiatric branch of the profession led the way by 'medically killing' some 80,000–100,000 hospitalised mental patients. The expertise that the Nazi psychiatrists acquired in killing off their mental patients was later applied to Jewish people.[41]

In modern democratic societies psychiatry treads a very fine line between benefiting and harming the exercise of human rights. While the basic principle of human rights is to set limits on the degree of social authority that is allowed to be imposed on individuals, the speciality of psychiatry is to fit 'difficult' individuals into the social fabric. In this way psychiatry can become opposed to human rights, even in the most benign political conditions.

When 'difficult' individuals acknowledge that they have a mental problem and seek treatment for it, psychiatry is not directly opposed to human rights. Article 12 of the International Covenant on Economic, Social and Cultural Rights (ICESCR) concerns 'the right of everyone to the enjoyment of the highest attainable standard of physical and mental health.' Signatory nations are instructed to provide for '[t]he creation of conditions which would assure to all medical service and medical attention in the event of sickness'.[42] These human rights are the basis for the 'right to treatment' which is often promoted by advocates of drug treatment as being the most important human right that relates to psychiatry.

But the 'right to treatment' can have a hollow ring to it when psychiatry is practised on people against their will. Involuntary mental patients often find themselves in a situation in which they are incarcerated for an indefinite period without being charged with a criminal offence. They can be interrogated, coerced into changing their thoughts and beliefs, subjected to painful and uncomfortable treatments if they cannot or will not make the required mental changes, and denied freedom until their self-identity has been sufficiently modified. It is in this context that questions arise about whether certain psychiatric practices might violate other human rights that are more fundamental than the 'right to treatment'.

Soviet Psychiatry

Perhaps the most widely recognised example of human rights abuse by psychiatry occurred in the Soviet Union. In the last couple of decades of the Soviet regime, the communist authorities viewed a growing epidemic of political dissidence as a malign social force, and Soviet psychiatrists were empowered to assist in dealing with it.

As early as 1974, psychiatrists in the West had become curious about reports of the high prevalence of schizophrenia in the Soviet Union: 5–7 per 1,000 population compared to 3–4 per 1,000 in the United Kingdom.[43] In due course, it was revealed that Soviet psychiatrists had discovered a unique form of mental disease to fit the profile of political dissidents. They called the condition 'sluggish schizophrenia, a form of schizophrenia where the symptoms are subtle, latent or only apparent to the skilled eye of the psychiatrist'. Soviet dissidents who 'wanted to reform the system and claimed that they had the personal vision to do it ... were exhibiting the textbook symptoms of sluggish schizophrenia.'[44] Soviet psychiatrists became so deeply involved in the control of political dissidents that a whole system of special mental hospitals was established, which they ran in co-operation with the KGB.

When this became apparent to the international psychiatric community, there was widespread condemnation of the Soviet practice. Pre-empting their inevitable expulsion from the World Psychiatric Association (WPA), the Soviet professional organisation, the All-Union Society of Neuropathologists and Psychiatrists, resigned in 1983.[45] The WPA responded by announcing that the Soviets would be welcome to return if they provided 'evidence beforehand of amelioration of the political abuse of psychiatry in the Soviet Union'.[46] It is worth noting that the WPA considered that 'amelioration' was all that was necessary to bring the Soviets back into line with international standards. The reason for this conciliatory approach may have been the general perception amongst Western psychiatrists that, despite the abuses, 'the concept of disease employed in the former USSR ... was similar to its counterpart in the UK and USA in being strongly scientific in nature.'[47]

United Nations' Principles on Mental Illness

The Soviet use of psychiatry for political purposes was the catalyst for a more general investigation into international psychiatric practices by the United Nations (UN) Commission on Human Rights. In 1977 the commission appointed a 'Sub-Commission to study, with a view to formulating guidelines, if possible, the question of the protection of those detained on the grounds of mental ill-health against treatment that might adversely affect the human personality and its physical and intellectual integrity'. The primary task given to the two Special Rapporteurs that the sub-commission subsequently appointed was to 'determine whether adequate grounds existed for detaining persons on the grounds of mental ill-health'.[48]

The UN Principles for the Protection of Persons with Mental Illness and for the Improvement of Mental Health Care did not emerge until more than a decade later.[49] Unfortunately, despite the brave start, the final document was so repeatedly rewritten and massaged by numerous committees dominated by psychiatrists that the primary tasks of attending to involuntary detention and the risks of treatment were largely buried by cross-referencing and other priorities.

The final version of the principles adopted by the UN General Assembly in 1991 was primarily designed to protect the rights of voluntary patients, not involuntary patients. Principle 1 begins with an assertion of the 'right to treatment'. This right thereafter becomes the basis for most of the other voluntary patients' concerns, such as confidentiality and protection against discrimination, addressed by the document.

Where the principles do address the problems of involuntary patients, it is done in a way that tends to undermine their rights rather than protect them. Principle 11, for instance, deals with 'Consent to Treatment' and specifies that 'No treatment shall be given to a patient without his or her informed consent, except as provided for in paragraphs 6, 7, 8, 13, and 15.' Paragraph 6, however, denies the right of informed consent to involuntary patients: '... treatment may be given to a patient without a patient's informed consent if the following conditions are satisfied: (a) The patient is, at the relevant time, held as an involuntary patient'.[50]

When the principles were introduced in 1991, they allowed for more psychiatric coercion than did much of the pre-existing mental health legislation in the signatory countries. In the early 1990s, for instance, the Mental Health Act[51] in the state of New South Wales required that a person be thought likely to cause serious physical harm to themselves or other people before involuntary commitment was permitted. But under the new UN principles, physical dangerousness is not required, and a person can be involuntarily committed merely because 'a qualified mental health practitioner' considers the person's condition is likely to deteriorate, or treatment will be prevented, without incarceration.[52]

The weakness of the UN principles in relation to the rights of involuntary patients makes them useless as a frontline defence against psychiatric abuse of fundamental human rights such as the 'right to liberty', the 'right to protection against torture, cruel, inhuman or degrading treatment', and the 'freedom of thought and belief'. In fact, the principles are so weak they probably wouldn't even deter the blatant Soviet-type of political abuse that brought them into existence. Although Principle 4 apparently stipulates that diagnosis 'shall be made in accordance with internationally accepted standards', and 'A determination of mental illness shall never be made on the basis of political, economic or social status',[53] these requirements effectively ask psychiatrists to be cautious in the language they use when they are describing the symptoms of their burgeoning array of mental disorders.

The Burdekin Inquiry

The UN Commission on Human Rights wasn't the only official human rights body to be galvanised into action by the Soviet example, only to end up burying psychiatry's darker side beneath a restatement of the 'right to treatment'. The Australian Human Rights Commissioner, Brian Burdekin, in his opening address to the Sydney hearings of the 1991–92 Inquiry into Human Rights and Mental Illness, said that Soviet human rights abuses in this area had been the catalyst for his own inquiry.[54]

Burdekin explained that human rights circles in the Western democracies had formed the view that investigations were required into the mental health systems of democratic countries, to ensure that they were beyond reproach, before a full human rights assault could be launched on the Soviet psychiatric system. He said that his own inquiry had been conceived as part of this project, but that while preparations had been under way to commence his inquiry the issue had gone off the boil because the Soviet Union had collapsed. This change of affairs might partly explain why the inquiry failed to fulfil one of its key terms of reference.

The inquiry's first term of reference clearly listed the classes of people it had originally intended to deal with: 'To inquire into the human rights and fundamental freedoms afforded to persons who are or have been or *are alleged to be* affected by mental illness, having due regard for the rights of their families and members of the general community'.[55] [my italics]

What is meant by 'alleged to be' affected by mental illness is not immediately apparent. An early usage of the term 'alleged mental illness' can be found in a published dialogue between United States' patient-rights activist Leonard Roy Frank and American Civil Liberties Union attorney and mental patient advocate Bruce Ennis. Ennis explained in the interview that he used 'alleged mental illness' because 'I personally have seen no evidence at all that there is such a thing as mental illness'.[56] It is possible that the inquiry, like Ennis, had originally intended to question the existence of all mental illnesses.

Alternatively, the inquiry might have only intended to indicate a level of uncertainty in the accuracy of diagnoses of mental illness. There are at least two ways the inquiry could have utilised this distinction. The first would have been to examine the issue of false positive diagnoses. This is a perennial problem for psychiatry: it arises from the subjective nature of psychiatric diagnostic techniques and the lack of laboratory tests to confirm diagnoses. The second would have been to review patients diagnosed with certain varieties of mental illness—such as the Soviets' sluggish schizophrenia—which are not generally recognised by international standards, but which some psychiatrists allege exist. Perhaps the inquiry had originally planned to investigate both problems. There are well-established concerns in both areas.

Regardless of what the inquiry's original interpretation of 'alleged' mental illness might have been, it was certainly appropriate for an inquiry into human rights and mental illness to investigate complaints from any person who had suffered the discomfort and humiliation of a psychiatric diagnosis, and possibly incarceration and imposed treatment, on the basis of a mere allegation. But despite the nomination of this category in its terms of reference, the inquiry completely ignored these people. They were not mentioned in the inquiry's report at all beyond a rehearsal of the terms of reference.

In fact, the definitions that were eventually adopted by the inquiry made it impossible to recognise people who are 'alleged' to be mentally ill. This is because the inquiry chose to use the term 'consumer'[57] to describe all of the people covered by the terms of reference—thereby implying that people who have been diagnosed with mental illnesses are all willing participants in a mental health service industry. This title of 'consumer' was an inappropriate description for people who are 'alleged' to be mentally ill. It appears that, some time between when the terms of reference were drafted and the hearings of witnesses began, a decision was made to prevent people who were 'alleged' to be mentally ill from influencing the outcome of the inquiry.

The failure to pursue one of its key terms of reference is a disturbing outcome for the Human Rights Commission. It reflects a general relaxation of civil liberties vigilance towards psychiatry in the post-Soviet new world order. This is an unfortunate development, because the same type of problem that overtook the Soviet system is now becoming apparent on a global scale. The problem arises because the natural boundaries of human diversity are far wider than the limited range of personality types needed by ideologically driven cultural systems. This is just as true for the new global culture of the market place as it was in the Soviet Union. Human rights advocates and civil libertarians who have not yet caught up with these developments may inadvertently be collaborating in repression by assisting in the expansion of psychiatric coercion.

Critics of psychiatry have long argued that a diagnosis of schizophrenia is the most frequent way in which psychiatry is used to control troublesome citizens. This is because 'schizophrenia' is considered a serious form of mental illness, and people with such a designation are, therefore, in urgent need of treatment and control. A further useful aspect of the schizophrenia label is that its symptoms are so vaguely defined that it can only be identified with authority by a psychiatric expert. This means that a diagnosis cannot be refuted by a non-psychiatrist. It is not surprising that Soviet psychiatrists used diagnoses of schizophrenia to persecute political dissidents.

There is little doubt that some people sometimes display the symptoms of schizophrenia. What is in doubt is whether these symptoms are really caused by an underlying 'disease' of the mind or brain accessible to medical analysis and treatment. Psychiatrists claim that it is a disease, and they have devised the medical model to explain schizophrenic symptoms.

2

The Medical Model:
schizophrenia as a disease

The medical model is the prism through which psychiatrists view the signs and symptoms of schizophrenia. It provides the 'disease' reason for explaining why a person might hear voices in his or her head and develop 'weird' ideas about life. Psychiatrists are trained as medical practitioners, and when they encounter people with psychological difficulties it is natural for them to apply their medical expertise and to assume that disease might be the cause. But this doesn't mean they are right. The medical concept of schizophrenia has two major deficiencies that undermine its scientific credibility. The first is an absence of scientific evidence supporting the assumption of an underlying disease; the second is the reality that diagnoses are made subjectively, without confirmation from laboratory tests or any other scientific evidence. Without any scientific confirmation, it is entirely possible that the disease—supposedly a collection of underlying schizophrenic symptoms—only exists in the minds of psychiatrists as a collective act of faith.

Early Thoughts on Schizophrenic Symptoms

The origins of the medical approach to schizophrenia can be traced in the history of the language used to describe the symptoms. The key words and terms that are currently used to describe the symptoms—such as delusions, hallucinations, thought disorder, and catatonia—all have long histories of usage, first to describe madness in general, and later as symptoms of earlier forms of mental disease that preceded the concept of schizophrenia.

Up to the middle of the nineteenth century the French word *délire* meant either madness or delusion, and when it was used for delusion the meaning was interchangeable with delirium.[1] This means that for several centuries in France the three concepts—madness, delusion, and delirium—were often indistinguishable. Influenced by religious beliefs, all three forms of *délire* were thought to be organic in nature because 'the soul is always in the same state and is not susceptible to change. So the error of judgement that is délire cannot be attributed to the soul but to bodily organs'.[2]

In pre-eighteenth-century Italy a similar view was expressed about the cause of delusion and delirium:

> Delirium was caused by organic changes for the soul cannot become diseased: 'How can delirium be called affection of the soul, in view of its [the soul's] unchangeable nature?' 'Where is the seat of delirium?' It is evident that true and basic errors of judgment and of reasoning, without any lesion in the organ of external senses, must be due to a physical disease of the brain.[3]

British thinkers appear to have had a more circumspect view of delusions and madness, sometimes being less willing to associate delusions with brain disease. Hobbes saw delusions as being the primary indicator of madness, but he was equivocal about the cause. He was unsure whether to adopt an ancient interpretation blaming 'Daemons, or Spirits, either good, or bad, which ... might enter into man, possess him, and move his organs in such strange, and uncouth manner,'[4] or whether to adopt the opinion current in his time that underlying 'passions' were the cause.

John Locke introduced the belief that delusions and madness were caused by associating inappropriate ideas: 'some of our ideas have a natural correspondence and connection with one another: it is the office and excellency of our reason to trace these, and hold them together in that union and correspondence'. However, to Locke, madmen 'do not appear to me to have lost the faculty of reasoning, but having joined together some ideas very wrongly, they mistake them for truths, and they err as men do that argue right from wrong principles.'[5]

Locke's view was amplified by eighteenth-century associationists such as David Hartley, and remained popular up to the middle of the nineteenth century. But Hartley believed, as did the French, that delusions and madness could also have organic causes:

> the causes of madness are of two kinds: bodily and mental. That which arises from bodily causes is nearly related to drunkenness, and to the deliriums attending distemper. That from mental causes is of the same kind with temporary alienation of the mind during violent passions, and with prejudices of opinionativeness, which much application to one set of ideas only occasions.[6]

In the late eighteenth century, French and German commentators agreed that hallucinations could be the cause of mental disorder, but they did not agree on the extent of this disorder. The Frenchman Dufor was of the opinion that 'The false impression of the external senses, then, must necessarily create disorder and confusion in a person's conduct.'[7] Crichton, a German, responded: 'that the diseases of the external senses produce erroneous mental perceptions, must be allowed; but it depends on the concurrence of other causes, whether delusion follows'.[8]

Disagreements such as these led on to a nineteenth-century debate about whether hallucinations could be a cause for insanity. Hallucinations were defined early in the debate: 'If a man has the intimate conviction of actually perceiving a sensation for which there is no external object, he is in a hallucinated state.'[9] The word 'hallucination' was closely linked with the word 'vision', and its usage caused some difficulties in dealing with false perceptions that were not connected with the sense of sight. But early psychiatrists found these difficulties were outweighed by the advantages:

> Hallucinations of vision have been called visions but this is appropriate only for one perceptual mode. Who would talk about auditory visions, taste visions, olfactory visions? ... However, the functional alterations, brain mechanisms and the clinical context involved in these three senses is the same as in visions. A generic term is needed. I propose the word hallucination.[10]

An important early debate about the nature of hallucinations was concerned with whether the fault was to be found in the external sense organs or whether it was in the 'central organ of sensitivity itself'.[11] Esquirol was of the opinion that 'hallucination is a cerebral or psychological phenomenon that takes place independently from the senses. The pretended sensations of the hallucinated are images and ideas reproduced by memory, improved by the imagination, and personified by habit ... visionaries are dreaming whilst awake'.[12]

Baillarger took up similar arguments after Esquirol died, and in 1811 presented his views to the Royal Academy of Medicine in Paris: 'The most frequent and complicated hallucinations affect hearing: invisible interlocutors address the patient in the third person, so that he is a passive listener in conversation ... the insane deaf is more prone to hear voices.'[13] But Baillarger's view was challenged by another of his countrymen named Michéa, who posed a complicated argument that 'hallucination consisted of a metamorphosis of thinking, was neither a sensation nor a perception but intermediate between perception and pure conception. It occupies the middle ground between these two facts of consciousness and participates in both.'[14]

In the middle of the nineteenth century an important debate broke out amongst French psychiatrists about the nature of hallucinations. According to Berrios, there were three main points to the debate: 'could hallucinations ever be considered as "normal" experiences? Did sensation, image and hallucination form a continuum? Were hallucinations, dreams and ecstatic trance similar states? A fourth issue (as Henri Ey noticed) "haunted everyone but was not made the base of the debate"—namely, whether hallucinations had a "psychological" origin.'[15]

All of these issues remain unresolved today. Indeed, they form much of the basis for the current controversy. It seems that although considerable progress has been made in the past century-and-a-half in categorising, identifying, and devising treatments for unusual mental phenomena, little progress has been made in understanding their underlying nature. This point is well illustrated by the example of thought disorder.

Thought disorder is indicated by disorganised or nonsensical speech. Although schizophrenic symptoms such as delusions and hallucinations are often recognised by the people who experience them, this is less likely with thought disorder. Usually this symptom must be identified by an observer. For a long time, therefore, thought disorder was considered as secondary in importance to delusions and hallucinations. It was not until the second half of the nineteenth century that psychiatrists began to form theories about the causes and nature of disordered thoughts.

Two broad theoretical frameworks emerged to explain such thoughts, both of which are now deeply embedded in psychiatric thinking about schizophrenia. One is faculty theory, which holds that 'the mind is a cluster of independent powers, capacities or faculties'.[16] After passing through dubious stages of development, such as the phrenology movement, based on the belief that personality could be revealed by measuring and mapping the pattern of bumps on the head, faculty theory is now largely at the base of current attempts to draw maps of the brain by identifying various mental functions with parts of the brain. This area of research, as will be discussed further on, is central to current scientific endeavours to link schizophrenia with defects in brain architecture.

The associationistic approach, on the other hand, 'was the legacy of British empiricism and started with Locke's description of simple and complex ideas'.[17] This theory had considerable influence on both Kraepelin and Bleuler, the two psychiatric researchers who are most commonly cited as being the pioneers, the inventors/discovers/definers, of the disease entity called schizophrenia. Through Kraepelin and Bleuler the associationistic approach has had an important influence on the selection of the primary indicators for schizophrenia that are found in modern diagnostic manuals.

The 'Discoverers' of Schizophrenia

Emile Kraepelin was a German psychiatrist practising in the late nineteenth century. In Kraepelin's time the psychiatric classification system was still very much in flux, and there was a shifting consensus about matching particular symptoms with specific mental diseases. This situation provided scope for individual psychiatrists to 'discover' new disease entities and then persuade their colleagues to recognise their new discovery. Kraepelin was the first psychiatrist to observe a certain pattern of madness that had an early onset and, as he falsely thought, led finally to a deteriorating condition. He called the new disease 'dementia praecox', dementia of early life.

Kraepelin's argument was that three psychiatric conditions, previously recognised separately, were actually different aspects of a single disease. The three pre-existing disease entities were 'hebephrenia', which was characterised by 'aimless, disorganised and incongruous behaviour; 'catatonia', in which the individual might be negativistic, motionless, or even stuporous or, at other times, extremely agitated and incoherent; and 'dementia paranoides', in which delusions of persecution and grandeur were prominent.'[18]

Kraepelin had to overcome professional opposition to gain recognition for his new interpretation. One of its central features was a clear distinction from other forms of madness, such as cerebral syphilis, that sometimes produced similar symptoms but had a demonstrable biological cause. He also sought to distinguish dementia praecox from other forms of mental illness that were clearly stress induced, and also from cyclical mood disorders. The description he gave of dementia praecox has become the foundation for the modern psychiatric description of schizophrenia.

Kraepelin worked as part of a highly successful team of psychiatric researchers that included Alzheimer, after whom Alzheimer's Disease takes its name. Kraepelin believed that dementia praecox was a 'brain disease and that its neuropathological substrates would be identified by the new techniques that he and his investigative team were developing.'[19] This focus on a search for a biological cause was largely based on what turned out to have been a false assumption that the disease necessarily takes a deteriorating course, from which sufferers do not recover.

In fact, as Kraepelin's research progressed, he began to find that the symptoms of a substantial percentage of the patients he had selected according to his new diagnostic criteria did not in fact follow a deteriorating course, and that 12 per cent of these patients actually made a complete recovery. This potential for recovery intrigued a Swiss psychiatrist named Eugen Bleuler, who realised that the new disease of dementia praecox had been misnamed: 'Stimulated by the psychoanalytical theories of his assistant, Carl Jung, Dr Bleuler formulated a new unifying concept for the condition and gave it a new name.'[20] Bleuler believed that the major identifying characteristic of the condition was not a progressive deterioration, but was instead a discontinuity and fragmentation between thinking and feeling. So he reformulated the description and called the condition 'schizophrenia', meaning 'split mind'.

In 1911 Bleuler published a monograph entitled *Dementia Praecox or the Group of Schizophrenias* in order to propagate his new description. Although this book was not translated into English for some thirty years, it is generally recognised as the foundation for the modern psychiatric understanding of schizophrenia.

In the first few pages of the book, Bleuler painstakingly explained why Kraepelin's description was unsatisfactory and why he found it necessary to rename the condition. His argument was that the term 'dementia praecox' inappropriately limited the disease to young people who progressively deteriorated. He said this had caused great confusion within the psychiatric profession in a number of countries, since it was readily apparent that many victims experienced the first onset later in life, and not all victims progressively deteriorated.

Bleuler went on to group the symptoms of schizophrenia into two categories. In the first group were what he called 'fundamental symptoms'. These were symptoms 'that are present in every case and at every period of the illness even though, as with every other disease symptom, they must have attained a certain degree of intensity before they can be recognised with any certainty'. According to Bleuler, the 'fundamental symptoms consist of disturbances of association and affectivity, the predilection for fantasy as against reality, and the inclination to divorce oneself from reality (autism).[21]

The second group of symptoms he called 'accessory symptoms'. These involved 'manifestations such as delusions, hallucinations or catatonic symptoms. These may be completely lacking during certain periods, or even throughout the entire course of the disease; at other times they alone may permanently determine the clinical picture.'[22]

As a 'disturbance of association', thought disorder was one of Bleuler's fundamental symptoms, which he described in an unusually candid fashion. He supplied numerous examples taken from conversations with his patients, as well as extracts from their letters, to demonstrate what he thought were the illogical and bizarre effects that could be produced by inappropriately associating ideas. The effect was to give an insight into psychiatric thinking that is rarely available in modern psychiatric writing.

One of Bleuler's examples, for instance, utilised quotations from a patient's written impression of ancient Egypt. According to Bleuler, the patient's writing demonstrated a failure to control impulses of fantasy which had opened the way for all sorts of incongruous material to be introduced. The writing referred to the habits and preferences of various national and religious groupings, including Parsees, Afghans, Jews, Moors, and Arabs, and finished with the assertion that 'China is the Eldorado of the Pawnees'.[23] Much of this material is clearly out-of-place in a factual account of ancient Egypt. But Bleuler's argument that the writing demonstrated clinical evidence of madness is also doubtful in a modern context. What might have been an excellent example of bizarre self-expression to a turn-of-the-century scientist is, to a contemporary reader, somewhat familiar as a variety of stream-of-consciousness writing.

Bleuler also gave examples of responses to questions that he asked his schizophrenic patients: the inappropriate answers were offered as clinical evidence to demonstrate the nature of disordered thinking. But, as Bleuler described his method, he seems to have been unaware that the patients might have given flippant or witty answers, or teased or joked with him, instead of expressing their most seriously held beliefs. What might be objectivity in other scientific research looks more like naivety—and a tendency towards the literal—in psychiatric research.

For instance, he gave the following as an example of schizophrenic symptoms: 'A female patient, supposed to help in the household work, is asked why she is not working. The answer, "But I don't understand any French", is logically related neither to the question nor the situation.'[24] Bleuler's assumption is that the woman's answer indicated disordered thoughts. However, it is possible to read a sophisticated retort into the answer. If, for instance, a similar dialogue were encountered in a novel, a reader might simply assume that the woman was protesting against being asked to do housework and, perhaps, with tongue in cheek, was asserting that she was not a French maid.

Throughout Bleuler's book there is an unsettling single-mindedness and inflexibility in the record of his interactions with patients. He gives the impression of functioning only as an investigative scientist in his personal interactions with patients, so that everything they say is scientific evidence before it is human communication. Patients might have encountered some difficulty in responding to this scientist who was talking to them as if they were all laboratory exhibits.

This same point has been raised by R. D. Laing in relation to Kraepelin's work. In *Lectures on Clinical Psychiatry*, Kraepelin described a clinical examination of a female patient he had conducted in front of a live audience of doctors to demonstrate dementia praecox. He described how the woman paced back and forth on a stage while he attempted to distract her. According to Kraepelin, the woman's indifference to his activities constituted the evidence of her condition. Laing made his point about Kraepelin by isolating all his actions in relation to the woman and printing them in italics:

> ... *On attempting to stop her movement* ... *if I place myself in front of her with my arms outstretched* ... *If one takes firm hold of her* ... *will not allow it to be forced from her* ... *If you prick her on the forehead with a needle* ... .[25]

Laing's purpose was to separate the psychiatrist's own actions in his account, and to demonstrate how extraordinary these actions were and how bizarre was the situation with which the woman had to deal.

Both Kraepelin's and Bleuler's works raise an important question about psychiatric research work in general. Is it possible for a patient's mind to be used as a laboratory exhibit for scientific investigation, and for it still to give responses that are considered normal? Perhaps another way of examining this problem is to ask the following question: if a psychiatrist assumes a patient's mind is diseased, and the patient perceives the psychiatrist's assumption, how should the patient behave?

This second question implies that patients might have choices about how to adapt to situations in which they find themselves. The possibility that schizophrenic symptoms are merely adaptive behaviour will be discussed more fully in Chapter 7. However, it seems apparent that the argument for a pathological cause relies heavily on the assumption that the indicators of schizophrenia are necessarily involuntary behaviours. The medical model tends to disregard the possibility that schizophrenic symptoms might sometimes be a deliberate strategy induced by the circumstances in which psychiatry is practised.

Regression Theories

Even if irrational and bizarre forms of behaviour are only adaptive strategies, the psychiatric profession is not alone in refusing to tolerate them. It is fairly obvious that there is a consensus amongst the general population which supports the psychiatric view that schizophrenic behaviour should be controlled. This cultural intolerance has its origins in eighteenth-century Enlightenment thinking which held that people who appear to lose control of their minds are thereby deprived of some essential aspect of their humanity. Enlightenment thinkers bequeathed to the people of contemporary industrial societies a belief that rational, self-controlled thought is the essential function of a fully developed human being. Mental activity that lacks rationality and self-control is viewed as harmful and as being less than fully human. Throughout the Enlightenment, people who were thought to be mad were usually treated as if they had lost their humanity and had reverted to an animalistic state. This Enlightenment view of madness allowed for mad inmates of institutions to be kept in chains and sometimes displayed as zoological exhibits.

It is from this treatment-as-animals that the medical profession claims to have rescued mad people around the turn of the nineteenth century by medicalising their condition and redefining it as mental illness. In doing so, however, some elements of the medical profession retained the notion that irrationality and loss of mental control are expressions of less than full humanity.

In relation to schizophrenic symptoms, modern psychiatry has developed two alternative regression theories. One explanation is that schizophrenic symptoms indicate a reversion to thought patterns that are believed to have prevailed in the minds of early or primitive human types. In this context, schizophrenic delusions have been referred to as 'paleological thinking' by some psychiatric theorists. This psychiatric hypothesis, however, is largely speculative and does not have a substantial following.

A second, more commonly accepted explanation was originally provided by early psychiatric theorists such as Freud. These early theorists assumed that 'psychotic processes reflected some regression to an earlier, and more "primitive" level of organisation'[26] found in children. Freud used the term 'primary process' to describe a child's first mode of thinking. He contrasted this with 'secondary process', which he thought was an adult way of thinking:

> Primary process thinking is, first of all, drive-directed. Its content and direction are determined by impulses rather than by considerations of external reality. Secondary process thinking is, instead, reality-oriented, having been developed to facilitate adaptation to the world outside the self.[27]

Using this formula, there are a number of ways that the inward focus of schizophrenic thinking can be likened to childish thought-processes. Delusions and hallucinations can be interpreted as wish fulfilment; schizophrenics can be observed to deny reality in the pursuit of their own goals in the way that demanding children do; and demonstrably infantile forms of behaviour, such as playing with faeces, can sometimes be observed in schizophrenics.

However, there is no universal pattern to these observations, and the same childish thinking and behaviour can be observed in various types of non-schizophrenic people. Prisoners, for instance, will sometimes smear faeces on the walls of cells as a form of protest, and many gamblers may attempt wish fulfilment by holding delusions about being in contact with forces that control the outcome of chance.

But the weaknesses of regression theories do not threaten to undermine the medical model. The assumptions of the medical model do not rest on either closely argued theory or empirical evidence. Instead they remain largely unformulated and mostly rely on affirmation provided by a widespread lay understanding, often gained directly through observation of family members, that the behaviour of people with schizophrenic symptoms is self-evidently caused by a weakness in the mind. Psychiatric textbooks even refer to popular knowledge to confirm psychiatric theory:

> Literary portrayals such as the madness of Orestes in the *Oresteia* of Aeschylus and the mumblings of Poor Tom in *King Lear* make it clear that serious psychoses have been recognised even by lay people for many years.[28]

The psychiatric profession prefers to focus most of its attention on the problem of standardising the diagnostic criteria for schizophrenia rather than going to the trouble of providing a persuasive philosophical rationale for pathology. This focus is necessary, since diagnoses have to maintain a semblance of consistency without the assistance of laboratory tests.

Diagnosing Schizophrenia

As mentioned in the previous chapter, there are two internationally recognised diagnostic systems for mental disorders that psychiatrists currently use in most countries of the world. One is the tenth revision of the *International Classification of Diseases* (ICD-10),[29] compiled and published by the World Health Organisation. The other is the *Diagnostic and Statistical Manual of Mental Disorders, Fourth Edition* (DSM-IV),[30] compiled and published by the American Psychiatric Association. The respective teams of psychiatric researchers responsible for compiling successive editions of the ICD and DSM systems have co-operated closely in their work to ensure that the two systems maintain a high level of compatibility.[31] Whereas the DSM system is dominant in English-speaking parts of the world such as North America and Australia, the ICD is the main diagnostic reference tool in European and developing countries.

Both manuals define schizophrenia by describing the symptoms. After giving general outlines of the disorder they go on to supply definitive lists of criteria that must be identified in order for a psychiatrist to make a diagnosis. To determine whether a person has schizophrenia, a psychiatrist will usually conduct an interview and listen to what the person says about his or her inner thoughts and beliefs. The psychiatrist will also make his or her own observations about the person's speech and behaviour. Reports and opinions of third parties, such as relatives, will also usually be considered. From these combined sources the psychiatrist will make a judgement about whether the person's mental state fits the criteria specified in one of the diagnostic manuals. No other evidence is required beyond the subjective opinion of the diagnostician.

The manuals define schizophrenia as a type of psychosis. However, the manuals themselves admit that there is some doubt as to what constitutes a psychosis: 'the term psychotic has historically received a number of different definitions, none of which has received universal acceptance.'[32] Nevertheless there seems to be a core understanding that when delusions, hallucinations, disordered thoughts, or extreme moods give rise to irrational behaviour, psychosis is likely to be present.[33]

DSM-IV specifies that time periods should be taken into account when diagnosing schizophrenia: 'The essential features of schizophrenia are a mixture of characteristic signs and symptoms (both positive and negative) that have been present for a significant portion of time during a 1-month period (or for a shorter time if successfully treated), with some signs of the disorder persisting for at least 6 months.' In conjunction with these signs and symptoms, there should also be a 'marked social or occupational dysfunction'.[34]

Although clarity of consciousness and intellectual capabilities might still be present, symptoms include 'characteristic distortions of thinking and perception'. These often take the form of delusions that 'supernatural forces are at work to influence the affected individual's thoughts and actions in ways that are often bizarre'.[35] In these circumstances, the person might believe himself/herself to be at the centre of world-shattering events that are taking place around him or her.

'Hallucinations, especially auditory, are common and may comment on the individual's behaviour or thought.'[36] This leads to disturbances in thinking patterns and particularly in behaviour. To observers of a person with schizophrenia, the person's thinking seems vague, and when it is expressed in speech it is sometimes impossible to understand. There are 'breaks and interpolations in the train of thought',[37] and the person's mood appears to be characterised by shallowness, ambivalence, and inertia.

Delusions can be of many types, and cover a variety of characteristic subject matter. Delusions may be persecutory, in which case the person might believe 'he or she is being tormented, followed, tricked, spied on, or subject to ridicule'.[38] Alternatively, delusions can be referential, meaning that the person interprets certain signs and signals in the surrounding environment, such as bill-board advertisements or newspaper headlines, as being directed specifically at themselves and containing hidden messages. Or the delusions might be bizarre. Examples of bizarre delusions can include 'a person's belief that his or her thoughts have been taken away by some outside force ("thought withdrawal"), that alien thoughts have been put into his or her mind ("thought insertion"), or that his or her body or actions are being acted on or manipulated by some outside force ("delusions of control")'.[39]

Hallucinations may be associated with any of the senses, but auditory hallucinations are particularly characteristic of schizophrenia. 'Auditory hallucinations are usually experienced as voices, whether familiar or unfamiliar, that are perceived as distinct from the person's own thoughts.'[40] These voices might present a running commentary on the person's thoughts and behaviour, or they might enter into dialogue with the person's own thoughts.

Disorganised thinking is also one of the definitive markers of schizophrenia. In diagnostic settings, psychiatrists have to rely on patterns of speech to indicate this symptom. Speech can indicate the presence of disorganised thoughts in a number of ways: 'The person may "slip off the track" from one topic to another ("derailment" or "loose associations"); answers to questions may be obliquely related or completely unrelated ("tangentiality"); and, rarely, speech may be so severely disorganised that it is nearly incomprehensible and resembles receptive aphasia in its linguistic disorganisation ("incoherence" or "word salad").'[41]

Disorganised thoughts and delusions may also affect a person's behaviour so that it becomes irrational: 'Grossly disorganised behaviour may manifest itself in a variety of ways, ranging from childlike silliness to unpredictable agitation.'[42] The person may find it difficult to carry out normal tasks necessary for day-to-day living, concerning such things as meals and personal hygiene. Dress may become eccentric, and behaviour may become inappropriate—in the form of indecent sexual displays, shouting, and unpredictable shows of anger and agitation—given the situations in which the observed person finds himself or herself.

One of the more extreme forms of behavioural disorder associated with schizophrenia is catatonia:

> Catatonic motor behaviours include a marked decrease in reactivity to the environment, sometimes reaching an extreme degree of complete unawareness (catatonic stupor), maintaining a rigid posture and resisting efforts to be moved (catatonic rigidity), active resistance to instructions or attempts to be moved (catatonic negativism), the assumption of inappropriate or bizarre postures (catatonic posturing), or purposeless and unstimulated excessive motor activity (catatonic excitement).[43]

All the symptoms discussed so far fall into the category of 'positive' symptoms. Juxtaposed to the positive symptoms are a range of 'negative' symptoms. There are three principal negative symptoms: flattened mood, poverty of speech, and avolition. Flattened mood 'is especially common and is characterised by the person's face appearing immobile and unresponsive, with poor eye contact and reduced body language.'[44] Poverty of speech is indicated by an inability to engage in useful communication while 'avolition is characterised by an inability to initiate and persist in goal-directed activities. The person may sit for long periods of time and show little interest in participating in work or social activities'.[45]

Most of these symptoms, both negative and positive, are aspects of human expression that are on a continuum with normality. Most of us, for instance, have experienced symptoms such as delusions at some time or other, simply by holding beliefs that proved to be false. This raises a problem for diagnosticians, in that they must individually decide the point on a highly abstract and arbitrary continuum—extending from rationality to irrationality—at which normal false beliefs turn into pathological delusions. Since each patient displays personal variations of the characteristic symptoms, the diagnostic process for schizophrenia is always at risk of inconsistency. To give some assistance to the standardisation of diagnoses, both the ICD-10 and DSM-IV supply diagnostic guidelines which act as ready references to help reduce the otherwise excessive subjectivity of the process.

DSM IV Diagnostic Criteria for Schizophrenia

The American Psychiatric Association's DSM-IV presents the symptoms of mental disorders in the form of grouped criteria. Here are the details of its diagnostic criteria for schizophrenia:

> **A.** *Characteristic symptoms:* Two (or more) for the following, each present for a significant portion of time during a 1-month period (or less if successfully treated):
> (1) delusions
> (2) hallucinations

(3) disorganised speech (for example frequent derailment or incoherence)
(4) grossly disorganised or catatonic behaviour
(5) negative symptoms, that is, affective flattening, alogia, or avolition

Note: Only one Criterion A symptom is required if delusions are bizarre or hallucinations consist of a voice keeping up a running commentary on the person's behaviour or thoughts, or two or more voices conversing with each other.

B. *Social/occupational dysfunction:* For a significant portion of the time since the onset of the disturbance, one or more major areas of functioning such as work, interpersonal relations, or self-care are markedly below the level achieved prior to the onset (or when the onset is in childhood or adolescence, failure to achieve expected level of interpersonal, academic, or occupational achievement).

C. *Duration:* Continuous signs of the disturbance persist for at least 6 months. This 6-month period must include at least 1 month of symptoms (or less if successfully treated) that meet Criterion A (that is, active-phase symptoms) and may include prodromal or residual symptoms. During these prodromal or residual periods, the signs of the disturbance may be manifested by only negative symptoms or two or more symptoms listed in Criterion A present in an attenuated form (for example, odd beliefs, unusual perceptual experiences).

D. *Schizoaffective and Mood Disorder exclusion:* Schizoaffective Disorder and Mood Disorder With Psychotic Features have been ruled out because either (1) no Major Depressive, Manic, or Mixed Episodes have occurred concurrently with the active-phase symptoms; or (2) if mood episodes have occurred during active-phase symptoms, their total duration has been brief relative to the duration of the active and residual periods.

E. *Substance/general medical condition exclusion:* The disturbance is not due to the direct physiological effects of a substance (for example, a drug of abuse, a medication) or a general medical condition.

F. *Relationship to a Pervasive Developmental Disorder:* If there is a history of Autistic Disorder or another Pervasive Developmental Disorder, the additional diagnosis of Schizophrenia is made only if prominent delusions or hallucinations are present for at least a month (or less if successfully treated).[46]

The above symptoms are meant to be guidelines for identifying the presence of schizophrenia in general. Once a diagnostician decides schizophrenia is present, the next task is to determine which of the various subtypes is the most appropriate label. DSM-IV provides a choice from five subtypes: Paranoid Type, in which the person is preoccupied with delusions or auditory hallucinations; Disorganised Type, characterised by disorganised speech or behaviour; Catatonic Type, involving abnormal movements or strange postures; Undifferentiated Type, in which the primary symptoms of schizophrenia are present but do not fit the criteria for Paranoid, Disorganised, or Catatonic subtypes; and Residual Type, for a person who has had at least one episode of schizophrenia and in whom residual indications of disturbance remain.

The various classifications of mental disorders relating to psychosis are presented in both DSM-IV and ICD-10 as if it is assumed there is a continuous spectrum of disorder that has to be broken up into recognisable segments. The result is that schizophrenia, as it is described in both manuals, shades into a number of descriptions of similar but supposedly clinically distinct disorders. The problem is that the symptoms do not always clearly demonstrate these clinical distinctions.

For example, in the DSM-IV system, Delusional Disorder is described as a psychotic condition which is distinguished from schizophrenia largely by an understanding that the 'delusions' of schizophrenia are usually 'bizarre' whereas those of Delusional Disorder are non-bizarre.[47] To facilitate this distinction, DSM-IV defines a 'bizarre' delusion as one 'that involves a phenomenon that the person's culture would regard as totally implausible.'[48] This leaves diagnosticians to assume that the non-bizarre delusions of Delusional Disorder must be delusions that the person's culture does find plausible.

Seven subtypes of Delusional Disorder are given in DSM-IV. The Erotomanic Type, for instance, defines unrequited love as a pathological symptom, and claims a diagnosis 'applies when the central theme of the delusion is that another person is in love with the individual. The delusion often concerns idealised romantic love and spiritual union rather than sexual attraction ... Most individuals with this subtype in clinical samples are female.'[49]

Similarly, a Delusional Disorder of the Jealous Type involves a supposedly non-bizarre sign of pathology which 'applies when the central theme of the person's delusion is that his or her spouse or lover is unfaithful'.[50] But how could the diagnosing psychiatrist possibly know with any certainty whether the patient's suspicion is a delusion or the truth? Is it simply a matter of consulting the suspected spouse? This kind of question is highly relevant when one considers the power vested in psychiatrists to lock up and force treatment on people diagnosed with delusional symptoms.[51]

Without any laboratory tests, a diagnostician can only rely on evidence provided by the speech and behaviour of the person in question, together with reports from third parties. The person's behaviour first has to be tested against the range of normal speech and behaviours that is within the diagnostician's experience. This will determine whether the person's mental state deviates too greatly from normal and is therefore pathological. Then, if it is judged to be abnormal, it has to be fitted into the correct point on the spectrum of mental disorders.

In regard to diagnosing schizophrenia, this would seem to be a task fraught with possibilities for inconsistency. If, for instance, a person expresses religious beliefs, the diagnostician must first determine whether they are delusional—that is, false beliefs not 'ordinarily accepted by other members of the person's culture or subculture'.[52] If they appear to be delusional, the diagnostician then has to decide whether the delusions are bizarre, and therefore indicative of schizophrenia. If they are non-bizarre, the alternative diagnosis might be Delusional Disorder—Grandiose Type: 'Grandiose delusions may have a religious content (for example, the person believes that he or she has a special message from a deity).'[53]

The risk of inconsistency is readily apparent, given the distinctly bizarre manifestations of many religious beliefs that are culturally acceptable and therefore not considered delusional (in the psychiatric sense). For example, thousands of people may practise a pseudo-cannibalistic ritual together, believing the biscuits and grape juice they consume to symbolise the body and blood of a god. But if the ritual belongs to a respectable mainstream Christian church, and is therefore culturally acceptable, psychiatrists by necessity must view it as being motivated by a non-pathological cause. However, if a solitary individual were to invent and practise a similar ritual it is unlikely that the same protection would be available. Such a person might easily be given a diagnosis of schizophrenia and, if so, would probably also be considered dangerous. This means that the level of popularity of certain kinds of thoughts and beliefs, rather than their type or quality, is a deciding factor in some diagnoses of schizophrenia. This is a fairly curious, although not unique, notion of disease.

Notions about the Meaning of Disease

The plausibility and credibility of the medical model largely relies on the assumption that the diagnostic indicators of schizophrenia fit into generally accepted notions of what constitutes a disease. But these notions are not stable; in fact, they sometimes change with fashion and public debate. To clarify this point, comparisons can be made between schizophrenia and a number of other human conditions for which the 'disease' label is also in dispute.

Baldness is a good comparison. Does baldness have an underlying pathological cause requiring medical attention? Is it a natural part of the aging process? Or is it merely a stylistic affectation some people express by shaving their heads?

Homosexuality also provides some interesting parallels. Is it a manifestation of mental disease requiring medical treatment?[54] Is it one of a variety of natural forms of sexual expression? Or is it an adaptation that some people—such as prisoners—choose to make when they are denied the companionship of the opposite sex?

In both cases it should be fairly apparent that the third interpretation most certainly applies to some people. But it obviously does not apply to all. Choosing between the other two positions—pathological and natural—is more difficult.

One approach to understanding what is and is not a disease is to consider how its manifestation relates to function. Function is an attractive approach, because the arguments can be made to appear objective.[55] If the function of hair on top of a man's head, for instance, is to provide insulation for his brain against extremes of heat and cold, and the climate demands this insulation so that a bald man must take special precautions, a lack of hair might be considered a malfunction and therefore a disease.

On the other hand, if the function of hair on a man's head is to attract sexual attention, and the baldness only develops after the man is no longer sexually active, lack of hair in an elderly man would hardly constitute a malfunction. But some human features have both function and accidental utility, and it is important to distinguish between them. A nose, for instance, 'has the function of heating and humidifying inspired air',[56] but it also has the accidental utility of being able to support spectacles. According to this line of thinking, a nose that functions properly, although it is unusually shaped, might be an oddity, but it would not be diseased simply because it was unsuitable for supporting spectacles.

The function test can also be applied to homosexuality, but there might be philosophical problems to solve in choosing between possible functions. Is the function of human sexuality to procreate, or is it to give pleasure? If it is to procreate, homosexual expression might be considered a malfunction. But such an argument would also render all other non-reproductive sexual expression—including contraception and bad timing—a malfunction, and therefore diseased as well.

The test of functionality is even more problematic when it is applied to schizophrenia. One of the functions of the human mind is the formulation of thoughts and beliefs. But the mere formulation of thoughts that appear to normal people to be unusual or bizarre, and beliefs (delusions) that are judged to be false is not enough in itself to indicate malfunction. A mind could only malfunction in this regard if it had first been clearly established that functional thoughts and beliefs must necessarily conform with social norms.

A converse problem with the functionality test occurs when it is agreed that a certain condition definitely indicates malfunction, but the cause of the malfunction is in dispute. Death, for instance, is a fairly definite indication of serious malfunctioning. Yet surveys of medical students, interns, and hospital resident doctors have shown that only 56–57 per cent of them can correctly identify causes of death on death certificates.[57] This converse approach to malfunction can be tested on a schizophrenic symptom such as hallucinations. It might be agreed that an hallucinating mind is definitely malfunctioning, but theories about the cause of the hallucinations might range from something essentially non-medical, such as fatigue, to a cause that is indisputably medical, such as malarial infection.

If the functionality test for distinguishing disease is problematic, there are several other tests to try. One involves discarding the pseudo-objectivity of functionality by adopting normativism, which defines diseases in terms of harm. On the surface, this is a simple premise: if a person is harmed in any way by having a certain condition, and is worse off than they would otherwise be, the condition can be described as a disease.

Many non-controversial disease descriptions, such as cancer and cholera, are easily accommodated by the test of 'harm'. But problems are soon encountered when the test of 'harm' is applied more widely. On the one hand, there are many conditions, such as ignorance and clumsiness, which apparently cause harm but are not usually described as diseases. On the other hand, a mild dose of what is clearly understood as a disease, in the form of a vaccination, for instance, can be good rather than harmful for a person.

The problem with using 'harm' as the criterion for determining disease is further exacerbated if we return to our three test cases: baldness, homosexuality, and schizophrenia. In each case there are circumstances in which a major aspect of the harm that can be caused by these conditions appears to come from cultural values, in the forms of aesthetics, prejudice, and discrimination, rather than from individual incapacity. If we were to allow social harm to determine what is and is not disease, we might leave the door open to claims that beautiful people are more healthy than ugly people; that light coloured skin in a predominantly black society, and vice versa, are diseases; and that personal traits that tend to give offence, such as vulgarity, loud voices, and excitable behaviour, are all symptoms of disease.

A further problem with the concept of 'harm' is that, from time to time, medical scientists develop notions that certain conditions are harmful, and forcefully propagate their view—only for a subsequent consensus view to develop that relegates this condition back to the status of a non-disease. There are a number of examples of this tendency, the more notable ones often being to do with reproductive organs. In 1856, for instance, 'T. B. Curling considered that the frequent emission of sperm gave rise to "constitutional symptoms of a serious character", and constituted the disease of "spermatorrhoea" ... However, frequent ejaculation is not harmful, and so there is no such disease.'[58]

Another approach to the nature of disease would be to consider the question of whether diseases are invented or discovered. To argue that diseases are discovered is to assume that disease classification is a continuing process after the fashion of biological and botanical classification systems. But there is a major problem with this assumption. Diseases derive their class identity from human values and human attitudes towards them. Two bacteria might share very similar properties and be both placed in the same biological family, but only the one that causes human disapproval, because it causes ill-health in humans, or to domesticated animals or food crops, will be classified as a disease-causing organism. When looked at this way, it seems apparent that human values play an essential part in the 'discovery' of any disease.

This leaves the question of whether diseases are invented. Most diseases satisfy one or another of the notions of disease and plausibly demonstrate that they are not inventions of the medical profession. But some, such as the disease of 'spermatorrhoea', look very much as if they might have been invented. To psychiatric sceptics, schizophrenia looks like one of these as well, and their doubts are continually fed by new reports of psychiatric fallibility. Only recently, delegates at an annual conference of the Royal College of Psychiatrists were told about research which found that British psychiatrists are strongly influenced in their diagnoses by the Christian names of their patients. The survey had found that because British psychiatrists were more attracted to the name 'Matthew' than to 'Wayne', patients named 'Matthew received a diagnosis of schizophrenia significantly more frequently than Wayne (77% vs. 57%)'.[59]

Unless medical researchers can find an underlying cause to show that there is more to schizophrenia than a psychiatric imperative to treat the symptoms, schizophrenia's disease-status will always be questioned. Unfortunately for the psychiatric profession—despite the concentration of money and energy that has been directed to this quest—the results so far have been very poor.

3

Theories Galore:
the quest for a cause

Research into the underlying cause of schizophrenic symptoms is based on a wide variety of psychiatric theories. These theories range from hard science to non-science, and the proliferation itself indicates a high level of confusion within the medical model. The theories essentially divide into two different types: those which assume a biological cause, and those which assume that the cause is in the person's past experience, and/or past/present environment. This dichotomy between biology and experience is an echo of the old nature/nurture debate about human psychological attributes. As with the nature/nurture debate, there is also a seemingly balanced and commonsense view which assumes that both sides of the dichotomy are partly right.

Psychiatrists who support biologically based theories normally hold the view that proper treatment requires some form of physical intervention, which usually means drug treatment. Subscribers to the environmental/experiential theories, on the other hand, usually prefer one of the many forms of talking therapy.

But the situation is not clear cut. Sometimes it seems apparent that the two psychiatric factions have adopted their beliefs about the cause of schizophrenia in order to justify the methods of treatment they have been trained to apply. That is, the psychiatrists whose training has favoured drug therapies have assumed a biological cause as a convenient rationale. Similarly, psychiatrists who have undertaken training in psychoanalytic and psychotherapeutic forms of talking therapy have little choice but to assume that the cause of the problem they have been trained to talk through can be found in the past experience or environment of the patient.

However, the actual practice of psychiatry does not follow such logical patterns. In practice, most psychiatrists are prepared to supervise treatment plans that mix both drugs and talk. But when psychiatrists supervise mixed-treatment plans, one form of treatment is usually seen as the essential therapy while the other is a convenient supplement.

For a biopsychiatrist—that is, a psychiatrist who favours a biological theory of cause and drug treatment—the supplement of talking therapy is most likely to be found useful when it involves teaching a patient some kind of living skills. This can be a useful supplement to drugs, because the efficacy of the medication in routine practice is generally measured by the ability of the patient to return to at least partial social functioning. While the drugs supposedly re-balance a patient's brain chemistry, so that he or she wants to return to normal, supplementary therapy in the form of living skills can supposedly teach the person how to be normal. If a semblance of normality is achieved, the efficacy of the medication is confirmed and the psychiatrist can claim a successful outcome.

Similarly, a talking therapist might find medication a useful supplementary tool to calm a patient as a necessary prelude to achieving a therapeutic relationship: that is, a relationship in which the patient submits to the dominance of the therapist. However, this type of convenience is not appreciated by all talking therapists, and an argument is often mounted that no useful talking therapy can be undertaken so long as the patient is under the influence of drugs. This sort of argument is most likely to be made by therapists who are seeking the cause of the schizophrenia in the past experience of the patient—where introspection and accurate recall are important—rather than by therapists who specialise in teaching adaptation skills.

Biochemical Hypotheses—and Associated Drug Treatments

The most influential biological theories assume that schizophrenic symptoms are caused by an imbalance in brain chemistry. Remarkably, at least to some non-medical observers, the dominance of this theory is not the result of laboratory work directly linking schizophrenic symptoms with a chemical imbalance. Rather it is derived from observations that drug treatment appears to blunt some of the outward displays of the symptoms. As a result, it has been deduced that the cause of the symptoms is a shortage of the chemicals contained in the medication.

This reasoning is, to say the least, not very sound. It could just as easily be argued that a person who counters shyness by drinking alcohol apparently has a shortage of alcohol in the brain. But the weakness in reasoning has not inhibited research based on this type of deduction. The most prominent of the biochemical hypotheses is the 'dopamine theory', under whose aegis a great deal of research has been undertaken to explore the relationship between the positive symptoms of schizophrenia and the supposed hyperactivity of the dopamine system in the brains of schizophrenics.

The dopamine hypothesis is principally derived from two kinds of observation. The first is that drugs which increase the supply of dopamine, such as amphetamines and L-dopa (which is used for the treatment of Parkinson's disease), can sometimes cause a person to enter a psychotic-like state. The second is that neuroleptic drugs used to treat schizophrenia have been observed to block dopamine neurotransmitter systems in the brains of laboratory animals. The hypothesis derived from these observations argues that untreated schizophrenics have hyperactive dopamine systems, and require neuroleptic medication to reduce dopamine activity in their brains.

An often-cited weakness with this theory is that, whereas the dopamine receptors in the central nervous system are blocked within twenty minutes of neuroleptic medication, the drugs usually take days, sometimes many weeks or even months, before they show any clinical effect.[1] A second weakness is that 'these drugs reduce psychotic symptoms regardless of the diagnosis'.[2]

In other words, just as alcohol affects garrulous people in much the same way as it affects shy people—and therefore makes improbable a 'lack of alcohol' theory to explain the cause of shyness—neuroleptics have much the same effect on people whether they have a prior diagnosis of schizophrenia or not. Everyone who is treated experiences 'some degree of (often total) indifference and apathy'.[3] This means that although neuroleptic medication might temporarily ameliorate some of the florid features of schizophrenia, it is not a cure, and therefore the dopamine hypothesis is doubtful.

There are many variables involved in the prescription of neuroleptic medication for schizophrenia. A match has to be found for a particular patient, through trial and error, with a particular type and brand of neuroleptic according to the individual tolerance of the patient; an appropriate dosage has to be determined for each individual patient, with the right combination of drugs to suppress any side effects; and the treatment has to be continued for an indefinite period to suppress psychotic symptoms, which tend to fluctuate over time.

The mainstream of the psychiatric profession was in a state of semi-denial until recent years regarding the seriousness of the side effects caused by neuroleptic medication. This situation has now changed, and DSM-IV even has an appendix with a detailed survey of medication-induced movement disorders caused by the use of neuroleptics. The list includes Neuroleptic-Induced Parkinsonism, which features a variety of tremors and muscle rigidity mimicking Parkinson's disease. (It afflicts some 50 per cent of patients on long-term neuroleptic treatment.) Neuroleptic Malignant Syndrome is an acute toxic reaction to the drugs, and occurs in 0.07–1.4 per cent of patients treated with neuroleptics. Of these, 10–20 per cent die from it.[4]

Neuroleptic-Induced Acute Dystonia features abnormal positioning of the head and neck in relation to the body, spasms of the jaw muscles, impaired swallowing, thickened or slurred speech, tongue protrusion, eyes deviated up, down, or sideways, and abnormal positioning of the limbs or trunk. Fear and anxiety are also often a symptom, and it occurs most commonly in young males.[5] If a person looked sane before treatment they certainly would not after developing this side effect.

Neuroleptic-Induced Acute Akathisia features symptoms of compulsive restlessness such as fidgety movements, walking on the spot, and inability to sit still. The reported prevalence of this side effect in people receiving neuroleptics varies widely from 20 per cent to 75 per cent.[6] Once again, a set of physical symptoms induced by the treatment contributes dramatically to the person's appearance of being mad. Agitation, aggression, and suicidal tendencies are a major problem for people suffering from akathisia, and most of the dangerous behaviour associated with schizophrenia is caused by the drug treatment, rather than the supposed underlying mental disorder.

But the most debilitating side effect of schizophrenia treatment is Neuroleptic-Induced Tardive Dyskinesia. The indications of tardive dyskinesia are involuntary movements that can be rapid and jerky, slow and sinuous, or rhythmic. They might involve the tongue, jaw, trunk, or extremities. Twenty to thirty per cent of people receiving neuroleptics—and up to 50 per cent of elderly people taking the drug—develop tardive dyskinesia.[7] This side effect is serious, because there is no supplementary drug treatment to mask its symptoms, and it appears to be an indication of permanent brain damage in many victims. If the neuroleptic treatment is discontinued, the symptoms of tardive dyskinesia remain permanently in 50 per cent of cases. This permanency is much higher in elderly people, in whom it remains unremitted in up to 95 per cent of cases.[8]

These neuroleptic-induced movement disorders are collectively known as the central nervous system extrapyramidal side effects (EPSEs). It is perhaps incorrect to call these disorders side effects, because they occur as a direct result of blocking the dopamine receptors, and most of the patients receiving neuroleptics develop EPSEs.

In fact, it is partly through the existence of EPSEs that scientists have been able to work out how neuroleptics affect brain chemistry.

Atypical Neuroleptics

Of the different types of dopamine receptors, the conventional neuroleptics under discussion have been shown to be most effective in blocking what are known as D2 receptors. But a new generation of neuroleptics called 'atypicals' have recently become available which target other types of receptors as well. It is claimed that the atypicals will prove to be safer than the conventional neuroleptics and will reduce the incidence of neuroleptic-induced disorders. At this stage the evidence for this claim is equivocal, since most of the atypicals are very new. It may take some years of usage before problems become fully apparent.

However, one of the atypicals, clozapine, is not a new drug, and some of the major problems attached to its usage have been known about for some time. In the early 1990s clozapine was the only atypical available, and for a time it had the aura of a wonder drug. But its origins were a lot earlier: 'clinical trials of clozapine were begun in the United States in 1972, but they were temporarily halted in 1975 following reports of clozapine-induced agranulocytosis'.[9] Agranulocytosis is 'a life-threatening blood disorder that reduces the white blood cell count',[10] and it was found that some 1–2 per cent of patients treated with clozapine were afflicted with this condition; of these, some 35 per cent died from it.[11]

Clozapine earned such a bad reputation from its early usage that a Reagan-era drug deregulation campaigner even blamed it for causing some of the legal restrictions that he claimed were inhibiting drug research. He described clozapine as being one of a number of 'major tragedies which have created public alarm and fear and which have led to the condemnation of drugs'.[12]

By the end of the 1980s, however, as the accumulation of evidence about disorders induced by conventional neuroleptics began to overwhelm the psychiatric establishment in the United States, clozapine was still the only neuroleptic medication with an atypical profile which gave hope for a resolution to the EPSE problem. And so, in some desperation, clozapine was rehabilitated. It was approved for clinical use in the United States in 1990 after Food and Drug Adminstration-controlled trials which 'lasted only six weeks'.[13]

When it first went back on the market, the manufacturer, Sandoz,[14] as a precautionary measure required that all the recipients undergo a weekly blood test conducted by the company's laboratories. This procedure was very expensive, and pushed up the price of treatment to about $9,000 a year. Under pressure from the consumer lobby, however, Sandoz was forced to make some concessions about the rigour of these blood tests, and the cost of clozapine treatment was soon lowered to about $4,000 a year in the United States.[15]

The combination of agranulocytosis risk, the inconvenience of regular blood tests, and excessive cost led to a situation in which clozapine was only being recommended for use with patients who did not respond to the traditional neuroleptics or who could not tolerate the adverse effects associated with these drugs. The clinical advice in the early 1990s was that 'a patient who has been unsuccessfully treated with three different antipsychotic drugs from different classes in sufficient doses, each for a least two months, is probably a candidate for treatment with clozapine'.[16]

During the period of its banning in the US, clozapine remained available in some European countries, where it continued to earn a bad reputation with some psychiatrists. Peter Breggin, a US-based psychiatrist critical of drug treatments for schizophrenia, claimed: 'Clinicians I have spoken to in Europe feel that clozapine produces a particularly profound lobotomy effect, adding to concern about long-term dangers of tardive psychosis and dementia.'[17]

This negative view was not shared by all European psychiatrists with long-term experience of clozapine. Two Russian psychiatrists who emigrated to the United States claimed that the drug had been used successfully in their home country for more than twenty years, where 'it was not reserved for neuroleptic-resistant disorders but instead was used with some success as a first-line treatment in acute disorders'. However, they admitted that their information was largely anecdotal and that 'the Russian studies did not include controlled clinical trials, standardised diagnostic criteria, random assignment, double-blind conditions, standardised rating instruments, and other methodological approaches that we associate with scientific rigour'.[18]

Clozapine survived the early scares, and is now generally considered to be less dangerous than was first thought. However, there have been reports of severe problems when people try to stop taking the drug.[19] Some people's brain chemistry adjusts so that they become dependent on regular dosing with clozapine, and when the drug is withdrawn they rapidly slide into psychosis.

Clozapine, unlike conventional neuroleptics, is claimed to reduce some of the negative symptoms of schizophrenia. This has led some researchers to focus their work on the serotonin levels in the brains of schizophrenics. The new line of research helped to spawn a growing array of atypical neuroleptics to complement clozapine, which share similar features.

One of the more recently launched atypicals is olanzapine (Zyprexa), made by Eli Lilly. Although quite a lot is already known about the effects of olanzapine on chemical receptors in the brain, it is not known whether any of these effects contribute in any way to the observed reduction in schizophrenic symptoms.

The binding properties of the atypicals are giving rise to wide speculation about the cause of schizophrenia which extend well beyond the old dopamine theory that was inspired by the conventional neuroleptics. Some researchers think that the mechanisms of the atypicals will eventually make it possible to trace the cause of schizophrenic symptoms, while others disagree.

Despite the claimed benefits for schizophrenics from these drugs, the enthusiasm of pharmaceutical researchers might be best understood in economic terms. By the end of the 1980s, as patents for the conventional neuroleptics expired and generics became available, a continued reliance on conventional neuroleptics threatened to undermine pharmaceutical profits. As a result, the quest for a new generation of schizophrenia drugs was driven at least as much by the need to ensure long-term drug profits as it was by the need to discover safer drugs that targeted the cause of schizophrenia more precisely. In fact, when the cost of the atypicals is compared to that of conventional neuroleptics, and the equivocal nature of some claims for atypicals is borne in mind, the significance of the economic factors is brought into perspective.

The table below shows the cost to pharmacists in the United States for thirty days' treatment for schizophrenia with a usual drug dosage, based on the average wholesale price in 1996 and January 1997:

Cost of some drugs for schizophrenia

Drug	Usual Dosage	Cost
Conventionals		
Thorazine* (SK Beecham)	200 mg	$ 64.65
Haldol* [Haloperidol**] (McNeil)	5 mg	$ 85.78
Generics		
Haloperidol**	5 mg average generic price	$ 36.01
Chlorpromazine**	200 mg average generic price	$ 8.89
Atypicals		
Risperidone** [Risperdal*] (Janssen	3 mg	$241.62
Clozapine** [Clozaril*] (Sandoz)	100 mg	$307.80
Olanzapine** [Zyprexa*] (Lilly)	10 mg once daily	$232.20

* Brand name   ** Generic name

Table adapted from: 'Olanzapine For Schizophrenia', *Medical Letter on Drugs and Therapeutics*, Vol. 38, No. 992, 17 January 1997, pp. 5–7.

Uncertainties in Schizophrenia Research

Most of the biological theories about the cause of schizophrenic symptoms can be explored using various methods of 'hard' science. But this type of scientific research, of necessity, always rests on swampy, very unscientific ground.

First, researchers assume that all the members of a schizophrenic cohort have a common denominator that makes them different from normal people. It is this assumed common denominator that researchers must rely on to point them to the cause of schizophrenia. However, the subjectivity of the diagnostic process and the absence of any definitive scientific tests to verify diagnoses means that, at the point of first diagnosis, there might not be any common denominator of abnormality amongst schizophrenics at all. Because each of them is likely to have been first diagnosed at different places and at different times, it is entirely possible that there will be no commonality between them besides the label and the subsequent treatment they receive.

The second problem arises from the history of neuroleptic medication of almost all schizophrenics who might be available to researchers. Routine psychiatric practice requires that a person be medicated immediately upon diagnosis. This means that any group of schizophrenics available to a scientific researcher will most likely be composed of people whose brain functioning has been modified by powerful chemicals. The subtle deviations from normal biochemistry and normal brain architecture that researchers sometimes claim to detect can usually be better explained as artefacts of neuroleptic medication than as pre-existing features of the supposed underlying schizophrenia.

This problem is readily apparent to researchers. While most of them choose to ignore it and to continue their research programmes as if it were not a factor, occasionally a researcher will claim to have carried out research on schizophrenics who have had no experience with neuroleptics. However, such claims usually avoid describing how the groups of 'never-medicated' schizophrenics were assembled, so there is inevitably some doubt about their validity. Occasionally, researchers suggest that their subjects were recruited prior to treatment on their first-admission entry to hospital. If this method of recruitment were actually used, it would raise an interesting question: would a hospital be acting ethically if it allowed people who were apparently in acute distress to undergo research testing before attention could be given to their problems? On top of this ethical problem, there are also practical grounds for doubt: how can a researcher accept, let alone confirm, a distressed person's claim of a lack of prior treatment at the point of the person's entry into hospital?

Scanning for Causes

Developments in brain-imaging techniques have given rise to a growing body of speculation that the cause of schizophrenia will be found in abnormalities in brain architecture. Brain scanning has revealed that the ratio of blood in the frontal lobes, between the front and the back, is lower in the brains of schizophrenics than in the brains of normal people. This has led to speculation that frontal-lobe dysfunction causes the positive symptoms of schizophrenia. Another theory that has developed out of apparent abnormalities detected by brain scans is that the cause of schizophrenia is to be found in some kind of trauma that has been experienced in the womb. Brain scans have revealed:

> increased amounts of cerebrospinal fluid (CSF) in the brain of many schizophrenics. A correspondingly slightly smaller brain volume has also been found. Since physical brain abnormalities do not progress further as the patient ages, levels of neuropathology may be present before birth. [20]

Apparent evidence from computed tomography (CT) scans of degeneration in a particular part of the brain called the cerebellar vermis has contributed to a brain-atrophy hypothesis for schizophrenia.[21] Magnetic resonance imaging (MRI) scans have also indicated that schizophrenic brains have a smaller average volume of total brain tissue than do the brains of normal people, and the smaller brain volume has been found to be offset by an increase in the volume of cerebrospinal fluid within schizophrenic brains. Specific decreases seem most apparent in the region of the frontal lobes. These findings have led researchers to conclude that:

> In addition to the generalised brain abnormalities observed in schizophrenia, a regional abnormality may be present in frontal regions. Since the frontal lobes integrate multimodality information and perform a variety of 'higher' cognitive and emotional functions that are impaired in schizophrenia, the frontal abnormality noted is consistent with the clinical presentation of the illness. Impaired frontal function and a disruption in its complex circuitry (including thalamocortical projections) may explain why patients with schizophrenia often have significant deficits in formulating concepts and organising their thinking and behaviour.[22]

However, there is no discussion in the description of this research as to whether the schizophrenics had been treated with neuroleptic medication prior to their MRI scans. It is therefore likely that the findings are simply artefacts of the treatment.

One group of researchers used MRI to scan the brains of fifteen pairs of identical twins, where one twin in each pair had schizophrenia. The schizophrenic twin in 14 of the fifteen pairs was found to have enlarged ventricles. (This correlates with increased amounts of cerebrospinal fluid and, it is thought, smaller brain volume.) To deal with the problem of prior neuroleptic treatment, the degree of ventricle enlargement was cross-checked to see if it correlated with the length of time that the schizophrenic twins had been on medication. It was found that, 'Brain abnormalities were not more severe among the schizophrenics with a long history either of the disorder or of antipsychotic drug treatment. Thus, the changes appear linked directly to schizophrenia.'[23]

These findings have led to speculations that early in brain development there might be some kind of viral infection, birth injury, or auto-immune disorder that underlies abnormal brain development in schizophrenics. These abnormalities could go unnoticed until late adolescence, when the central nervous system undergoes maturational changes. This is the time of life when the symptoms of schizophrenia most commonly emerge.

One problem with this is that the possible contribution of neuroleptic medication to the abnormalities is not properly discounted. The approach presupposes that, if neuroleptics do play a role, there would be a dose-response relationship between the abnormalities they caused and the length of time they were used; that is, the abnormalities would be greater the longer the neuroleptics were taken. But no evidence is supplied to support this assumption.

Another problem is that some schizophrenics do not have large ventricles. One investigation found that it was only the males in a group of schizophrenics who had large ventricles. As well, it has been found that some people with Alzheimer's disease and others with manic depression also have large ventricles. So this abnormal feature is neither necessary for schizophrenia, nor is it associated solely with schizophrenia.[24]

Despite the enthusiasm of some research reports, proponents of the enlarged ventricle theory remain on the margins of mainstream psychiatry. In fact, 'a simple statement that "schizophrenics have larger ventricles than controls" will be marked wrong in an MCQ examination of the Royal College of Psychiatrists, as the ventricles of the brains of most schizophrenics have scores within the normal range'.[25]

Infection Theories

The belief that infectious organisms might be the cause of many mental diseases is not new. In the early decades of the twentieth century between one-quarter and one-third of patients admitted to mental hospitals in industrialised countries were suffering from general paresis, a condition produced in the tertiary stage of syphilis.[26]

The discovery of penicillin, and its success in treating syphilis, has implanted a belief amongst some psychiatric researchers that an infectious cause and medical remedy can also be found for schizophrenia. Viral theories of aetiology are particularly attractive to some researchers, because they can tie up a number of loose ends—such as the perceived seasonality of schizophrenic births,[27] the difficulties some schizophrenic women are said to have in childbirth, the frequency of auditory hallucinations, and an assumed genetic component of the disease.[28]

The viral theories are essentially of two types: those which postulate an active but undetected virus that directly affects the brain and gives rise to unusual psychological phenomena; and theories which postulate a past infection that, although no longer active, caused abnormalities in brain development. Retroviruses have been suggested as the likely culprit for the first type of possibility, but researchers have been unable to find any positive link between schizophrenia and this type of virus.[29] Borna disease was recently discounted as a virus that might be active in schizophrenics.[30]

One explanation for the second type of possibility is that schizophrenics might be part of a sub-population with special resistance to disease. Although the resistance itself may not be a factor in the development of schizophrenia, it might result in foetal vulnerability to hormonal disturbances during prenatal viral infection. This vulnerability might in turn lead to neurodevelopmental damage. It is further argued that, if this were so, schizophrenia could be seen as a price that a population has to pay for surviving epidemics.[31]

Enthusiasm for the viral epidemic theory has recently focussed on polio. There are a number of attractive features to the polio theory: a claimed decrease in numbers of schizophrenics coinciding with the advent of polio vaccine; a higher number of winter births, confirming the possibility of second-trimester infection in summer months, when polio is most active; and a higher incidence of schizophrenia amongst immigrants to the United Kingdom whose countries of origin also have a higher incidence of polio. Once again, it is postulated that prenatal infection with polio might cause developmental problems in the brain that do not emerge until sexual maturity.[32] But no significant evidence has been found yet to provide confirmation for the polio hypothesis.

Nutrition

Another area of speculation with a substantial following is concerned with nutrition. The nutritional theories divide in the same way as the viral theories. Some postulate prenatal nutritional deficiencies which have caused developmental abnormalities, and others argue that schizophrenia is caused by a deficiency in the current diet of the patient. Whereas the first group of theories generally do not have a direct remedy, the second group often does.

A considerable amount of research has focussed on historically recorded famines, which have been used to explore a hypothesised link between the starvation of pregnant mothers and schizophrenia in offspring.[33] The Dutch winter famine of 1944–1945 has provided Dutch researchers with the opportunity to explore this connection, and one group has concluded that starvation during pregnancy can be a factor in the development of schizoid personalities in offspring.[34]

Researchers give four reasons for supporting the prenatal nutrition hypothesis: the known effects of prenatal starvation are not incompatible with the observed features of schizophrenia; brain abnormalities can develop as a result of these events; general malnutrition has also been observed to cause abnormalities in areas of the brain that have been linked to schizophrenia; and it is known that proper prenatal nutrition is essential for the correct development of the foetal nervous system.[35] But no hard evidence has yet been found to support this type of hypothesis. Indeed there appears to be no evidence of a relatively high incidence of schizophrenia in countries where malnutrition has been endemic for generations. Nevertheless this area seems particularly attractive to some researchers, and the Dutch winter famine has been linked statistically to a two-fold increase in the risk of schizophrenia.[36]

Amongst the second group of nutritional theories, which argue that schizophrenia is caused by deficiencies in the diets of adult schizophrenics, one theory claims that schizophrenia can be rectified with a high wheat diet.[37] But this recommendation is directly contradicted by another theory that recommends avoiding wheat products:

> The kinds of cereal grain from products customarily eaten may be a factor in the production of psychiatric symptoms. There might be a relationship between schizophrenia and coeliac disease, a disease of known sensitivity to wheat and sometimes to milk. The wheat and rye-eating areas of the world have the highest incidence of schizophrenia, with oats and barley areas next, followed by the rice-eating areas (with approximately 60% of the incidence of the wheat areas). In sorghum and maize-eating areas the incidence of schizophrenia was approximately 25% of the wheat areas and in the highlands of New Guinea a practically nil incidence is found. Here no grains are eaten. William Philpott, an American psychiatrist, found that half his sample of schizophrenic patients could not tolerate milk and 64% were wheat sensitive.[38]

The confusion over whether wheat might have a beneficial or detrimental effect on people inclined towards psychosis is fairly typical of the many contradictions that surround schizophrenia. Perhaps this particular area of confusion might in part be explained by the well-known relationship between vitamin B12 deficiency and pellagra—a disease that affects the skin, and the digestive and nervous systems—and which commonly presents with schizophrenia-like symptoms:

In 1937, Elvehjen identified niacin deficiency as the cause and niacin the cure for pellagra, after which large numbers of pellagra psychotics recovered and were found not to be schizophrenic. As a result of this discovery, niacin is now routinely added to bread.³⁹

Despite the length of time over which this association between vitamin B12 deficiency and psychotic symptoms has been known, contemporary researchers still occasionally announce its rediscovery. One recent example from Singapore reported a case study involving an observed link between vitamin B12 deficiency, anaemia, and schizophrenia, and recommended supplementing neuroleptic medication to compensate.⁴⁰

Genetic Theories

Genetic theories underlie many of the biological theories, since it is often assumed that only those people with a genetic vulnerability will manifest the neuropathological condition that causes schizophrenia, or succumb to the virus or the malnutrition that causes the neuropathology that in turn causes schizophrenia. Indeed, a genetic factor is necessary to give credibility to any biological explanation of the cause, because one of the few uncontested features of schizophrenia is that it tends to run in families. Without a plausible genetic argument, the phenomenon of family propensity for schizophrenia might be better explained by environmental causes.

The idea that a single dominant genetic component might be solely responsible—that there could be a 'schizophrenia gene'—is a highly attractive notion to researchers that, I believe, has to be discounted by other observable phenomena. Breggin argues that when geneticists go in search of a dominant gene as the cause for a disease such as Huntington's chorea, the quest makes sense because there is prior knowledge from the set pattern of family inheritance that a dominant gene is responsible.⁴¹ But this is clearly not the case with schizophrenia. Although there is a family association with schizophrenia, there is no set pattern of inheritance.

However, some genetic researchers have not been deterred from embarking on the quest for the schizophrenia gene. Indeed they have even occasionally announced their success. In 1988, for instance, Chromosome 5 was announced to be the site of the gene: 'For the first time, scientists have obtained evidence that a specific chromosome mutation contains a gene predisposing its bearers to schizophrenia and closely related mental disorders'. The announcement was made in the 10 November 1988 issue of *Nature*, but a refutation came so swiftly that it was published in the same edition of the journal.

More recently, the search for the schizophrenia gene has concentrated on Irish families. In 1995 a team of scientists from the United States

> headed by Scott Diehl of the National Institute of Health found a specific region of Chromosome 6 that appears to contain a gene for the disorder. 'If our finding holds up, it means that, contrary to what a lot of researchers have thought, there is at least one major gene that predisposes a person to schizophrenia,' said Diehl.[42]

The equivocal statement, 'If our finding holds up,' was a definite warning that Diehl himself was uncertain about the claims he was making for Chromosome 6. Ten days later, the reason for this uncertainty was revealed. It seems that Diehl had published the results of work he had been engaged in as a junior research scientist at the Medical College of Virginia under the direction of Dr Kenneth Kendler. But Diehl had moved on to another research facility in 1993. A simmering dispute had continued between Diehl and Kendler between 1993 and 1995 over whether Diehl had any rights to the research he had undertaken while working for Kendler. Diehl's 1995 announcement of having discovered the schizophrenia gene turned out to be a pre-emptive strike to claim ownership of the intellectual property. It seems that he had only completed 10 per cent of the gene mapping work envisioned in Kendler's research scheme, and Diehl's article only described preliminary findings. At stake were millions of dollars of research funding to complete the project.[43]

Many genetic researchers are not convinced that Kendler and Diehl are even on the right track in pursuing Chromosome 6. Some researchers have targeted Chromosome 22 as being the most likely site for the schizophrenia gene.[44] Most genetic research, however, now assumes that there is no single schizophrenia gene, and that a variety of separate genetic factors are involved.[45]

The basis for the genetic theory is a well-observed family association with schizophrenia.[46] Psychiatric textbooks often misleadingly present this association as concordance rates indicating established genetic risk factors for schizophrenia:

Genetic Risk for Schizophrenia

Identical twin affected	50%
Fraternal twin affected	15%
Brother or sister affected	10%
One parent affected	15%
Both parents affected	35%
Second-degree relative affected	2–3%
No affected relative	1%

Source: Norman L. Keltner, 'Schizophrenia and Other Psychoses', in Norman L. Keltner, Lee Hilyard Schwecke and Carol E. Bostrom, eds., *Psychiatric Nursing*, Mosby, St Louis, 1995, p. 368.

These concordance rates, however, can also support arguments for an environmental cause. In cases, for instance, where one or both parents have schizophrenia, it can be argued that it is not the transmission of genes that passes the condition on to offspring but rather the parental role model. Similarly, if one child develops schizophrenia due to an environmental cause in family life, it is likely that other children in the family will be affected in the same way.[47]

This exploitation of concordance research by advocates of an environmental cause has prompted genetic researchers to explore the concordance rates of siblings who have been reared separately. The adoption studies that are most frequently cited are quite old, dating back to the 1960s and 1970s. Of these, the most important was published in 1975 by a team led by Seymour Kety.[48]

The Kety study was sponsored by the National Institute of Mental Health in the United States: it involved locating Danish schizophrenics who had been adopted as children, before their schizophrenia had become apparent. Denmark was chosen because of the efficiency of its official system of record-keeping. The second step in the investigation required locating and psychiatrically assessing the biological relatives of the adopted schizophrenics to see if there was a higher incidence of schizophrenia amongst them than amongst the relatives of a control group of non-schizophrenic adoptees. The findings, which revealed that schizophrenia and 'schizophrenia spectrum' disorders were more prevalent amongst the relatives of the schizophrenic adoptees, were taken to be positive evidence of a genetic link for schizophrenia.[49]

However, even this apparently conclusive study has been severely and persuasively criticised. Claims have been made that there was a double sleight-of-hand involved in the presentation of the results.[50] It has been pointed out that the Kety study could not find any increase in schizophrenia amongst the close relatives of the adopted schizophrenics—mothers, fathers, sisters, and brothers—and that the only significant increase it found was amongst paternal half-siblings. Furthermore this increased incidence amongst paternal half-siblings was all contained within one large family.

As well, the distantly related association with schizophrenia was largely due to the inclusion of 'schizophrenia spectrum' disorders in the comparative study. The Kety study used the second edition of the *Diagnostic and Statistical Manual of Mental Disorders* to define the relevant range of disorders. As it happens, this edition of the manual included a category that has since been dropped, called 'latent schizophrenia'. This was a supposed tendency towards schizophrenia without a history of psychosis. It was similar to the Soviet concept of 'sluggish schizophrenia', and almost anybody could be fitted into it. Fourteen out of a total of 18 half-siblings diagnosed with 'schizophrenia spectrum' disorders had only this latent form.

Breggin argues that the four cases of full-blown schizophrenia within the one family could be best explained by an environmental cause—perhaps sexual abuse. He dismisses the cases of latent schizophrenia as irrelevancies.

Adoption studies have also been severely criticised because of concerns that adoption practices may have been influenced by eugenics policies in the countries where the most influential adoption studies were carried out. Jay Joseph has analysed the development of eugenics policies, and their translation into laws sanctioning sterilisation of mentally ill people, in Denmark, Finland, and Oregon.[51] He argues that a number of adoption studies undertaken in Denmark in the 1960s and 1970s, others undertaken in Finland in the 1970s and 1980s, and another in Oregon in the 1960s all used schizophrenic adoptees who were placed for adoption at a time when eugenics legislation was in force.

Jay's argument is that adoption agencies would have been influenced by eugenics policies in regard to the type of families children were placed into. If a child who was given up for adoption had a natural mother who had schizophrenia, or if there was any known mental illness in the family of the mother or father, the child would most likely have been placed in a family of lower socio/economic status. This in turn would have increased the likelihood that these children would have been reared in a more stressful environment, and they would therefore have been more likely to develop schizophrenia.

The most persuasive evidence for a genetic link comes from the study of concordance rates in twins. The twins method is widely used to determine whether a particular trait has any connection with genetic inheritance. The method involves comparing the concordance rates of monozygotic (MZ) twins (one egg, identical) with concordance rates of dizygotic (DZ) twins (two egg, fraternal). In schizophrenia studies these comparisons are confined to twins where both members have been reared together. The object is to determine whether the 100 per cent genetic concordance of monozygotic twins, compared to the 50 per cent genetic concordance of dizygotic twins, reflects in similarly divergent concordance rates for schizophrenia. The results are quite impressive.

When the results are pooled of 14 twins' studies conducted between 1928 and 1998 the pooled concordance rates for monozygotic twins is 44 per cent compared to 9 per cent for dizygotic twins.[52] At first glance, this offers convincing evidence for a genetic factor in schizophrenia. However, critics of the studies point to two major problems with this approach. The first is that the studies themselves all have methodological problems. The most serious of these problems are the familiar ones concerning diagnostic criteria and subjective methods of diagnosis for schizophrenia. Critics have pointed out that all of these studies were undertaken by researchers who set out to confirm the genetic hypothesis, and that in most cases non-blinded diagnostic procedures were used. Given the subjective nature of schizophrenia diagnosis, this gives rise to concerns that diagnoses might have been inflated for one group and deflated for the other.

The other major problem concerns the possibility that concordance rates might have been confounded by environmental factors. Analysis of the studies has shown that, although there is no sex-link to the genetic hypothesis for schizophrenia, the twin studies show a distinct pattern of sex-linked concordance. In summary, 'female MZ pairs were more concordant than male MZ pairs; female DZs were more concordant than male DZs; DZ same-sex twins were more concordant than opposite-sexed DZs; and DZ twins were more concordant than ordinary siblings, despite sharing the same genetic relationship'.[53]

These results suggest that something other than genes is responsible for the concordance patterns. Critics suggest that the most likely explanation is that family environments tend to compress the identities of twins so that they experience a phenomenon called 'ego-fusion'. This occurs as a result of families endeavouring to treat them equally, which often means duplication of clothing and experience. The more similar the twins are, whether MZs or same sex, the more duplicated their experience tends to be. The result is that if one twin experiences madness the other will have a propensity to follow, depending on their history of duplicated experience: 'It is therefore concluded that there is no reason to accept that the twin method measures anything other than the environmental differences distinguishing identical and fraternal twins'.[54]

It is not only the gene sceptics who warn about excessive optimism pervading the genetic quest. Some of the leading researchers in the field also find it necessary to keep the issue in perspective:

> The search for genes of major effect in schizophrenia, however, is premised not so much on hard evidence that they exist, as on the absence of evidence that they do not ... Recent work suggests that such genes of major effect exist in other common disorders, but linkage studies in schizophrenia must still be regarded as acts of faith.[55]

Theories of an Environmental/Experiential Cause

Environmental/experiential theories are very different to biological theories, and begin from an altogether different premise. Biological theories largely disregard or discount any concept of mind, preferring instead to assume that abnormalities of thought are caused by abnormalities in brain functioning. Environmental/experiential theories, on the other hand, assume that the symptoms of schizophrenia are manifestations of a person's mind, rather than of his or her brain.

An individual's experience within the family environment is the matrix from which many environmental/experiential theories arise. Family life, particularly during infancy and early childhood, is often seen as the environment in which the fundamental characteristics of a person's mind are formed. Accordingly, environmental determinists blame malformations of mental characteristics as causes of schizophrenia.

A variety of talking therapies have been used for treating schizophrenia when it is thought to be caused by environmental influences. There are therapies which assume that the fault is a problem of intrapsychic development (that is, that it is in the psychological make-up of the schizophrenic), and that it can be corrected by making the affected individual more aware of the problem; there are therapies which assume that the fault is with the schizophrenic's family, or a particular member of the family, and can be corrected by making adjustments to family structures; and there are therapies which assume that the fault is in a competitive/hostile social environment to which the schizophrenic is maladapted.

Developmental Theories

The first type of therapy is often based on some kind of developmental theory about the cause of schizophrenia, in many cases stemming from Sigmund Freud's ideas about schizophrenia. Freud in turn based many of his ideas about the subject on his analysis of a distinguished jurist named Daniel Paul Schreber, who developed a psychosis in mid-life.[56] Schreber's psychosis involved paranoid delusions of persecution, which Freud interpreted as manifestations of Schreber's latent homosexual attraction to his father.

Freud theorised that because the homosexual attraction was too unbearable for Schreber to acknowledge, it had instead been transformed into hatred for his father. Hatred for his father, in turn, caused Schreber to see him as a persecutor. This simple rationale became the basis for Freud's general explanation of the paranoia that is commonly associated with schizophrenia. Similarly, the equally common phenomenon of hallucinations was explained conversely as 'wish fulfilment of unbearable ideas rejected by the ego'.[57]

Freud observed that problems with interpersonal relationships were associated with schizophrenia, and he applied his libido theory to find an explanation. He speculated that a schizophrenic's inability to properly relate to other people is caused by the withdrawal of libido into the self. This withdrawal of libido is a regression to the infantilism of primary process thinking, and the ensuing focus on the self gives rise to delusions and hallucinations as compensation for the deficit in interpersonal relations.

Freud believed that schizophrenics could not be treated by psychoanalytical means, because their inability to form interpersonal relationships meant they were unable to engage in transference— which is essential to the process of psychoanalysis. This declaration of untreatability led to the marginalisation of Freud's theories on schizophrenia and to a quest by successive theorists for a developmental hypothesis that would support some form of therapeutic intervention.

Harry Stack Sullivan's theories extended Freud's considerably. Although Freud and Sullivan had similar approaches to schizophrenia, they came from very different cultural backgrounds that led them to different conclusions. Freud came from a Jewish, middle-class, sophisticated Viennese background that gave him a detached, scholarly perspective, with an observer's status that was not so much a personal attribute as one he had inherited with his ethnic identity. Sullivan, on the other hand, had grown up as a lonely outsider in a rural area of the United States.[58]

Sullivan's personal struggle through childhood and adolescence with a cold, rejecting mother and a shy, distant father gave him a certain empathy with the schizophrenics he encountered in his adult career as a psychiatrist from the 1920s to the 1940s. Although he began his career accepting many of Freud's beliefs, his technique of closely observing and empathising with his patients led to many revisions.[59]

Sullivan came to believe that many psychiatric problems were due to the fraud and hypocrisy which he thought were endemic to society. He believed that the Oedipus complex, for instance, on which Freud's theory of schizophrenia was based, 'must be recognised as a distortion, not a biological development, in the normal male child. It is a fraudulent symbol situation commonly the result of multiple vicious features of our domestic culture'.[60]

Sullivan's version of the developmental theory conceived by Freud was that schizophrenia is the outcome of interpersonal problems. To Sullivan, personality development is dependent on a person monitoring the appraisal of him or her by significant people. When significant people are perceived to have a negative opinion, or when there are no significant people in a person's life, there is a risk of developing a personality deficit or schizophrenia. Sullivan's theory contributed to a change in the focus of the developmental theories, so that schizophrenia was no longer seen as an intra-psychic problem but instead became a problem associated with a person's family or social environment.

The Family Environment

On the non-biological side of the psychiatric dichotomy, theories that have evolved about environmental causes for schizophrenia usually focus either on the family or the larger social environment. Those which focus on the family environment demonstrate a clear pattern of evolution. At first, mothers were the focus of research, on the assumption that some fault in mother/child bonding was the cause of schizophrenia. Then the focus of research moved on to marital relationships between mothers and fathers, based on the assumption that some kind of distortion in these relationships might impact on children and cause schizophrenia. Finally, researchers began to take account of the family environment as a whole, theorising that any member of a family, or all the members of a family together, might somehow create conditions of stress that produced schizophrenia in a family member.

The term 'schizophrenogenic mother' was first coined in 1948 by a psychiatrist named Frieda Fromm-Reichman. 'The schizophrenic,' she wrote, 'is painfully distrustful and resentful of other people due to the severe early warp and rejection he encountered in important people in his infancy and childhood, as a rule mainly the schizophrenogenic mother.'[61] There were two ideas embodied in Fromm-Reichman's concept of the schizophrenia-inducing mother that made her terminology a powerful message for the times—the notions of maternal rejection and maternal overprotection.[62]

The post-World-War-II period was one of rapid cultural change, in which attention was often focussed on the relationship between mothers and children.[63] Uncertainty had developed about the quality of mother–infant bonding in industrialised countries as a result of a variety of factors, including a rising divorce rate, adolescent pregnancies, and working mothers who left their babies with minders. The satisfying pre-war cultural image of a young mother successfully nurturing an infant was being eroded.

Social commentators often blamed mothers for any troubles children had with social adjustment, and also for any problems the society might have with maladjusted or delinquent children, and other social stresses. As a result, the suburban housewife was often stereotyped as a frustrated, repressed, disturbed, martyred, never-satisfied, unhappy woman; a demanding, nagging, shrewish wife; and a rejecting, over-protecting, dominating mother.[64]

This changing cultural identity of women enhanced the significance of the role of motherhood in the eyes of psychiatrists. As faith in the competence of mothers declined, advice was increasingly sought from professionals on matters concerning nurturing and child care. But mothers remained powerful. Although they might be perceived as failing to produce healthy, well-adjusted children, they could still wreak social havoc by producing deviants.[65]

As well, at the same time as women were increasingly seen as becoming dominant, masculine power was thought to be on the decline. Popular literature complained about the emasculation of men due to factors such as the bureaucratisation of work, the rise of the corporate 'man in the grey flannel suit', and the demise of individualism. The newly enfeebled men of the 1950s had castrating women waiting for them in every suburban home.[66]

The significance of these cultural trends for the development of the idea of the schizophrenogenic mother, despite the originator herself being a woman, is that most of the psychiatric researchers who pursued this line of research were men. The general notion they were pursuing was of a dominating, over-protective, but basically rejecting mother who somehow induced a schizophrenic reaction in her offspring.[67] A considerable number of uncontrolled studies were undertaken that seemed to confirm this premise. These were usually in the form of interview studies or case-record studies without control groups.

However, by the early 1980s the concept of the schizophrenogenic mother had run its course. A researcher could argue in 1982, after reviewing the literature on the subject, that '[t]he most plausible explanation is that there is no *sui generis* schizophrenogenic mother; instead, there is a parental type distinguished by hostile, critical, and intrusive style and it is not particularly over-represented in the parents of schizophrenics'.[68] With further shifts in cultural values over the intervening years, it had become apparent that only a small percentage of women who might arguably fit the criteria of schizophrenogenic mother had actually produced schizophrenic children. Conversely, many schizophrenics were found to have mothers who did not fit the criteria.

By the early 1980s some psychiatric researchers were ready to include the schizophrenogenic mother on a list with other 'dangerous psychosocial hypotheses' that supposedly had retarded the progress of psychiatry.[69] Yet despite the hostility that had developed against the idea within the psychiatric profession, and despite the lack of evidence to support it, the schizophrenogenic mother was still being presented as a viable concept in psychology textbooks up to the end of the 1980s.[70]

Double Bind Theory

The schizophrenogenic mother was only one of a number of possible complications in the childhoods of schizophrenics that might account for the disorder. The search for a distortion in family experience that could be described in finite terms, measured, and positively connected with schizophrenics was something of a holy grail for psychiatrists in the decades following World War II. Perhaps the most seductive idea that arose from this quest was the 'double bind' theory.

In 1956 Gregory Bateson and his colleagues at Stanford University published a 'report on a research project which has been formulating and testing a broad, systematic view of the nature, etiology, and therapy of schizophrenia'.[71] The double bind theory that arose from this research was based on communications theories. Although many relationships have double bind potential, Bateson preferred to illustrate the theory by depicting the mother-child relationship:

> we hypothesise that the mother of a schizophrenic will be simultaneously expressing at least two orders of message. These orders can be roughly characterised as (a) hostile or withdrawing behaviour that is aroused whenever the child approaches her, and (b) simulated loving or approaching behaviour which is aroused when the child responds to her hostile and withdrawing behaviour, as a way of denying she is withdrawing.[72]

Bateson gave an example of the double bind situation taken from observations made during clinical practice. This example is much cited, and has been frequently used by other writers to illustrate in summary the mechanism of the double bind:

> A young man who had fairly well recovered from an acute schizophrenic episode was visited in the hospital by his mother. He was glad to see her and impulsively put his arm around her

shoulders, whereupon she stiffened. He withdrew his arm and she asked, 'Don't you love me any more?' He then blushed, and she said, 'Dear you must not be so easily embarrassed and afraid of your feelings.' The patient was able to stay with her only a few minutes and following her departure he assaulted an aide and was put in the tubs.[73]

Bateson's view was that the inner turmoil experienced by schizophrenics is associated with a habit of routinely thinking and communicating in metaphorical language without fully comprehending that they are doing so: 'The peculiarity of the schizophrenic is not that he uses metaphors, but that he uses *unlabelled* metaphors'.[74] In normal speech, a labelled metaphor transfers a word to an object to which it does not properly belong, in order to make an implied comparison. A statement such as 'That man is a snake' is a normal figure of speech when clearly labelled in the minds of both the speaker and the hearer as a metaphor. But if it has not been so labelled, and it appears to have been uttered literally, it is likely to induce confusion in the mind of the speaker and to be taken for a schizophprenic delusion by the hearer.

Bateson argued that there are numerous classes of ideas used in human communication which each dictate different modes of communication within their fields of influence. According to the theory, it is imperative that a discontinuity prevails between the class and the members:

> Although in formal logic there is an attempt to maintain this discontinuity between a class and its members, we argue that in the psychology of real communications this discontinuity is continually and inevitably breached and that *a priori* we must expect a pathology to occur in the human organism when certain formal patterns of the breaching occur in the communication between mother and child. We shall argue that this pathology at its extreme will have symptoms whose formal characteristics would lead the pathology to be classified as a schizophrenia.[75]

The description of the double bind situation, from which schizophrenics were assumed to contract their mental pathology, was persuasive and logical. Bateson specified six ingredients for a double bind:

(1) The 'victim', that is, the schizophrenic person, must have had a childhood relationship with one or more family members whose communication techniques induced inner conflict.

(2) The double bind communications were a repeated rather than a single traumatic experience. The repetition is necessary in order to induce in the victim a habitual expectation of double bind forms of communication.

(3) The double bind communication first takes the form of a primary negative injunction. 'This may take either of two forms: (a) "Do not do so and so, or I will punish you", or (b) "If you do not do so and so, I will punish you".' The punishment that is threatened might take the form of either withdrawal of love or the expression of anger.

(4) The primary negative injunction is followed by a secondary injunction which conflicts with the first. The secondary injunction is on a more abstract level and, although like the first it is enforced by an implication of punishment, it is usually communicated in a more subtle fashion which might involve nonverbal means such as posture, gesture or tone of voice.

(5) A tertiary negative injunction prevents the victim from escaping from the situation.

(6) When the victim has learned to anticipate double bind patterns in all communications the complete set of ingredients is no longer necessary and 'almost any part of the double bind sequence may then be sufficient to precipitate rage or panic. The

pattern of conflicting injunctions may even be taken over by hallucinatory voices.'[76]

The simplicity of the double bind argument was very appealing However, while many schizophrenics appeared to have a history of some kind of double bind situation,[77] so did many non-schizophrenics. In fact, the popularity of the idea might be attributable to the fact that most people have experienced the frustration of a double bind relationship with a person of authority at some time in their lives, and can easily recognise the problem. This only begs the question: if the double bind is a factor in the causation of schizophrenia, why are only some people vulnerable? The answer to this question proved to be elusive,[78] and by the end of the 1970s researchers had largely moved on to focus on other hypotheses.

Family Stress

Another line of research, explored over the same time-period as the schizophrenogenic mother and the double bind, concerned theories that distortions in the marital relationship of a mother and father might impact adversely on a child and cause schizophrenia. Theodore Lidz was one of the leading researchers in this field. Lidz hypothesised that there are two different kinds of distortion in parental marital relationships which had the effect of alternatively selecting boys and girls as candidates for schizophrenia.

The first kind of distortion Lidz called 'marital skew'.[79] This occurs when one parent yields to the idiosyncrasies and over-bearing dominance of the other. This situation was thought to be particularly relevant to the cause of schizophrenia in male children.[80] In families with marital skew, the dominant parent was usually the mother, and in contrast to her the father was perceived as being a weak, passive type of person who provided a poor role model for his son. In these families, the mother was believed to turn away from her husband as a source of emotional comfort and to fixate on her son in a search for solace. The combination of a poor paternal role model and a fixated, dominant, and often eccentric mother was thought to be a frequent cause of schizophrenia in male children.[81]

Schizophrenia in female children was thought to be usually caused by a variation on this theme, due to a condition called 'marital schism'. Marital schism occurred when there was conflict between the mother and father, but neither party yielded to the other.[82] In this situation, each partner was constantly striving to satisfy his or her own needs while ignoring the partner's needs. This perpetual battle for ascendancy between parents inevitably involved the children as the parents competed for their affections and enrolled them as supporters. The schismatic family was thought to be far more selective in causing schizophrenia in females than in males.[83]

In both the skewed and schismatic types of family, Lidz hypothesised that children are reared in an abnormal environment because there is an absence of parental cooperation, and the normal delineations between generations are not observed. He believed that these conditions could lead to anxieties in children involving the induction of incestuous feelings. Lidz's basic approach to schizophrenia was similar to Bateson's, in that he believed it was the manifestation of inappropriate behaviour that had been learned in the family environment.[84]

Although a considerable amount of research has been conducted over the years to test Lidz's theories, most of the results have not supported them. The American researcher S N Sharan undertook a particularly thorough study in the mid-1960s which involved twelve families with a schizophrenic son, and twelve with a schizophrenic daughter. Each of these groups of families were symmetrically balanced by dividing them into six families with a healthy sibling of the same sex as the schizophrenic, and six families with a healthy sibling of the opposite sex to the schizophrenic.[85]

The core of the study required each family to complete a questionnaire. This was done under tape-recorded supervision with the family members assembled in groups of three, firstly comprising the two parents and the schizophrenic child, and secondly comprising the two parents and the healthy child. Different questionnaires were used each time, and answering the questionnaires required discussion amongst each separate group. The objective was to score the individual parents for indications of dominance by assessing how often one parent's answers became the group's decision. Support between individuals was also scored by recording how often supportive and non-supportive remarks were directed at individual family members.

Sharan could find no clear pattern confirming Lidz's theories about either the relationship of parental marital skew to schizophrenia in male children or the relationship of marital schism to female schizophrenia. Nor could he uncover any clear pattern of parental support or non-support for schizophrenic children as compared to their healthy siblings.[86]

Another line of research that assumed an environmental cause involved studying the families of schizophrenics as whole units, to see if the cause of schizophrenia could be found in group deviance rather than in the deviations of individual members.[87] One influential hypothesis postulated that when there are mutual expectations amongst family members of reciprocal fulfilment which have no basis in reality, the false atmosphere in the family is often accompanied by disjointed forms of communication and irrational shifts in the focus of family attention. This situation was thought to give rise to conditions in which all family communications were polarised between superficiality at one pole and fragmented, disjointed thinking at the other. These conditions in turn influenced the cognitive development of children who were subjected to them. Schizophrenia was thought to be one of the outcomes.

More recently, deviance in the language of schizophrenic patients has been compared to similar deviations in the language of their parents, in the hope that some light may be shed on the cause by understanding how the language deviations of schizophrenia are learned.[88] Research is now also turning to focus on positively identifying a link between genetic vulnerability and environmental stresses in family life that might trigger schizophrenia. One recent study compared adopted children of schizophrenic mothers, who were thought to have an enhanced genetic risk, with a control group of adoptees with normal genetic risk profiles, to see whether there were any consistent patterns of thought deviation in the two groups of children that might be associated with environmental triggers. However, no clear pattern has emerged from this research yet.[89]

Stress in the family environment has been extensively researched as both an originating cause of schizophrenia and as a factor in relapse. Two types of stresses have largely been the focus of attention: the ambient stresses of everyday life, and abnormal stresses brought on by important life events such as a death in the family.[90] Ambient stresses are often measured in the form of 'expressed emotion' (EE). Schizophrenics are thought to come from families with higher than normal levels of EE, and some researchers claim that a high level of EE between a mother and child, for instance, deepens the emotional bond but also puts the child at a higher risk of developing schizophrenia.[91] Comparisons have been drawn between the key components of EE research—that is, critical comments and the over-involvement of family members in the schizophrenic's life—with the rejection and over-protection that was formerly attributed to the schizophrenogenic mother.[92] This suggests that EE researchers might be merely extending the schizophrenogenic concept from the mother to the whole family.

One type of important event that has attracted research attention is the death of a grandparent within two years of the birth of a schizophrenic person. Researchers found that a grandparent of 41 per cent of a large sample of schizophrenics had died within this period. This rate was significantly higher than the rate in a control group of normal people, and it was hypothesised that the additional stresses introduced into family life by two major events—a birth followed by death, or vice versa—might confuse the parenting and mourning roles. In this situation, a bereaved parent might be emotionally unavailable to an infant and a spouse or, alternatively, a child might be used as a distraction from mourning and as a result could inadvertently absorb the painful feelings of the bereaved parent.[93]

Social Stress

Comparisons have been made between schizophrenic and non-schizophrenic people to determine whether personal experience of negative life-events is a significant factor. It has been found that schizophrenics have a higher incidence of these negative experiences in the areas of work, health, family, and social relationships.[94] It has also been observed that the incidence of schizophrenia is higher in urban centres, but recent research has been unable to confirm that the stress of city living is implicated as a cause.[95]

Stresses arising from social class have also been a subject for research into the cause of schizophrenia. There has been consistent evidence of a higher incidence of schizophrenia amongst people of lower social classes. Two principal hypotheses have been presented to account for this. The first is that stresses induced by social conditions such as poverty, unemployment, and welfare dependency can cause schizophrenia. The second is that the confused state of mind experienced by schizophrenics makes them socially uncompetitive, which in turn leads them into a downward social drift.

Stresses arising from racial identity have also been explored as possibly contributing to the cause of schizophrenia. A recent study conducted in the United Kingdom compared the incidence and outcomes of schizophrenia amongst whites, Afro-Caribbeans, and Asians. Afro-Caribbeans and Asian women were found to have a higher incidence of schizophrenia, and Afro-Caribbeans were more disabled by the experience. The only significant variable the researchers could find to explain these results, other than racial identity, was a higher level of unemployment amongst the Afro-Caribbeans.[96]

Theories Galore

In recent years, there has been an increasing trend amongst psychiatric practitioners to advocate an end to the mind/brain dichotomy and to argue that a more sophisticated approach to schizophrenia can be based on the assumption that the cause has both biological and environmental components. This is sometimes called a biopsychosocial approach, and it is often endorsed by psychiatrists who are currently treating schizophrenics with a mixture of drugs and talking therapy. However, it is not a position that appears to be particularly attractive to researchers seeking the cause of schizophrenia, because it tends to multiply the already vast field of possibilities.

The sheer number of past and present theories, on both sides of the biology/environment dichotomy, is evidence of deep confusion within the medical model about the cause of schizophrenia. In turn, this confusion is reflected in the proliferation of therapies. And yet it does not seem to have had any negative effect on the high confidence-levels of individual psychiatrists, even when they are imposing dangerous drug treatments on involuntary patients.

In the early 1990s, Theodore Sarbin reviewed his long career in pursuit of definitive evidence that might explain the cause of schizophrenia. He related how, in the early 1970s, he had analysed the various theories that had been postulated up to that time. He said that 'the rise and fall of theories of schizophrenia led me to conclude that such theories have a half-life of about five years. The conclusion applied to somatic theories and psychological theories alike.'[97] Sarbin went on to cite more recent research that confirmed his own findings, but which also found that biological theories have shorter life spans than psychological theories.

4

Behind The Medical Model:
interest groups and human rights

Constant movement in the fashion of ideas is a central feature of the psychiatric view of schizophrenia. Without these changing fashions it would be far more difficult to maintain high confidence-levels amongst supporters about the verities of the medical model. As most of the psychiatric ideas about the cause and the treatment of schizophrenia are simply guesswork—sometimes wild guesswork—a consistent strategy has evolved to cover up the doubtful nature of these ideas. First, loud cheering is heard as new theories are conceived and imminent breakthroughs are predicted. Then, after reality intervenes but before failure becomes apparent, the theories and predictions are disposed of, and new ones are adopted to the accompaniment of a new set of triumphant noises.

This strategy encourages supporters to continually focus their gaze optimistically on the near future. By anticipating imminent breakthroughs,[1] supporters are able to tolerate current anomalies and human rights problems as temporary aberrations that will soon be corrected. The anticipation of breakthroughs also distracts supporters from the wreckage of past psychiatric theories and practices.

A powerful coalition of interest groups supports the medical model. Apart from psychiatrists, it includes other mental health professionals such as psychologists and social workers, consumers of mental health services—that is, voluntary patients and patients' relatives—the pharmaceutical industry, and the State.

People who manifest schizophrenic symptoms are often seen as being socially disruptive and potentially dangerous, both to themselves and to other people.[2] In past times and in other cultures, the State attempted to control such people by a variety of means, usually through banishment or some form of incarceration. The current method is for the State to provide mental health services, and for disturbed people who are thought to be potentially disruptive or dangerous to be controlled by applying psychiatric treatments to them. To facilitate this form of control, the State enacts and enforces mental health legislation that empowers medical practitioners to identify such people—and, if the newly diagnosed patients are unwilling to co-operate, to incarcerate them involuntarily in mental hospitals and impose forced treatment on them.

These arrangements have one major advantage and one major disadvantage for the State. The advantage is that human rights complaints, which inevitably arise from a situation in which a large number of non-criminal citizens are stripped of their civil liberties, can be deflected by assertions that the control is really care and treatment provided for a medical condition. The disadvantage is that the State has to underwrite the cost of most mental health expenses.[3]

The costs of schizophrenia are substantial. Over ten years ago, researchers working for the National Institute of Mental Health in the United States estimated the total annual cost of schizophrenia at $65 billion. This estimate was based on an assumption that the lifetime prevalence of schizophrenia for adult Americans was 1.5 per cent. The costs were broken down into direct and indirect components. Direct costs were related to expenditures on treatment for both inpatients and outpatients, as well as costs incurred by the criminal justice system that were estimated at $19 billion. Indirect costs were based on estimates of lost productivity: they were broken down into $24 billion for wage earners; about $4 billion for homemakers; about $4 billion for individuals in institutions; $7 billion for people who commited suicide; and $7 billion for people who could not work because they were required to take care of schizophrenic family members.[4]

The cost of research and training in relation to schizophrenia is also substantial. In 1991 it was estimated at $71 million in the United States. This figure was composed of $51,302,000 in direct grants from the National Institute of Mental Health, and approximately $20 million from state governments, private institutions, and pharmaceutical companies.[5] The size of this schizophrenia research industry has allowed psychiatric researchers to become an influential interest group supporting the medical model.

Psychiatrists are trained in medicine before they begin to specialise. Although the training of psychiatrists produces two branches of treatment—the talking therapies and the biomedical treatments—all students of psychiatry are taught, as a matter of course, that the symptoms of schizophrenia have a pathological cause; and most psychiatrists find that their professional interests give them little cause to question this teaching. Psychiatry continues to hold a dominant position within an increasingly competitive mental health industry. However, the medical training of psychiatrists will only continue to provide them with a competitive edge over rival professionals such as psychologists as long as medical explanations for abnormal psychology prevail.

Like the psychiatric profession, the pharmaceutical industry has strong commercial interests in ensuring the continued dominance of the medical model for schizophrenia. The medical model provides the rationale for drug therapy and, in turn, the pharmaceutical industry provides an extensive range of neuroleptic drugs from which prescribing psychiatrists can choose. In the United States the pharmaceutical industry openly funds the main psychiatric professional organisation, the American Psychiatric Association, which receives '30% of its total budget from drug company advertising in its many publications':[6]

Pharmaceutical companies pay through the nose to get their message across to psychiatrists across the country. They finance major symposia at the two predominant annual psychiatric conventions, offer yummy treats and music to conventioneers, and pay $1,000–$2,000 per speaker to hock their wares. It is estimated that, in total, drug companies spend an average of $10,000 per physician, per year, on education.[7]

The pharmaceutical industry also selectively funds scientific research into the side effects of neuroleptic drugs, as well as research and development of new products. Drug company sponsorship of clinical trials is a major source of revenue for many psychiatric researchers. This flow of money provides strong incentives for further promotion of the medical model, but it also casts doubt on the quality of the findings:

> This spring, the *New York Post* revealed that Columbia University has been cashing in. Its Office of Clinical Trials generates about $10 million a year testing new medications—much of which is granted to the Columbia Psychiatric Institute for implementing these tests. The director of the institute was being paid $140,000 a year by various drug companies to tour the country promoting their drugs.[8]

Pharmaceutical companies advertise their products in psychiatric journals, often alongside scientific research reports in the same areas of treatment for which their own drugs are being recommended. Because these drug companies are driven by the normal market concerns for the promotion of product sales, there is often a certain amount of confusion concerning the difference between scientific findings and sales promotion.

This point can be illustrated by a recent report of research undertaken into the efficacy of an atypical neuroleptic called risperidone, which was approved for use in the United States in 1994. The pre-approval research used a sample of 388 people diagnosed with schizophrenia. Some were treated with the conventional neuroleptic haloperidol, some were given a placebo, and some were given risperidone. After eight weeks, the researchers found that the patients given risperidone were more improved than those in the other two groups.[9]

But there was a serious problem with the report of this research. The methods used to assess patient improvements were highly subjective, and one of the authors, Richard Meibach, was identified in a subsequent article as being an employee of Janssen Pharmaceutical Research Foundation, the research arm of the manufacturer of risperidone.[10] This type of conflict of interest is a constant feature of pharmaceutical-industry involvement in discussions about schizophrenia.

Consumer Support Groups

The appellation of 'consumer' of mental health services has come to be used in recent years to describe a fairly diverse interest group. Consumers divide into primary consumers (that is, patients or people in receipt of psychiatric treatment), and secondary consumers (usually meaning the relatives of patients). However, the patients themselves can also be divided into voluntary and involuntary patients. Involuntary patients sometimes complain that they are held hostage within the collective description of 'consumers', and many former involuntary patients prefer to differentiate themselves by using the title 'psychiatric survivors'.

The importance of relatives as an interest group lies in their closeness to the problems that arise when a person manifests unusual thoughts and beliefs. It is usually the relatives who are the first to know when a family member begins to experience unusual mental phenomena. They are often alarmed at a sudden change in the person, and frequently become confused and fearful about the situation—fearful both for themselves and for the person displaying the symptoms. The first inclination of relatives is to seek help and advice, and this is readily available from the medical profession. Relatives usually see themselves as managing a crisis situation, and medical treatment can be highly attractive because it quickly pacifies the person and provides a causal explanation of 'disease' which satisfies normal scrutiny.

In the United States, the consumer lobby is well organised, and the National Alliance for the Mentally Ill (NAMI) operates nationally and has more than 210,000 members. NAMI's enthusiasm for lobbying on behalf of the medical model is encouraged by large donations from drug companies:

> The National Alliance for the Mentally Ill, which is pushing to have mental health laws rewritten so that people can be involuntarily hospitalised for refusing to take their medications, received nearly $1 million in 1995 from more than 13 drug companies.[11]

Since 1995, NAMI's drug company funding has increased dramatically. The magazine *Mother Jones* recently did an exposé of this development:

> According to internal documents obtained by *Mother Jones*, 18 drug firms gave NAMI a total of $11.72 million between 1996 and mid-1999. These include Janssen ($2.08 million), Novartis ($1.87 million), Pfizer ($1.3 million), Abbott Laboratories ($1.24 million), Wyeth-Ayerst Pharmaceuticals ($658,000), and Bristol-Myers Squibb ($613,505).
>
> NAMI's leading donor is Eli Lilly and Company, maker of Prozac, which gave $2.87 million during that period. In 1999 alone, Lilly will have delivered $1.1 million in quarterly instalments, with the lion's share going to help fund NAMI's 'Campaign to End Discrimination' against the mentally ill.
>
> In the case of Lilly, at least, 'funding' takes more than one form. Jerry Radke, a Lilly executive, is 'on loan' to NAMI, working out of the organization's headquarters. Flynn explains the cozy-seeming arrangement by saying, '[Lilly] pays his salary, but he does not report to them, and he is not involved in meetings

we have with [them].' She characterizes Radke's role at NAMI as 'strategic planning.'[12]

In Australia, an organisation called Schizophrenia Australia was established some years ago to lobby governments and educate the public about the medical-model view of schizophrenia. The organisation also uses an alternative business name, SANE Australia. In 1998 the focus of their campaign was 'Help for Families'.[13]

Schizophrenia Australia/SANE has a glittering array of entertainment, legal, and business celebrities listed as patrons. However, like NAMI, the Australian organisation is largely funded by pharmaceutical companies. Its 1996 'Carers Handbook' states that Schizophrenia Australia's community education program was 'proudly supported' by Janssen Cilag, Sandoz, ICI Pharmaceuticals, and Eli Lilly. The drug companies' logos are all prominently displayed.[14] Successive editions of SANE News, the organisation's newsletter, carry advertisements stating that 'SANE News is proudly sponsored by Janssen Cilag—Supporting care of mental illness in the community'.[15] SANE letterheads state that it is sponsored by yet another drug company, Pfizer.

Laurie Flynn, the executive director of NAMI in the United States, summed up what she called the 'synergy' between relatives' support groups and drug companies this way: 'The drug companies want more and greater markets, and we want access and availability to all scientifically proven treatments. We don't think drugs are everything, but for the vast majority they are important.'[16]

In both the United States and Australia in recent years, organisations purporting to represent the interests of relatives have been in the forefront of campaigns that have successfully persuaded governments to alter mental health legislation so that involuntary commitment and forced drug treatment is made easier. Relatives' groups often complain that civil liberties protections, which restrict the unnecessary and unfair use of involuntary hospitalisation, interfere with the need to incarcerate schizophrenic relatives in times of crisis. But the revelations that these organisations have been funded by drug companies that are seeking to expand their markets raises an important question: do these organisations only represent the interests of relatives, or have they become unwitting front groups for the pharmaceutical industry?

A recent campaign by secondary consumers to modify the involuntary commitment procedures specified in the New South Wales (NSW) Mental Health Act might serve as a useful illustration of campaign tactics.

The Campaign to Extend Involuntary Treatment in New South Wales

On 26 May 1995, a letter from a Dr Inge Southcott was published in the *Sydney Morning Herald*. Dr Southcott's letter told about her anguish as 'the mother of a 20 year old schizophrenic man who now lives on the streets'. The purpose of Dr Southcott's letter was to appeal for changes to be made to the NSW Mental Health Act so that her son, who she said was 'harmless and not suicidal', could be involuntarily incarcerated in a mental hospital and given treatment. Dr Southcott's proposal was to have a stipulation removed from the Mental Health Act which required that a person had to be thought likely to cause serious physical harm to himself or herself, or other people, before they could be committed to a hospital involuntarily.

Her letter was followed five days later by an article in the same newspaper written by Anne Deveson. Deveson began with a reference to Dr Southcott's letter and then proceeded to review her own similar experience with a schizophrenic son who, she says, 'killed himself from an overdose of alcohol and sedatives while living on the streets, psychotic, malnourished, vulnerable'.[17] Deveson's article went on to endorse Southcott's concern about the difficulties that the requirement of 'dangerousness' causes to the relatives of mentally ill people.

Shortly afterwards, two letters from doctors, written on the day Southcott's letter was published, appeared in the *Sydney Morning Herald*. They were both supportive of Dr Southcott's proposal to amend the Mental Health Act. One doctor argued that 'the criteria for instituting compulsory treatment should be widened'[18] while the other, after affirming the difficulty of committing involuntary patients under the existing conditions, went on to demand more mental health resources.[19]

Five days later, Dr Peter Macdonald, an independent member of parliament and himself a medical practitioner, made a speech in the NSW Legislative Assembly outlining his intention 'to lead a crusade'[20] on certain mental health issues over the next few years. He indicated that amendments to the Mental Health Act to widen the criteria for involuntary treatment would be central to his plan.

Macdonald complained to the parliament that the existing criteria for involuntary treatment gave patients too much right to determine for themselves whether they needed any treatment. He said the existing situation 'caused significant suffering to families'. He went on to explain his reasoning by describing what he called 'an ironic situation': 'psychotic patients do not learn from their mistakes ... have no insight and do not realise that they need treatment. By denying that they have an illness they are depriving themselves of the very treatment that will restore their capacity to recognise their illness'.[21] This was more of an irony than Dr Macdonald seemed to appreciate.

The Minister for Health, Dr Andrew Refshauge, also a medical doctor, responded sympathetically, proposing to collaborate with Macdonald in his crusade to expand the use of forced treatment. However, in reference to drug treatments, further irony was added when Refshauge admitted to his parliamentary colleagues that 'we do not have the answers to mental illness at the moment'.[22]

Several months later, on 26 October 1995, Macdonald introduced into the NSW parliament the Mental Health Amendment Bill 1995, which proposed to replace the requirement of dangerousness for involuntary hospitalisation with loosely worded criteria that would have allowed involuntary procedures to be invoked if a person were thought to be incompetent and in need of treatment.

To support his argument, Macdonald referred to Dr Southcott's letter to the editor, and quoted extensively from another letter she had written to him. In this correspondence Dr Southcott carefully detailed changes she wanted made to the Mental Health Act, and said she had 'last worked in psychiatry in Adelaide in the late 1970s'.[23]

If we examine this sequence of events in human rights terms, Inge Southcott's campaign for legislative changes might be a matter of some concern. Whilst she had a legitimate role as an anxious mother, she was also campaigning as a medical professional who was part of a co-ordinated effort to expand psychiatric coercion. Her letter indicated that she was a member of a support group for relatives called the Schizophrenia Fellowship and that this organisation planned to set up a discussion group 'to look at further amendments to the Act especially the scheduling clauses'.[24] The scheduling clauses are the parts of the Act which relate to involuntary incarceration.

It should be noted that Anne Deveson, the author of the *Sydney Morning Herald* article which supported Dr Southcott, helped to establish the NSW Schizophrenia Fellowship and then became the vice chairperson of the national organisation, Schizophrenia Australia.[25] This is an organisation supported by drug company money. Ms Deveson has been engaged in high-profile activity on mental health issues in NSW since the 1980s. She chaired a government-appointed committee set up in 1988 to review the Mental Health Act 1983, the findings of which 'were integral to the final draft' of the amendments to the 1983 Act.[26] She was also the initial chair of the implementation monitoring committee of the Mental Health Act 1990 that was set up by the NSW government to report on the efficacy of the new mental health legislation.[27]

Deveson stands out as one of the most influential figures directing recent NSW initiatives in mental health legislation. By occupation a film-maker and writer, her expertise in the mental health area is largely based on her experience as the mother of a schizophrenic son, who died in 1986. The story of her relationship with this son is poignantly told in her book *Tell Me I'm Here*.

Deveson's subsequent zeal to reform public policy on mental health issues is outlined in the proceedings of a symposium on schizophrenia and human rights that was jointly sponsored by the Human Rights and Equal Opportunity Commission and the Schizophrenia Australia Foundation, held in Brisbane in February 1989.[28] At the time there were daily newspaper reports emanating from the Chelmsford Royal Commission[29] exposing psychiatric malpractices. Yet, curiously, most of the speakers at the symposium chose to focus attention on a perception that 'the right to treatment' should have precedence over 'patients' rights'.[30] This was despite the fact that the human rights principles summarised in the opening address by the Human Rights Commissioner, Brian Burdekin, as being the principles most closely related to mental health issues neither included a right to treatment nor rights for relatives to arrange for involuntary treatment. They were all concerned with the rights of the individual to avoid coercion and discrimination.[31]

Deveson's contribution to the symposium largely consisted of detailed advice about how members of support groups for relatives of schizophrenic people might be able to campaign in the mass media. She advised that 'you can plan over a year the numbers of stories that you plant, you seed, on that particular topic. It's no use just doing a one-off story. It's an ongoing campaign that you have to plan and stage ... there is a need for something to be done about the image of psychiatrists ... we can lobby governments; so we can change political awareness ... we need to start setting a national agenda, and state agendas'.[32]

Given the linkages in the sequence of events leading up to the tabling of Macdonald's amendment bill, it might be fair to assume that Macdonald's 'crusade' was closely associated with Deveson's 'ongoing campaign'.

On 29 November 1995, Macdonald arranged a meeting at Parliament House with a number of representatives from organisations with an interest in mental health issues. The purpose of the meeting was for Macdonald to consult with stakeholders in order to gauge community support for his amendments. The Bill was still lying on the parliamentary table, and Macdonald had to decide whether to bring the matter on for debate during the pre-Christmas session of parliament.

During the course of this meeting, Macdonald acknowledged that he had drafted his amendments in consultation with the Schizophrenia Fellowship. A representative of the Fellowship was at the meeting, and presented an argument in support of the amendments by claiming that the removal of the requirement for dangerousness was necessary in order to save people from suicide. He argued that people who had suicidal relatives with mental illness were consistently failing to have them committed to mental hospitals. Being present, I observed that the urgency of his presentation seemed calculated to induce a belief that the requirement for dangerousness was causing a virtual epidemic of suicide.

However, there was already a provision in the Mental Health Act that dealt with suicidal people and permitted involuntary hospitalisation 'for the person's own protection from serious physical harm'.[33] In fact, this was the very clause that Macdonald was proposing to amend. If it were true that people were having difficulty in committing their genuinely suicidal relatives to hospital, a more plausible cause would have been the inability of relatives to convince doctors and hospital medical superintendents that suicide was intended.

But even this possibility was not supported by statistical evidence. Normally a person is involuntarily committed to a mental hospital under the direction of a doctor's certificate. But in emergencies, when there is no doctor close at hand to make the order, there is provision in the Mental Health Act for relatives and friends to take mentally ill people directly to hospital and ask for them to be involuntarily admitted.[34] In the years 1993, 1994, and 1995 a total of 174 people were presented at NSW mental hospitals in this way by relatives and friends.[35] Of this number, only one person failed to be admitted for not meeting the existing criteria of being both mentally ill and dangerous.³⁶ It therefore seems likely that the issue of suicide was inappropriately raised in support of Macdonald's Amendment Bill, in order to give it more urgency.

Macdonald decided not to risk putting his amendments to the vote in the busy pre-Christmas session of parliament in 1995. Instead his plan was to negotiate support for the proposal over the New Year break, and to bring it to a vote when the parliament sat again in April 1996. But he was overtaken by events.

Under instructions from the Labor government, which had observed the lobbying of Macdonald by secondary consumer groups, the NSW Department of Health set about drawing up its own plans for reform of the Mental Health Act. In May 1996, a public discussion paper including proposed amendments was circulated, and comments from stakeholders and the public were sought.³⁷ When the government had determined that there would be no serious opposition to the erosion of civil liberties it proposed, legislative amendments were prepared which made it much easier to institute involuntary commitment and longer periods of forced medication in the community. In 1997, a government-sponsored amendment bill was passed which now allows involuntary treatment of people who are thought likely to cause 'serious harm' to themselves or others. The change had been effected by simply removing the word 'physical' from the prior stipulation of 'serious physical harm' and then loosely defining 'serious harm' as being harm to a person's social identity, including such matters as finances and reputation.³⁸ This perceived risk of harm can now be applied to either the mentally ill person or others.

The changes in New South Wales are typical of a world-wide trend to provide conditions that will expand the numbers of people under the control of psychiatric drugs. The essential features of the NSW campaign are also apparent in similar campaigns in other parts of the world. These features include relatives' support groups campaigning with drug company funding, outspoken doctors, and psychiatrists, and politicians responding to what they think is community pressure. The central argument which all these players use is that mentally ill people are being denied their human rights because there are not enough coercive powers available to ensure that they all receive treatment.

Human Rights Supporting the Medical Model

The human rights that support psychiatric practice within the medical model relate to mental illnesses in general. These generalised human rights have been codified in recent years, and all the most relevant ones are now specified in the United Nations (UN) Principles for the Protection of Persons with Mental Illness and for the Improvement of Mental Health Care.[39] National governments have been encouraged by the UN to ensure that their mental health systems are compatible with the UN objectives. In Australia, the commonwealth government is advising state governments on any changes that might be necessary to bring mental health legislation into line with the UN principles.[40]

Principle 1.1 sets out the right to treatment as being the primary human right on which other rights are based: 'All persons have the right to the best available mental health care, which shall be part of the health and social care system.' A number of 'Fundamental Freedoms and Basic Rights' are then listed, including the 'right to be treated with humanity and respect', 'protection from exploitation and discrimination', and 'the right to exercise all civil, political, economic, social and cultural rights as recognised' in other UN human rights declarations and covenants.[41]

The UN principles then go on to list a total of 25 areas of human rights protection. These include the right for people with mental illness 'to live and work, as far as possible, in the community' (Principle 3). This right gives rise to a further 'right to be treated in the least restrictive environment with the least restrictive or intrusive treatment appropriate to the patient's health needs and the need to protect the physical safety of others' (Principle 9).

There is a stipulation that 'a determination that a person has a mental illness shall be made in accordance with internationally accepted medical standards' (Principle 4). Confidentiality is protected (Principle 6), standards of care are specified (Principle 8), 'medication shall meet the best health needs of the patient' (Principle 10), and informed consent to treatment is required—although, paradoxically, only from voluntary patients. The principles specify that informed consent to treatment is not required from involuntary patients, patients who are thought to be incapable of giving their consent, or patients who unreasonably withhold their consent (Principle 11).

A list of 'Rights and Conditions in Mental Health Facilities' are specified (Principle 13), along with the required 'Resources for Mental Health Facilities' (Principle 14). 'Admission Principles' are at first covered in a general way in Principle 15: for example, 'Access to a mental health facility shall be administered in the same way as access to any other facility for any other illness'. More specific conditions are given for 'Involuntary Admission' in Principle 16. The need for a review body, procedural safeguards, patient access to information, and a complaints procedure are also specified in various other principles.

Most of these specifications are straightforward, aiming to provide a regulatory framework that minimises the social exclusion of voluntary mental patients and ensures that they receive humane treatment. But the simplicity of these ideas does not always extend to involuntary patients, and the standing of the principles is largely dependent on the willingness of practitioners and proponents of the medical model to ignore the paradoxes that are thereby created for involuntary patients.

There are two human rights specified in the principles—the 'right to treatment' and the 'right to informed consent'—that are worth analysing in some detail. When these rights are used to guide psychiatric practice on voluntary patients, they appear merely to enforce routine procedures that have long standing in other branches of medicine. But unlike other areas of medicine, psychiatry is frequently practised on involuntary patients. In fact, more than half the people who receive psychiatric treatment for schizophrenia are involuntary patients. Consequently, these two human rights have special connotations when they are used to guide coercion in psychiatric treatment.

The Right to Treatment

The principle of the right to treatment implies that people in need of psychiatric treatment might otherwise be denied it. That is, they might go in search of medical treatment but, because of lack of money, a shortage of services, professional incompetence, rejection by the service providers, or perhaps because of a discriminatory policy, they might fail to get the necessary psychiatric attention.

In this respect, the right to psychiatric treatment is an example of the right that all people are assumed to have for any kind of urgently needed medical attention. This basic human right, and its limitations, are instantly recognisable when cases of medical denial are given publicity. A homeless man might be left injured in the street because it is assumed he has no money to pay for hospital expenses and is unlikely to have any medical insurance. Or doctors might publicly debate the ethics of withdrawing expensive life-support from terminally ill patients. As with other human rights, the right to treatment is meant to support the needs of the individual when he or she is threatened by the exercise of social or professional expedience.

However, it is not only the sufferers who are likely to complain about a supposed violation of the right to treatment. Complaints about violations of this right are also made by the relatives of mentally ill people. These complaints by relatives do not always arise from situations where a mentally ill person has approached a mental hospital voluntarily and has been refused admission. They also arise from a situation in which the person who is said to be mentally ill denies it and refuses to volunteer for treatment.

When a person's unusual behaviour and thinking patterns give rise to a perception that a mental illness such as schizophrenia might be the cause, and the person is unwilling to volunteer for treatment, it is common for relatives and mental health professionals to argue that the person's refusal of treatment is a manifestation of the mental illness. That is, the presence of mental illness has clouded the person's thinking and prevented him or her from discerning the urgent need for treatment.

In this situation, the person who is said to be mentally ill is handled as if he or she were unconscious. A person who has been seriously injured in a motor accident and rendered unconscious is assumed both to want treatment and to have a right to it. Similarly, a person who has been diagnosed with schizophrenia, and who refuses treatment, is frequently assumed to be so out of touch with reality that the 'real' person has been obscured by the mental illness. In such a situation, relatives often undertake decision-making roles on the mentally ill person's behalf, and assume that if the 'real' person were present he or she, like an unconscious motor accident victim, would both want treatment and have a right to it. This assumption is often made in the face of vigorous objections by the person concerned.

The 'right to treatment' has become deeply entrenched in the ethical consensus of the mental health system, including those on the periphery of it. It is argued by social workers in the United States, for instance, that the profession is required to advocate the right to treatment whenever its members encounter a mentally ill person who is going untreated:

> if there are means (medications) to treat unrelieved psychosis, failure to use these means is opposed to social work principles. Similarly, failure to advocate for a patient's right to treatment runs counter to fundamental social work principles and the right to due process. There are legal case precedents that ensure the right to treatment for people confined in public psychiatric hospitals. In the 1966 case of Rouse v. Cameron, the D.C. Circuit Court ruled that confining a person in an institution for treatment and failing to provide treatment is a violation of the due process clause of the Fourteenth Amendment.[42]

The lack of distinction in this ethical position between the advocacy of treatment for voluntary and involuntary patients brings the paradox of the right to treatment clearly into perspective. The practice of this ethical position apparently requires social workers to advocate psychiatric treatment for people who do not want to be treated. Even if the comparison of a mentally ill person to an unconscious person is acceptable, the quality and efficacy of the psychiatric treatment generally on offer also has to be considered.

In the case of an accident victim who is unconscious with serious injuries, it can generally be assumed that medical attention will more likely be beneficial to the person than detrimental. In fact, the imposition of medical treatment on an unconscious person who has not given prior consent imposes on the medical practitioner an expectation that the patient's condition will not be made worse by the treatment. A patient who recovers from such a condition could be expected to show gratitude to the doctor.

However, the limitations of the analogy become clear when these criteria are applied to the post-crisis mental patient. Unlike recovered accident victims, many former involuntary schizophrenic patients have complained that neuroleptic drug treatment did them far more harm than good. Rather than showing gratitude to the psychiatrists involved, they are inclined to argue that the coercive interpretation of their 'right to treatment' violated their more fundamental 'right to refuse treatment'.

Informed Consent

The right to refuse treatment is embodied in the standard medical procedure of obtaining a patient's informed consent before treatment.[43] In turn, the origins of this medical concept of 'informed consent' are to be found in a complex arrangement of cultural inheritance involving moral, ethical, and legal considerations. The moral element is concerned with notions of individual autonomy and a person's right to determine what is allowed to be done to his or her own body by a doctor. The ethical part involves the relationship between an individual and a professional expert who has been consulted by the individual, and concerns the expectations of duty and trust that surround such a relationship. The legal aspect is concerned with the contractual arrangements that have been entered into by the two parties.[44]

The binding together of these separate concepts into a formally stated principle did not occur until after World War II. The trials of Nazi war criminals had revealed many atrocities in the name of experimental science, most of which were performed by qualified doctors, and the Nuremberg Code was adopted by the United Nations General Assembly in 1946 as an international standard to ensure that these atrocities were never repeated. The first principle of the code states that '[t]he voluntary consent of the human subject is absolutely essential' when conducting medical experiments.[45] Although this code is considered by many to lack the necessary detail for enforcement, it is the seminal document for international law in this area, and has been subsequently used as a basis for other international agreements of a similar nature.

From these beginnings, 'informed consent' has been developed into a fully fledged doctrine to guide the delivery of professional medical services. Although the procedures appear simple, there are hidden complexities concerning the notion of 'informed' and the notion of 'consent'.

To satisfy the 'informed' half of the doctrine, the doctor is required to tell the patient why the treatment is necessary and what its expected outcome is, and to describe any possible side effects and, if failure is a possibility, the likelihood of failure and its consequences. Alternative treatments should also be canvassed.

Although this might seem straightforward, doctors frequently complain about problems they face in properly implementing this procedure. From the doctor's point of view the problem is deciding how much detail is necessary to satisfy a particular patient. Some patients would rather not be told any more than is strictly necessary, preferring to trust in the wisdom of their doctor. Others want all the information they can get.

The problem for the doctors is in knowing which sort of patient they are dealing with. Doctors argue that giving too much information to patients who don't want it does them harm by increasing their anxiety. Doctors also complain that they are too busy to waste time educating patients who want to know everything. But neither of these arguments is sufficient when doctors have to defend themselves against litigation for having failed to satisfy the procedure.

Clinical trials of psychiatric drugs are particularly problematic in regard to informed consent. People who have been diagnosed with serious mental disorders such as schizophrenia are usually assumed to be incapable of making rational decisions. This assumption is the basis for the involuntary treatment that many of them receive in the first place. However, pharmaceutical companies are constantly developing new products that have to be tested by clinical trials before they may be released onto the market. These conditions produce a paradoxical situation whereby people who are deemed by medical/legal procedures to be unfit to make decisions in regard to their need for treatment in the first instance are, all the same, frequently assumed to be rational enough to give their informed consent to participate in medical experiments.

The notion of 'consent' does not generally cause as much anxiety for the medical profession as does the notion of 'informed'. Even so, 'consent' still involves many areas of contention. The main problem area concerns people who are considered unfit to give their consent. When a medical patient is unconscious and needs urgent medical attention, it is normal practice to assume 'the notion of *presumed consent,* namely that it is a safe assumption that patients would want whatever is medically indicated to minimise or prevent injury, stop the progression of disease, sustain life, relieve pain and suffering, and so forth'.[46]

This presumption of consent can extend into more controversial areas. These include *proxy consent*, which is the form of consent given by a third party, usually a relative on behalf of children and elderly people, and 'the doctrine of *parens patriae*, which provides that the State has the duty to care for those individuals who are not able to do so themselves'.[47] The right to give involuntary treatment to mental patients, without their informed consent, is often drawn from the doctrine of *parens patriae*.[48] However, routine involuntary treatment is not found in other branches of medicine, and its practice in psychiatry still necessitates a certain amount of duplicity in the interpretation of human rights, despite these legal devices.

In summary, psychiatry's overall tactic is to justify involuntary treatment by assuming that a person who resists treatment lacks sufficient insight to comprehend the need for it. This assumption clears the way to assert that the person would assent to treatment if the need were properly understood, and that the person's 'right to treatment' would be violated without the imposition of involuntary treatment. In this way the medical model can satisfy the perceived need to control certain people while at the same time appearing to respect their human rights.

But there are at least two classes of people who are regularly diagnosed with schizophrenia and forced into treatment when they clearly do not have medical problems. These are people undergoing spiritual/mystical emergencies and people who have problems of living arising from social or occupational dysfunctions. When these types of people attempt to resist forced treatment it is not because they lack 'insight' into their supposed mental illness. Rather it is because drugs are simply inappropriate as a method of dealing with their problems. When 'lack of insight' and the 'right to treatment' are invoked to justify overriding their wishes, these concepts turn into expressions of extreme cynicism.

The response from supporters of the medical model to these claims is usually to deny that such people exist. The medical model views everyone diagnosed with schizophrenia, by definition, as being mentally diseased. A person with a diagnosis who claims to have a healthy mind is seen to be exhibiting a symptom of the disease. This simple logic of denial has been central to the consensus-building around the structure of the medical model, and has added greatly to its strength. But despite this structural strength it is built on very unstable ground. This is because it is fairly easy to demonstrate that another cultural consensus exists, outside the medical model, which agrees that mystics and people with social problems do exist—and that their deviations from normal are not necessarily due to mental disease.

These anomalies are even apparent to some psychiatrists. There have been a number of dissident psychiatrists who have rejected the medical explanation of schizophrenic symptoms and who have adopted alternative non-medical interpretations instead. These alternatives are usually based on assumptions of either a spiritual/mystical emergency or social alienation as the cause. Needless to say, the few psychiatrists who pursue these non-medical explanations are viewed with distrust by their peers and are professionally marginalised. But their writings are often very attractive to interested lay people who are sceptical about the medical explanation. They also supply credible evidence to support a person's right to refuse medical treatment when it seems inappropriate.

5

Non-Medical Models:
schizophrenia as a spiritual/mystical emergency

Many people are diagnosed with schizophrenia when they are in the midst of an intense, inner experience that is loaded with religious content. It is quite common for schizophrenics to report that they have been in communication with God or a higher being, and have been given some kind of messianic mission to fulfil.[1] Personalised religious beliefs and fantastic stories of internal conversations with deities and saints are common signs that lead to diagnoses. But the psychiatrists who make these diagnoses are often mistaken. These are not necessarily signs of mental illness; they may well be signs of a spiritual/mystical emergency. Unfortunately, psychiatrists are not trained to understand these phenomena.

In fact, psychiatrists are poorly equipped by their training to understand any kind of speculative thinking about the meaning of life. This psychiatric knowledge-deficit is particularly evident in areas associated with religious thinking, and it presents distinct dangers for naive patients. Some psychiatrists have recognised this, and have written despairingly about their colleagues:

> I am quite convinced that a most certain way for a person to acquire a label of schizophrenia is to come before a clinician and talk about certain kinds of topics, these include the occult, ESP,

religion, God, and the general range of metaphysical phenomena. I do not really think that *how* one talks about these things has much to do with whether or not he is given the diagnosis. He can be quite coherent and ordered in his speech, follow the rules of grammar and logic, and yet if he expresses serious concern with, or some kind of excitement in, these topics, he is on his way to winning the label.[2]

Many traditional mystical practices and even conventional religious observances can easily fit the symptoms of schizophrenia. Ordinary Christians, for instance, quite commonly demonstrate thinking patterns and behaviours that are very similar to schizophrenic symptoms when they hold conversations with God in the form of prayer. This raises questions about the competency and the consistency of psychiatrists when they are required to make assessments of peoples' religious beliefs.

Psychiatrists are scientists, or so they claim, and their professional training could be expected to lead them to the view that all religious beliefs are irrational superstitions hanging over from pre-scientific times. But a closer look at psychiatric attitudes shows that the profession is deeply confused on the issue of religion. On the one hand, there is evidence that individual psychiatrists are strongly influenced in their professional decision-making by their own religious upbringing.[3] On the other hand, there are indications that, despite having respect for religious institutions, psychiatrists remain true to their scientific identity and show little respect for the beliefs that drive those institutions.

A survey of Melbourne psychiatrists has found that religious upbringing influences psychiatrists in their treatment decisions. Researchers set out to determine whether the differing theological perspectives of the Catholic, Protestant, and Jewish faiths might be reflected in decisions by psychiatrists when choosing between somatic or talking forms of therapy.

Their hypothesis was that if the psychiatrists' religious beliefs included a source for the control of human experience that is external to the individuals concerned, these psychiatrists would be disinclined to encourage patients to take personal responsibility for their mental state by using talking therapy. Instead they would use somatic treatments such as drugs and electroconvulsive therapy.

In comparing theological perspectives about internal and external controls for human behaviour, the researchers found 'that both Protestantism and Judaism are paradoxical here, whereas Roman Catholicism much more clearly places the locus of responsibility as external to the individual'.[4] They predicted that Catholic psychiatrists would therefore favour somatic forms of treatment, while Jewish and Protestant psychiatrists would prove to be statistically ambivalent in their choices of treatment. The survey covered 74 per cent of all Melbourne psychiatrists. Of those surveyed, it found that 100 per cent of Catholics, 53.3 per cent of Jews and 55.5 per cent of Protestants practised somatic forms of treatment.

If psychiatrists are so dramatically influenced by religious affiliation in their treatment decisions, it is fair to assume they are similarly influenced in their diagnostic decisions. However, in regard to diagnosing schizophrenia, neither DSM-IV nor the ICD-10 makes any provision to safeguard against this bias. There are no differential diagnostic guidelines to distinguish normal religious/mystical practices from schizophrenia.[5] That is, the manuals do not give detailed descriptions of authentic religious beliefs and mystical experiences—nor do they show how these differ from the symptoms of schizophrenia.

The only attempt at differentiation in DSM-IV is a definition of 'delusion' that excludes beliefs which are ordinarily accepted by the person's culture as articles of religious faith. It seems that, if religious beliefs are ordinarily accepted by others, the person's mind is healthy; if they are not, it is diseased. In distinguishing mental health from mental disease by taking notice of the popularity of religious beliefs instead of the authenticity of the ideas behind the beliefs, psychiatrists imply that the substance of mainstream religious beliefs is indistinguishable from schizophrenic delusions.

They also imply that they are unwilling to antagonise

mainstream churches by diagnosing ordinary followers, and that they are only interested in diagnosing solitary individuals. This means that the relationship of candidates-for-diagnosis to their churches is sometimes critical. It puts people who undergo mystical experience directly in line for diagnosis.

Historically, mystics have had ambivalent relationships with the religious movements to which they have been affiliated. This is particularly true of monotheistic religions such as Christianity. Mystical experience has been traditionally associated with spiritual guidance, the discovery/uncovery of religious knowledge, communion with a deity, healing, the arts, and prophecy. But perhaps more often it has also been viewed as heresy.

Reports of mystical experience to religious peers can be greeted alternatively as a welcome refreshment for collective faith or as a threatening sign of corruption. The reception seems to depend more on the place and the time, and the preparedness of peers to receive the messages, than with the content of the experience. This perennial ambivalence towards mystics makes the psychiatric test of soundness—whether religious beliefs are ordinarily accepted by the person's culture as articles of religious faith—somewhat arbitrary. Should a disease be indicated by whether or not Christianity is currently in need of mystical inspiration? This type of test, which is implicit in the diagnostic procedures for schizophrenia, is not the way hard-nosed scientists normally go about their work.

Nevertheless most people who come in contact with psychiatry, and who are subsequently diagnosed with schizophrenia, usually do so because they are undergoing acute psychological distress, and/or are causing distress to others. It is probably fair to assume, therefore, that most people who are diagnosed and treated when they are undergoing a spiritual/mystical emergency demonstrate a low level of competency in handling a mystical experience. But this concession still does not mean that they have a mental disease, or that they require any form of psychiatric attention.

In comparing modern schizophrenics with mythological heroes, Joseph Campbell, the great mythologist, summed up his opinion this way: 'our schizophrenic patient is actually experiencing inadvertently that same beatific ocean deep which the yogi and saint are ever striving to enjoy: except that, whereas they are swimming in it, he is drowning'.[6]

Swimmers and non-swimmers might both be in the same waters, and their splashing might look the same to an untrained observer. But what is pleasurable exercise to one could be a life-or-death struggle for the other. The modern tragedy, however, for both swimmers and non-swimmers alike, is that all of them are now routinely drowned by the rescue efforts of an over-zealous and incompetent life-guard. This incompetence is largely due to ignorance about the nature of mystics and the mystical experience.

Background to the Mystical Tradition

Definitions of mysticism and descriptions of mystical experience range widely through literature. The word itself 'has its origin in the Greek mysteries' and 'mystery (mysterium) comes from the Greek verb muo, to shut or close the lips or eyes'.[7] In this original sense, a mystic was a person who had been 'initiated into the esoteric knowledge of Divine things, and upon whom was laid the necessity of keeping silence concerning his secret knowledge'. But the priests of the ancient mystery religions lost control of the term when philosophers began to use it to describe aspects of their own speculations. From the Greek philosophers it was passed on to 'the Christian Church, which held itself to be a body of initiates into a truth not possessed by mankind at large'.[8]

Modern uses for terms such as 'mystic', 'mystical' and 'mysticism' range far beyond the ancient applications to pagan and Christian ritual. Most of the contemporary major religions of both east and west have recognised practices that can be understood in these terms. There are also contemporary anthropological observations of traditional tribal practices such as shamanism to which the terms can be applied.

Mysticism in the modern sense refers to a psychological

experience involving a conscious transcendence of the normal self-identity. The mystic usually believes that he or she has entered into a higher state of consciousness, has made contact with a deity, or has entered into some form of communion with the object of devotion of the religious or philosophical tradition concerned.

There is a tendency amongst some religiously inclined academic analysts to divide mystical experience into different types, according to the religious or philosophical tradition to which the mystic is allied. For instance, it is sometimes argued that monistic, theistic, and nature mysticism are qualitatively different.[9]

One leading theorist has divided mysticism into two broad types, extroversive and introversive: 'The extroversive way looks outward and through the physical senses into the external world and finds the One there. The introversive way turns inward, introspectively, and finds the One at the bottom of the self, at the bottom of the human personality.'[10] The language of mysticism is often difficult, 'ineffability' being one of its characteristics, and 'the One' is usually interchangeable with 'the Absolute', 'God', 'nirvana' or some other transcendental objective (see below).

The general consensus seems to be that psychological phenomena that follow certain broad principles can be described as mystical experience. All mystical experience has validity, regardless of the particular path by which it has been approached. One exception is that the mystical validity of drug-induced experience is sometimes disputed:

> There is hardly any soil, be it ever so barren, where Mysticism will not strike root; hardly any creed, however formal, round which it will not twine itself. It is, indeed, the eternal cry of the human soul for rest; the insatiable longing of a being wherein infinite ideals are fettered and cramped by a miserable actuality; and so long as man is less than an angel and more than a beast, this cry will not for a moment fail to make itself heard. Wonderfully uniform, too, whether it come from the Brahman sage, the Persian poet, or the Christian quietist, it is in essence an enunciation more or less clear,

more or less eloquent, of the aspiration of the soul to cease altogether from self and to be at one with God.[11]

Essentially, a mystical experience involves an altered state of consciousness. A metaphor that repeatedly appears is of a house or structure with many rooms in which human consciousness abides. Normally these rooms have to be explored in the dark; but when a person consciously enters a certain room, usually in the highest part of the house, a bright light is switched on which variously blinds, confuses, or inspires a person with the inner scene that is revealed.

Plato's simile of the cave is one of the clearest descriptions of this idea. In *The Republic* he has Socrates describe the normal human condition as one in which most people live out their lives chained up at the bottom of a dark cave. The reality perceived by the inhabitants is limited to a view of distorted shadows projected on the opposite wall of the cave, which the prisoners habitually misinterpret. The exceptional person who escapes this bondage, and who climbs out of the cave, is at first dazzled by the sunlight but eventually learns to view a different, properly illuminated reality:

> connect the ascent into the upper world and the sight of the objects there with the upward progress of the mind into the intelligible region ... the final thing to be perceived in the intelligible region, and perceived only with difficulty, is the form of the good; once seen it is inferred to be responsible for whatever is right and valuable in anything, producing in the visible region light and the source of light, and being in the intelligible region itself the controlling source of truth and intelligence.[12]

Plato also discusses the difficulties encountered by a person who returns to the cave after a sojourn in the light. Such a person has to learn once again to live in the dark and to successfully compete with other people at the bottom of the cave in an elaborate game of misinterpreting reality:

> Nor will you think it strange that anyone who descends from contemplation of the divine to human life and its ills should blunder and make a fool of himself, if, while still blinded and unaccustomed to the surrounding darkness, he's forcibly put on trial in the law-courts or elsewhere about the shadows of justice or the figures of which they are shadows, and made to dispute about the notions of them held by men who have never seen justice itself.[13]

People who describe their mystical experiences can be divided into two types: those who were trained for the experience and those who were not. Training methods vary as widely as the mystical traditions that teach them, and are as various as the names of the final goal: 'in all the great spiritual traditions is a relatively rare but universal and liberating experience either of self-oblivion or nirvana as in Buddhism or of a special relationship with the Deity, whether this remain unnamed or named as God, the Absolute, the Ultimate Reality, the All-Holy and Almighty, Cosmic Reality, the Ground of Being, the Transcendent or the One'.[14]

Underlying them all is a fairly simple common principle: normal human consciousness has evolved into an awareness of individual mortality, from which there is a need to escape. At some time in the distant ancestry of humanity a threshold of consciousness was crossed, since when individual humans have had to endure constant anxiety about personal death. The ancients variously referred to the crossing of this threshold as a fall from grace, a descent from a Golden Age, or an eviction from a garden of easy living. Modern people are more likely to see it as an advancement or an evolutionary step, rather than a fall, which has provided the fundamental distinction between humans and other animals.

Dealing with the Knowledge of Mortality

Whether the development of the knowledge of personal mortality is viewed as a descent or an ascent does not matter a great deal.

Either way, it produces the effect of what is now generally referred to as self-consciousness. The awareness of personal mortality, combined with the understanding that the lives of others, and the physical reality in which they abide, will all continue independently after one's own death, causes individual humans to see themselves as separate and alienated from the physical and social environments in which they live. Each person understands that death has to be faced alone, which leads to the awareness that life is also faced alone. Consciousness is thus focussed on the individual self, and on the need to prolong its survival. In this way, existence can become an uncomfortable and futile experience:

> And God has so arranged this existence that it is impossible in this world to be related in truth to truth without coming to suffer—and eternity judges everyone according to whether he has been related in suffering to truth.[15]

Mysticism appears to be a somewhat novel method of dealing with this harsh reality, and it is normally only utilised by individuals who find the traditional strategies unsatisfactory. The traditional methods involve reinforcing the self, rather than transcending it, through procreation and/or social status. Children are seen as extensions of the self and, since it can be anticipated that children will further extend a person's procreative chain of existence, people who have children are able to reassure themselves with the thought that their own being is a link in a chain of immortal existence.

But there is large scope for disappointment for those who rely on this strategy. Infertility, the premature death of offspring, the failure of children themselves to marry and procreate, or simply inter-generational conflict can all create conditions in which the immortal chain appears to break. The most basic problem with this strategy for men is uncertainty over paternity.[16] When men adopt tactics designed to ensure the security of paternity, such as imposing binding marriage contracts on women and restricting their freedom, the stress is passed on from men to women.

To combat the anxieties caused by the knowledge of personal mortality, and also to ameliorate the further stresses caused by the 'cure' of procreation, a further cultural strategy involves a competitive struggle for social status and power. The principle here is simple: people who can gain power over others can command them to provide services in the task of preserving the wellbeing of the person holding power. Men who pursue this strategy believe that if they can dominate male rivals, and gain ascendancy over a particular woman, exclusive sexual access will be guaranteed and procreative certainty will be assured. Surplus wealth, which can be accumulated by the exercise of power, can also be used to insulate the person in power against premature death from accident, disease, war, exposure, or hunger.

The obvious flaw in the status strategy is that it can only work for the benefit of a minority of people at the expense of the majority. Mystics are usually drawn from the ranks of the majority for whom the quest for status offers little comfort. The pursuit of mystical experience can be seen as a further attempt, beyond the more normal strategies of procreation and status, to combat anxiety over mortality by escaping from the consciousness of self altogether.

Attaining Mystical Experience

Mystical experience which is deliberately intended, rather than spontaneous, is usually attained through the practice of spiritual exercises. These take the form of meditation and yoga, as in Buddhist and Hindu traditions; Christian prayer; dancing in Sufism; or even the repetition of the mystic's own name, as the nineteenth-century English poet Alfred Lord Tennyson found:

> I have never had any revelations through anaesthetics, but a kind of waking trance—this for lack of a better word—I have frequently had, quite up from boyhood, when I have been all

alone. This has come upon me through repeating my own name to myself silently, till all at once, as it were out of the intensity of the consciousness of individuality, individuality itself seemed to dissolve and fade away into boundless being, and this not a confused state but the clearest, the surest of the surest, utterly beyond words—where death was an almost laughable impossibility—the loss of personality (if so it were) seeming no extinction, but the only true life.[17]

The intuitive inventiveness Tennyson describes is not unusual amongst mystics who are independent of organised disciplines. But most descriptions of mystical technique are more likely to follow the proven formula of a tradition. These formulas often have common elements: that is, the novice mystic should follow a lifestyle committed to humility (transcendence of the status quest) and, following the example of celebrated mystic role-models, should usually be celibate as well (detachment from fertility). Once the novice has correctly arranged his or her lifestyle, which might require residence in a monastery, convent, or spiritual community, mental exercises are learned and practised, usually using a combination of techniques. Variations of Tennyson's name repetition are often found as components under the name of 'mantra' or 'prayer'.

Meditation, in one form or another, is usually the centrepiece of mystical practice. The essential component of all meditative practice is for the practitioner to develop an ability to observe his or her own flow of thoughts. This involves the establishment of an aspect of identity that looks inward and relates to mental phenomena, and is distinguished from self-identity by being its observer. This deliberate effort to consciously observe the mental activity of the self, rather than to participate in existence through the expression of self-identity, can produce an effect in which the person's mind is split so that consciousness is catapulted in a trajectory above and beyond the existential anxieties of self consciousness.

Different experiences of transcendence have a number of common components. The most notable of these involve emotional perceptions—the transcendence of fear and the experience of love—and non-sensory communications, perceived directly in the mind as voices or visions:

> Imaginary visions may appear with the intensity of actual sensations ... It is as if the images and symbols normally restricted to the unconscious are released when the mind first penetrates into the unknown depths of itself ... The mystical vision structures this 'unconscious' material according to its own intentionality.[18]

It is not normal for mystics to refer to these thought patterns as hallucinations, though clearly this is the psychological terminology that most appropriately describes them. The term 'hallucination', as has already been discussed in the description of the medical model, was given its special psychiatric meaning about the middle of the nineteenth century. Mystics are generally inclined to perceive and describe their experiences in terms of the particular discipline in which they have trained, and many of these predate the nineteenth century by a considerable margin.

Academic analysts have some difficulty in finding the right terms with which to describe the voices and visions of mystics: 'intellectual visions are not visions proper, since they do not consist of perceptions or images. Nor are they intellectual in the ordinary sense, since they are entirely nondiscursive and contribute nothing to the subject's "understanding" of himself and his world. Nevertheless, their main impact is one of insight and even of all-surpassing insight.'[19]

Some analysts deal with the problem by focussing on the emotional aspects of mystical experience, so that the 'consciousness of close communion with God' is presented as being the primary aspect of mystical experience. Seemingly hallucinatory experience is relegated to a secondary role of lesser importance:

> Among these symbols we must reckon a large number of the secondary phenomena of mysticism: divine visions and voices,

and other dramatisations of the self's apprehensions and desires. The best mystics have always recognised the doubtful nature of these so-called divine revelations and favours, and have tried again and again to set up tests for discerning those which really 'come from God' i.e. mediate a valid spiritual experience.[20]

However, some of the 'best mystics'—that is, those whose mystical experiences have been incorporated into the lore of mainstream religions—have been unequivocal about the significance of their voices and visions. John of Ephesus, for instance, the author of the Book of Revelation in the New Testament, relates how he was on the Isle of Patmos and

> was in the Spirit on the Lord's day, and heard behind me a great voice, as of a trumpet, saying, 'I am Alpha and Omega, the first and the last', and 'What thou seest, write in a book, and send it unto the seven churches ... ' And I turned to see the voice that spoke to me. And being turned, I saw seven golden candlesticks; and in the midst of the seven candlesticks one like unto the Son of Man, clothed with a garment down to the foot, and girt about the paps with a golden girdle. [21]

Mohammed, the founder of the Islamic religion, spent many years in contemplation before a mystical experience gave him the necessary insights to launch a major religion. He saw a vision of the angel Gabriel, who asked Mohammed to read instructions that had been written on cloth:

> He was passing the month of Ramadan in the cavern of Mount Hara, endeavouring by fasting, prayer and solitary meditation to elevate his thoughts to the contemplation of divine truth. As Mohammed lay wrapped in his mantle he heard a voice calling upon him. Uncovering his head a flood of light broke upon him in such intolerable splendour that he swooned. On regaining his senses he beheld an angel in human form, which, approaching

from a distance, displayed a silken cloth covered with written characters.[22]

Moses' inspiration to lead the Hebrews out of slavery in Egypt came from a mystical encounter with God as he tended his flock of sheep in the desert:

> he came to the mountain of God, even to Horeb. And the angel of the Lord appeared unto him in a flame of fire out of the midst of a bush: and he looked, and, behold, the bush burned with fire, and the bush was not consumed. And Moses said, 'I will now turn aside, and see this great sight, why the bush is not burnt.' And when the Lord saw that he turned aside to see, God called to him out of the midst of the bush, and said, 'Moses, Moses'.[23]

Moses' 'hallucinations' covered a considerable range in this encounter with God. He was given a messianic mission, and as evidence that he would have the persuasive power necessary to fulfil the role he was led to believe that he had a magical ability to turn his rod into a snake and to induce the symptoms of leprosy by putting 'his arm into his bosom'.[24]

The New Testament provides ample evidence that the 'best mystics' are not immune to encountering visions and voices in their mystical experiences. John the Baptist had been instructed by a mystical presence to baptise people in the River Jordan, and to persevere in this task until he encountered a person 'upon whom thou shalt see the Spirit descending'[25]

> And it came to pass in those days, that Jesus came from Nazareth of Galilee, and was baptised of John in Jordan. And straight away coming up out of the water, he saw the heavens opened, and the spirit like a dove descending upon him: and there came a voice from heaven, saying, 'Thou art my beloved Son, in whom I am well pleased.'[26]

George Fox, the founder of the Quaker religion, left a journal with many accounts of his mystical experiences, some of which involved visions and voices. He relates how, on one occasion, he separated from friends to pay a solitary visit to the city of Lichfield in England:

> I was commanded by the Lord to pull off my shoes. I stood still for it was winter: but the word of the Lord was like a fire in me. So I put off my shoes and left them with the shepherds; and the poor shepherds trembled, and were astonished. Then I walked on about a mile, and as soon as I got within the city, the word of the Lord came to me again, saying: Cry, 'Wo to the bloody city of Lichfield!' So I went up and down the streets, crying with a loud voice, Wo to the bloody city of Lichfield! It being market day, I went into the market-place, and to and fro in the several parts of it, and made stands, crying as before, Wo to the bloody city of Lichfield! And no one laid hands on me. As I went thus crying through the streets, there seemed to me to be a channel of blood running down the streets, and the market-place appeared like a pool of blood.[27]

In *The Varieties of Religious Experience* William James shows considerable respect for George Fox's mystical accomplishments and his contribution to religious understanding. James returns repeatedly to Fox's journal to demonstrate finer points of religious understanding. By way of explaining Fox's unusual behaviour in Lichfield, James writes:

> No one can pretend for a moment that in point of spiritual sagacity and capacity, Fox's mind was unsound. Everyone who confronted him personally, from Oliver Cromwell down to county magistrates and jailers, seems to have acknowledged his superior power. Yet from the point of view of his nervous constitution, Fox was a psychopath or *détraqué* of the deepest dye.[28]

James was a medical practitioner and a psychologist, and *The Varieties of Religious Experience* came out of a lecture series he gave at Edinburgh University in 1901–02. His assessment that Fox had soundness of mind in regard to spiritual judgement but that his nervous constitution, as indicated by the Lichfield behaviour, was psychopathic, supports the argument that mental health professionals are predisposed to label mystics with mental illnesses. In James's case this is done in spite of the recognition given to the value of Fox's mysticism. This raises the impossible but tantalising question of whether James would have offered treatment to Fox, at the possible risk of undermining his mystical capacity, had the two men lived at the same time.

Mysticism and Psychiatry

James was not the only mental health professional living around the turn of the twentieth century who made a link between mysticism and mental illness. Richard Maurice Bucke was a late-nineteenth-century Canadian psychiatrist whose book *Cosmic Consciousness* (1901) outlined a theory about the evolution of consciousness that he had developed from various sources—including observations of his patients, analyses of literature, and self-examination of his own mental functioning. His theory not only linked mysticism with the psychiatric concept of 'mental illness', but also fitted them both into an evolutionary context.

Bucke's hypothesis was that human consciousness is engaged in an evolutionary process and is slowly moving through three distinct phases of development. The first stage he called 'simple consciousness', which he described as being concerned with sense perceptions. This primary level of consciousness is shared with other animals, and was the only kind of consciousness available to our humanoid ancestors.

According to Bucke, humans became distinguished from other animals by growing into a second level of development that he called 'self consciousness'. While most people live on this second level of consciousness, a third level is also available. He argued that the attainment of this higher level of understanding, which he called 'cosmic consciousness', is an evolutionary step above the current human status.

Bucke believed that only a select few individuals had so far experienced cosmic consciousness. Unusually, he thought that some of these were his own mental patients. He also claimed to have had first-hand experience of it himself. Speaking disconcertingly of himself in the third person, he wrote the following description of his own mystical experience:

> He was in a state of quiet, almost passive enjoyment. All at once, without warning of any kind, he found himself wrapped around as it were by a flame-coloured cloud. For an instant he thought of fire, some sudden conflagration in the great city; the next, he knew that the light was within himself. Directly afterwards came upon him a sense of exultation, of immense joyousness accompanied or immediately followed by an intellectual illumination quite impossible to describe. Into his brain streamed one momentary lightning-flash of the Brahmic Splendour which has ever since lightened his life; upon his heart fell one drop of Brahmic Bliss, leaving thence-forward for always an aftertaste of heaven. Among other things he did come to believe, he saw and knew that the Cosmos is not dead matter but a living Presence, that the soul of man is immortal, that the universe is so built and ordered that without any peradventure all things work together for the good of each and all, that the foundation principle of the world is what we call love and that the happiness of everyone is in the long run absolutely certain.[29]

At the time of writing, Bucke was at the height of a successful career. Between 1876 and 1890 he held posts as superintendent of the Provincial Asylum for the Insane at Hamilton and superintendent of the London (Ontario) Hospital. He was also made professor of mental and nervous diseases at Western University

(London, Ontario), and elected president of the psychological section of the British Medical Association and president of the American Medico-Psychological Association. In his time he was considered 'one of the foremost alienists' on the North American continent. The description of his mystical experience, far from being an embarrassment to him, was written up separately as a scientific account of unusual psychological phenomena, and appeared in the *Proceedings and Transactions of the Royal Society of Canada*.[30]

Bucke's book is divided into six parts, the first three of which lay down the foundations of his theory. Part IV aims to demonstrate that a number of historical figures, most of whom were poets or the founders of major religions, had experienced unusual mental phenomena which Bucke claims were instances of cosmic consciousness. He largely relies on interpreting their writings, or accounts of their lives and experiences, to provide the evidence. The list includes Gautama the Buddha, Jesus, Mohammed, Dante, Francis Bacon (also known as William Shakespeare, according to Bucke), and William Blake.

Part V of the book is a similar examination of a longer list of 'Additional—some of Them Lesser, Imperfect, and Doubtful Instances' of cosmically conscious individuals.[31] This list also largely comprises poets and religious figures, but it also includes thirteen people who were contemporaries and whose identities Bucke concealed by referring to them by their initials only. Some of the accounts given of their lives and experiences indicate that they had sought medical advice, and it is fairly certain that they were Bucke's own patients.

Bucke observed that people who had undergone mystical experiences often developed difficulties relating to other people. He noted that, throughout history, they have been 'either exalted, by the average self conscious individual, to the rank of gods, or, adopting the other extreme, are adjudged insane'.[32] Bucke believed that he had found a solution to this problem by defining them as ordinary people who had simply taken an evolutionary step that all humans would inevitably take, sooner or later.

Anti-Psychiatry, Laing, and the Mystical Approach

The widespread interest in psychic and mystical interpretations of mental phenomena which was apparent around the turn of the twentieth century later faded into indifference. In fact, the realisation that a spiritual/mystical emergency could be mistaken for mental illness did not properly surface until the 1960s. This was largely born out of the spirit of anti-establishment protest that characterised the era. The wide-ranging rebellion against conventional psychiatric models utilised 'key ideas of the time, combining Sartre, Jung and Gregory Bateson into a perfect model of Rousseallian humanism for the counter-culture of the 1960s'.[33]

The unifying principle of what became known as the anti-psychiatry movement was the view that psychiatric practice is a form of social control. However, although there was agreement on the need to curb this aspect of psychiatry, there were still a number of diverse positions taken within the movement on the interpretation of schizophrenic symptoms. The mystical interpretation was only one of these positions.

The two leading polemicists associated with the anti-psychiatry movement were both psychiatrists: Ronald D. Laing in England and Thomas Szasz in the United States. A mystical interpretation of schizophrenic symptoms, in so much as it confirms the reality of abnormal mental experience, is anathema to Szasz. His view is that the symptoms are manufactured. (I will examine Szasz's theory closely in Chapter 7.) R. D. Laing, on the other hand, became the godfather and chief advocate for misunderstood mystics:

> Certain *transcendental experiences* seem to me to be the original well-spring of all religions. Some psychotic people have transcendental experiences. Often (to the best of their recollection), they have never had such experiences before, and frequently they will never have them again.[34]

Laing was deeply influenced by something Gregory Bateson

wrote in what Laing described as a 'brilliant introduction to a nineteenth-century autobiographical account of schizophrenia'.[35] Bateson likened a person experiencing schizophrenic symptoms to an explorer 'embarked on a voyage of discovery which is only completed by his return to the normal world, to which he comes back with insights different from those of the inhabitants who never embarked on such a voyage'.[36]

Laing's own favoured metaphor begins with a dichotomy that he sees as having given rise in the human condition to 'the split of our experience into what seems to be two worlds, inner and outer'. The outer world is the world of normal experience, whereas the inner world is the venue for the unusual experiences encountered by schizophrenics and mystics. To Laing, any separation of these two worlds is artificial, and 'the process of entering into the other world from this world, and returning to this world from the other world, is as natural as death and giving birth or being born.'[37]

Taking up Bateson's motif of a journey to describe the mystical/schizophrenic experience, Laing himself speculated that:

> The journey is experienced as going further 'in', as going back through one's personal life, in and back and through and beyond into the experience of all mankind, of the primal man, of Adam and perhaps even further into the being of animals, vegetables and minerals.
>
> In this journey there are many occasions to lose one's way, for confusion, partial failure, even final shipwreck: many terrors, spirits, demons to be encountered, that may or may not be overcome.
>
> We do not regard it as pathologically deviant to explore a jungle, or to climb Mount Everest ... We are far more out of touch with even the nearest approaches of the infinite reaches of inner space than we now are with the reaches of outer space. We respect the voyager, the explorer, the climber, the space man. It makes far more sense to me as a valid project—indeed as a desperately urgently required project of our time, to explore the

inner space and time of consciousness. Perhaps this is one of the few things that still make sense in our historical context. We are so out of touch with this realm that many people can now argue seriously that it does not exist. It is very small wonder that it is perilous indeed to explore such a lost realm.[38]

Speaking about people who have inadvertently lost themselves in this mystical realm, and have been diagnosed with schizophrenia, Laing says: 'This is where the person sitting in a chair labelled catatonic has often gone. He is not at all here: he is all there. He is frequently very mistaken about what he is experiencing, and probably does not want to experience it ... There are very few of us who know the territory in which he is lost, who know how to reach him, and how to find the way back.'[39]

Laing was very concerned with the approach of normal psychiatric practice, which he called 'a degradation ceremonial'. He believed that a new approach, an 'initiation ceremonial', should be developed for 'those who are about to go into a schizophrenic breakdown'. Laing argued that psychiatrists and psychiatric treatment should be replaced by guides who have themselves been on the inner journey: 'Psychiatrically, this would appear as ex-patients helping future patients to go mad.'[40]

Laing likened people returning from these inner experiences to lost explorers of the Renaissance who eventually found their way home. He argued that they deserved no less respect than was accorded to these explorers. But there is also a pessimistic streak behind some of Laing's thinking, as when he implied a belief in a forthcoming apocalypse, with schizophrenic experience playing some kind of preparatory role for post-apocalyptic renewal: 'If the human race survives, future men will, I suspect, look back on our enlightened epoch as a veritable age of Darkness ... They will see that what we call "schizophrenia" was one of the forms in which, often through quite ordinary people, the light began to break through the cracks in our all-too-closed minds.'[41]

Laing was scathing in his criticism of psychiatric practice when it is informed by a belief in a biological cause for schizophrenia:

> The ways of losing one's way are legion. Madness is certainly not the least unambiguous. The counter-madness of Kraepelinian psychiatry is the exact counterpart of 'official' psychosis. Literally, and absolutely seriously, it is as *mad*, if by madness we mean any radical estrangement from the totality of what is the case.[42]

Laing himself was not very popular amongst his psychiatric peers, and most of his following came from the anti-establishment new left of politics: 'We may see the growth of his ideas as a progressive and serial challenging of the whole catalogue of schizoid "symptoms" that is customarily presented in psychiatric textbooks.'[43]

Laing not only viewed his schizophrenic patients as mystical voyagers, but was himself personally engaged in mystical pursuits. Appended to the Penguin edition of his 1967 book *The Politics of Experience* was a short autobiographical fragment entitled *The Bird of Paradise*. This piece was written in the first person, and described an inner journey. Commentators have speculated that it may have been either an experimental attempt to describe the schizophrenic experience of one of his patients or, alternatively, it could have been an account of a brief psychotic experience that Laing had actually undergone himself.

In 1971 Laing surprised both his psychiatric colleagues and his new left followers by withdrawing from psychiatric practice and departing for Sri Lanka, where he set about devoting himself entirely to the mystical pursuit of Buddhist meditation. An academic from the anthropology department of Syracuse University, who encountered him there towards the end of 1971, wrote that Laing

> has virtually broken his bridges with things British and psychiatrical. He is not only doing Theravada Buddhist meditation there—he does it seventeen hours a day, for the past five months. He spent six weeks in a training monastery in Kandubodda, in central Ceylon, and the senior monk there told

me that Laing has been doing better, much better, than long-time meditation experts, Singhalese Buddhist as well as foreign.[44]

But Laing was back on the lecture circuit in the United States and Europe in less than a year. In his meditations he had been visited by a vision of a new solution to the problem of the human condition. Adults, he claimed, are haunted throughout their lives by fragmented memories of their own conception, foetal life, and birth experiences. He preached a new panacea in the therapeutic 'rebirthing experience'. Of his own birth, he said:

> I can remember it happening to me as a body blow, a searing pain, a complete total organismic reflex ... which took my breath away before I got my breath, and produced a triple red light ... quite suddenly the only status quo I knew was, within seconds—the time it took for the scissors and clamp to sever that connection—abruptly ended ... being born was an experience I certainly wouldn't like to repeat.[45]

Psychiatric theories are subject to changing fashions in social thought, and Laing's approaches to psychiatric issues have now become decidedly unfashionable. One observer of psychiatric trends, writing in the mid-1990s, had difficulty in understanding why anybody had taken Laing seriously in the first place:

> But how, how could intelligent and literate college students, professors, and physicians take such nonsense seriously? It had to be the times. Large public mental hospitals were an abomination. Vietnamese were being bombed into smithereens to 'free' them from oppression. Heads of government lied to their peoples cavalierly. Reason had not worked in an age of unreason; perhaps mysticism, raw emotion, transcendental experiences, primal screams, or rebirthing would.[46]

It is true that some of Laing's hyperbole looks very dated now.

But this does not necessarily reflect adversely on the argument that a spiritual/mystical emergency can be mistaken for mental disease. Like all psychiatrists, Laing was trained in medicine. He had no substantial training in the history of ideas, comparative religion, anthropology, the philosophy of mysticism, or even the school of hard knocks. Any of these might have better prepared him than medical psychiatry to understand and describe the meaning of mystical experience when it is mistaken for mental disease.

These deficiencies in training seem to have prevented Laing from making sound rational arguments out of his intuitive insights that could stand the test of time. Even his year of Buddhist training in Sri Lanka seems to have failed quite completely, if it can be judged by the absurd, literal interpretation of the mystical rebirth metaphor with which he emerged. But Laing had a conscience, and it told him that something was seriously wrong with the way in which many schizophrenics are treated by psychiatrists.

Laing's difficulties in articulating the meaning of mystical experience is fairly typical of psychiatrists who attempt to do so, though some are more successful than others. The more successful ones often practise under the banner of 'Jungian'. This is somewhat ironic, because Jung himself had doubtful notions about the nature of the mystical problem in schizophrenia.

The Development of Jungian Thought

Carl Gustav Jung was born in Switzerland in 1875. Although he made his reputation as an innovative psychiatrist pioneering religious/mystical approaches to the explanation of unusual psychological phenomena, he remained for the most part fairly conventional in his attempts to explain schizophrenic symptoms. In fact, he spent most of his long career wavering within the medical model. At first he favoured the biological explanation of the cause, and then he favoured the environmental approach. Finally, towards the end of his career, he found a way to integrate both as causal agents. But in this synthesis he also included observations of mythological phenomena in schizophrenic thinking that are essential components of mystical experience.

The full complexity of Jung's theorising is often not adhered to by modern Jungians. By selecting only certain parts of his theories, Jungians find that they can accommodate themselves to both medical and mystical interpretations of schizophrenic symptoms.

As a young man, Jung studied under Professor Bleuler at the Burgholzli hospital in Zurich, where he was an assistant physician. Under Bleuler's guidance, Jung chose for his doctoral dissertation to 'investigate experimentally the disintegration of ideas in schizophrenia'.[47] In 1907 he published a paper entitled 'The Psychology of Dementia Praecox' in which he set forth the knowledge he had accumulated on the subject.[48] (This was shortly before Bleuler gave the condition its modern name of schizophrenia.) The publication of Jung's paper established his reputation as a psychiatric researcher, bringing him to the attention of Freud.[49]

In this paper, Jung continued Kraepelin's work of delineating the boundaries of the mental disease that was soon to become known as schizophrenia, and which was then generally assumed to have a biological cause. Some of Jung's most interesting assertions are concerned with a symptom he called 'affectations'. He argued that affectations involved phenomena such as 'mannerism, eccentricity, and mania for originality', and were often encountered in people who were out of their social element:

> A very common form of this affectation is the pretentious and artificial behaviour of women of a lower social position—dressmakers, nurses, maids, etc.—who mix with those socially above them, and also of men who are dissatisfied with their social status and try to give themselves at least the appearance of a better education or a more imposing position.[50]

What is noteworthy here is that brain dysfunction was indicated, according to Jung, when people belonging to the lower class, but not the upper class, used affectations that were inappropriate for the class to which they belonged.

Jung's cavalier attitude towards power relationships, and his belief that a reluctance to adopt submissive postures was indicative of mental disease, is evident elsewhere in this paper. At one stage he discusses 'the characteristic lack of *emotional rapport* in dementia praecox', which he compares to that which is found in hysteria, and explains that it is only through having this emotional rapport that an analyst can penetrate the mind of the patient and gain moral power over them. He likens this process of gaining moral power over a patient to that of 'ordinary confessions'. But he goes on to lament that dementia praecox 'patients cannot feel their way into the mind of the doctor, they stick to their delusional assertions, they attribute hostile motives to the analyst, they are and remain, in a word, uninfluenceable.'[51] Quite possibly it was Jung's inability to influence this type of person that contributed to his belief at the time in a biological cause for the condition.

By 1914 Jung's thinking had advanced beyond his original class-oriented view. In a paper entitled 'The Content of the Psychoses'[52] he observed that 'psychiatry is a stepchild of medicine' and that, unlike other branches of medicine, it did not have ready access to the scientific method. This was because psychiatry had to deal with problems that lie beyond the brain in the 'psyche, as indefinable as ever, still eluding explanation, no matter how ingenious'.[53]

Jung was now ready to scoff at the 'dogma which you will find repeated in every text-book of psychiatry: "Mental diseases are diseases of the brain".[54] This critique was reiterated in a 1919 paper entitled 'On the Problem of Psychogenesis', in which he called the brain disease interpretation 'materialistic dogma'.[55]

In a 1928 paper, 'Mental Disease and the Psyche', Jung was able to state firmly that 'schizophrenia has a "psychology", that is, a psychic causality and finality, just as normal mental life has'.[56] But by 1939 he was beginning to waver in his certainty that there was no biological component in schizophrenia. In a paper entitled 'On the Psychogenesis of Schizophrenia' Jung began by agreeing with his former mentor, Bleuler, that there are primary and secondary symptoms for schizophrenia. Jung argued that, while the secondary symptoms 'are due chiefly to psychic causes', he was less certain about the cause of the primary symptom, which Bleuler had nominated as being 'a peculiar disturbance of the association-process'.[57]

Musing over the lessons of his youth, Jung wrote: 'My teacher, Eugen Bleuler, used to say that a psychological cause can produce only the symptoms of the disease, but not the disease itself.' Jung summed up his equivocation at this time by arguing that 'it is well-nigh impossible to prove, even approximately, that schizophrenia is an organic disease to begin with. It is equally impossible to make its exclusively psychological origin evident'.[58]

It was not until 1956 that his equivocation between a biological and a psychological origin produced a synthesis that could also take into account mystical considerations. In 'Recent Thoughts on Schizophrenia' Jung categorically asserted that 'this condition has two aspects of paramount importance, biochemical and psychological'.[59] He added that he had proved fifty years before that it could be treated by psychotherapy. He argued that the contents of schizophrenic experience were like those of a significant dream, what he called a 'big dream':

> Unlike ordinary dreams, such a dream is highly impressive, numinous, and its imagery frequently makes use of motifs analogous to or even identical with those of mythology. I call these structures *archetypes* because they function in a way similar to instinctual patterns of behaviour.[60]

Jung believed that the archetypes are probably 'the psychic expressions or manifestations of instinct', and that schizophrenia is caused when they are released into consciousness by the effect of an unknown toxin in the brain. He further argued that future research into schizophrenia would require a two-pronged effort:

Whereas the problem of a specific toxin presents a task for clinical psychiatry on account of its formal aspects, the question of the *contents* of schizophrenia and their meaning presents an equally important task for the psychopathologist as well as the psychologist of the future.[61]

Jung's view, which he further elaborated in another paper presented the following year, entitled simply 'Schizophrenia',[62] was essentially that stress triggered the release of a toxin, which he described as 'a kind of mistaken biological defence-reaction'.[63] When this happened the toxin could act in a way similar to hallucinogenic drugs such as mescalin and, by penetrating a biological storage area in the brain, unlock the person's instincts and flood the conscious mind with archetypal images.

Jung's final theory is comprehensive, to say the least. It bridges the two main branches of the medical model, and it also recognises mystical experience in the form of archetypal images. It says that in the first instance the symptoms of stress are caused by environmental pressures, and that when these are not addressed a toxin is released which switches the condition into a biological mode. But it goes on to recognise a pattern of mythological archetypes in the phenomenological content of schizophrenic experience.

This is unlike the conventional medical model that generally prefers to view the visionary content of schizophrenic symptoms as a random procession of delusions and hallucinations produced by a malfunctioning brain. Jung's recognition of mythological material might have allowed him to see schizophrenic symptoms as essentially non-medical religious phenomena. But he was prevented from adopting this position because he also believed that these archetypes are actually the raw material of instincts which, in normal circumstances, are locked away from conscious access in an unconscious biological storage-area of the brain. The implication of Jung's composite theory is that the release of archetypes through the agency of a toxin is unnatural, and it is therefore a symptom of disease.

However, considering the central role of mystical knowledge in the development of religious thinking and, in turn, the central role of religion in the development of civilisation, the corollary of accepting the disease interpretation of mystical experience is to assume that the project of civilisation is the outcome of mental disease. The full scope of Jung's theory is therefore rather doubtful. At this stage the 'toxin' theory is no more than an aging, unconfirmed hypothesis without any evidence to support it.

Some contemporary Jungian psychiatrists tend to ignore the implication of disease in Jung's theories on schizophrenia. Focussing only on the part of his theory that explains the phenomenology of schizophrenic visionary experience in terms of archetypes, they have successfully treated schizophrenia as an essentially non-medical problem associated with a spiritual/mystical emergency. One interesting Jungian theorist who practised this way was John Weir Perry.

John Weir Perry

Perry trained at the C. G. Jung Institute in Zurich. In the early 1970s he was engaged in a programme sponsored by the US National Institute of Mental Health looking at innovative methods of handling schizophrenia. Under this programme, Perry established a treatment centre in San Francisco called Diabasis that gave him an opportunity to test some of his theories.

In his 1974 book *The Far Side of Madness* Perry gave an unequivocal account of schizophrenia as a mystical experience, and criticised conventional psychiatric approaches for their 'interdiction against listening to the "patients' " nonrational concerns'.[64] Perry recounted how a relative with personal experience of psychosis had told him early in his career that the most essential requirement of somebody experiencing schizophrenic symptoms was to have another person listen to a description of the internal experience. Perry appears to have listened to his patients much more closely than have other psychiatrists, and as a result he has found consistent patterns of mythological material in the symptoms.

But he hints at also having had the advantage of some first-hand experience of his own. He recounts some details of a conversation with a patient in which the woman described her descent into madness as being 'a little like dying'. Perry recalls how he:

> leapt at this statement to assure her that dying was just the point, that it is what has to happen when there is an urgent need for change. She responded, 'Have you been through all this yourself? I've never met anyone as wise as you about these things.' I answered her question. I said, Yes, in a fashion I'd been through this, too; but my way was not in the involuntary experience of being overwhelmed by it as she was, but in intentionally dipping down into this same inner life to explore it; the inner experiences in that process were much the same, though.[65]

Perry is probably referring to his own experiences in psychoanalysis when he talks about 'dipping down' to the inner life. It is evident he believes that some schizophrenic symptoms can be experienced voluntarily, and that this can be beneficial.

Perry believes that the human condition requires people to simultaneously live in two different dimensions. One is the familiar territory of the ego that deals in the mundane affairs of everyday life. The other is a reservoir containing 'the great basic metaphors of the human experience', through which a person's emotions can engage with worldly matters that are not yet fully conscious:

> The latter is the mind into which one plummets when seized with madness. As Plato told us, it might be the divine frenzy of the seer or the revelation of the founder of religious forms, the inspiration of the artist or possession by a great love. And it might be a 'schizophrenic' episode.[66]

Perry theorised that schizophrenia manifests as a combination of the unconscious activating and the ego collapsing. This assessment fits closely with mystical practice, in which the mystical aspirant deliberately activates the unconscious through techniques such as word repetition and visualisations, while denying expression to the conscious self-identity (ego) through ascetic practices such as seclusion, celibacy, and fasting.

The Far Side of Madness documented Perry's findings after analysing in depth the psychic experiences of twelve patients over a twelve-year period. The book identified consistent patterns of myth, ritual, messianism, and mysticism in the schizophrenic experiences of his patients. According to Perry, the origins of these patterns are to be found in the kingship rituals of ancient Mesopotamia: 'the ceremonial death and renewal of the year and of the sacral king and his kingdom, out of which other religious forms have differentiated and evolved in the centuries since'.[67]

The essence of Perry's theory is that the earliest civilisations required the invention of specific rituals and myths in order to give them collective guidance and continuity. These rituals and myths became buried in the collective unconscious of the original city-dwellers. After civilised culture was launched in Mesopotamia, the people of other cultures, learning from this model, absorbed in some osmotic manner, along with the urban way of life, the original Mesopotamian collective unconscious.

These rituals and myths now lie buried in the collective unconscious of all modern people, where they act as a common denominator to give coherence to social organisation based around life in cities. When the individual ego of a person collapses—often because the person has not been properly integrated into civic society—these archetypal myths and rituals flood into his or her consciousness. When this process is successful the effect is to reinvent the person's individual ego so that it can find a role that is better adjusted to the requirements of civic society.

In a more recent interview, Perry made clear his approach to the treatment of schizophrenia. He said that he agreed with Jung's belief that schizophrenia is not really amenable to psychiatric control (although Jung clearly came to believe that it could be treated with psychotherapy), and that for therapeutic purposes the best interpretation of the condition is that it is itself a spontaneous healing process. In his opinion, the term 'sickness' should only be applied to the pre-psychotic personality, which can be seen as standing in need of reorganisation:

> The way 'schizophrenia' unfolds is that, in a situation of personal crisis, all the psyche's energy is sucked back out of the personal conscious area, into what we call the archetypal area. Mythic contents thus emerge from the deepest level of the psyche, in order to re-organise the Self. In so doing, the person feels himself withdrawing from the ordinary surroundings, and becomes quite isolated in this dream state ... The whole schizophrenic turmoil is really a self-organising, healing experience. It's like a molten state. Everything seems to be made of free energy, an inner free play of imagery through which the alienated psyche spontaneously re-organises itself—in such a way that the conscious ego is brought back into communication with the unconscious again.[68]

Perry claimed that, in the absence of psychiatric intervention, the acute phase of the schizophrenic experience normally only lasted six weeks. He argued that this was confirmed by the biblical tradition of forty days in the wilderness. He said that in his experience this pattern was so universal that he had formed the opinion that chronic schizophrenia, in which a person had recurring crises over a lifetime, was socially constructed by intolerance encountered during the first acute phase.

Perry was surprised to discover that people experiencing these symptoms were usually more concerned with cultural and social issues than with their own personal affairs. He says that his Freudian training in medical school had not prepared him for this, and that when Jung had informed him about it he had at first been sceptical. But after he observed the phenomenon for himself, he says it became the primary reason for developing his alternative methods of handling people in acute crisis:

> Our new understanding shows that the process of re-connection to the unconscious, which these millions of people go through in a way that's usually so very hazardous, isolated and uncreative, is nonetheless made up of the same stuff as seers, visionaries, cultural reformers and prophets go through.[69]

When traditional societies are overtaken by a crisis of confidence in their established cultural patterns, according to Perry, they are likely to produce messiahs, seers, and prophets who have caught a glimpse of a new myth-form and who endeavour to transmit it to the people at large. If the new myth-form is successful it will give new direction and purpose to the society. Most modern societies are constantly changing and are therefore in constant crisis, at least in mythological terms.

To Perry, people in modern societies who manifest schizophrenic symptoms are struggling to fulfil the same function as the seers in traditional societies: 'I am not suggesting that all persons in the "psychotic" form of visionary state should be considered prophets, but rather that the program of the visionary experience and its imagery is the same in well-known 'prophets' as in our little-known "patients"'.[70]

To support this view, he cites the observation that the specific nature of the opposing forces of good and evil, and the messianic function perceived by schizophrenic individuals, has been changing from one decade to another in accordance with the shifting cultural crisis of modern America. In the 1950s, for instance, the primary schizophrenic concern was with the preservation of democracy in the face of a challenge from communism. In the 1960s it was the preservation of peace against the constant threat of an enlargement of war. By the 1970s the focus had shifted dramatically to a concern about environmental issues and the need to defend the global ecology against destructive forces.

The therapeutic approach practised by Perry at Diabasis was to give emotional support while encouraging the person to plumb the depths of the experience. This is basically the opposite of the conventional psychiatric approach, which seeks to abort the experience, usually by the application of drug treatment, as soon as possible. Perry says that in the fully supportive environment of Diabasis it was not uncommon for a person to emerge from the schizophrenic crisis prematurely. When this happened, he says, it was necessary to encourage the person to re-enter psychosis so as to complete the process. In regard to the success of his method, and indeed of the healing properties of schizophrenia itself, Perry claimed of his former patients that 'the outcome of their stay at Diabasis was that their life after the episode was substantially more satisfying and fulfilling to them than it had been before!'[71]

Perry's observation, that without medical treatment his patients could re-emerge from a psychological crisis with improved mental health, is confirmed by research of an entirely different kind. Joseph Campbell has made similar observations about spiritual/mystical emergencies by analysing folk heroes in mythological traditions.

Mythological Heroes and Schizophrenia

Campbell had written extensively on the subject of mythology, but only became interested in schizophrenia in 1968, when he was asked to give a series of lectures on the condition at the Esalen Institute.[72] Campbell has recounted how, when he told the organiser that he knew nothing about the subject, he was put in contact with Perry in order to learn. Perry sent him a paper he had published in 1962. Upon reading it, Campbell said he discovered 'that the imagery of schizophrenic fantasy perfectly matches that of the mythological hero journey, which I had outlined and elucidated, back in 1949 in *The Hero with a Thousand Faces*'.[73]

Campbell was then engaged in a vast project involving a cross-cultural comparative study of mythology.[74] He had paid no attention in researching this project to specific problems of psychopathology or personalised mystical visions, and was mainly concerned with analysing ideas he found to be common to all mythologies:

> According to my thinking, they were the universal, archetypal, psychologically based symbolic themes and motifs of all traditional mythologies; and now from this paper of Dr. Perry I was learning that the same symbolic figures arise spontaneously from the broken-off, tortured state of mind of modern individuals suffering from a complete schizophrenic breakdown.[75]

The usual pattern of the mythological hero journey uncovered by Campbell in his own research involved three stages: separation, initiation, and return. An individual separates from the established social order and goes on a long inward and backward journey, deep into the psyche, and is confronted there by chaotic and terrifying forces. If the person is fortunate a centre of harmony is found, and new courage discovered, before a return journey of new birth is completed:

> A hero ventures forth from the world of common day into a region of supernatural wonder; fabulous forces are there encountered and a decisive victory is won: the hero comes back from this mysterious adventure with the power to bestow boons on his fellow men.[76]

Campbell drew an analogy between schizophrenia and the mythological mystical journey that he had been researching. He compared the fortunes of two divers, one who could swim and one who could not: 'The mystic, endowed by native talents for this sort of thing and following, stage by stage, the instructions of a master, enters the waters and finds he can swim; whereas the schizophrenic, unprepared, unguided, and ungifted, has fallen or has intentionally plunged, and is drowning.'[77]

It is not uncommon for theorists to position mystical experience in the context of some kind of evolutionary process. As has been discussed above, Bucke had a theory about an evolutionary potential he called cosmic consciousness. Perry also developed an evolutionary theory, of sorts. In his book *Roots of Renewal in*

Myth and Madness,[78] Perry elaborated on the themes he had developed in his earlier works, and articulated a theory about the evolution of the Semitic/Judeo/Christian religious ideas in which he found most of his patients to be drowning.

Perry argued that there is indeed an evolutionary process under way involving the faculties of consciousness of individual participants. His view was that this process was initiated by a breakthrough in the development of human consciousness that occurred with the establishment of the first city states in ancient Mesopotamia. The specialised social roles that became necessary with the establishment of civilisation required new forms of social organisation that fundamentally altered the way in which individual people related to one another and to life in general. Life in cities required clearly defined structures of social authority. Hierarchies of power emerged from these conditions, which in turn led to individual identity being largely vested in the social ranking of the individual concerned.

The collective and individual focus on status at first removed ordinary people from the possibility of finding a solution to the problem of personal mortality. All power was at first transferred upwards to the king and, in the early centuries of these ancient city-states, the king was thought to be the only person capable of fulfilling the evolutionary potential by transcending the problem of death. The king was so powerful he was given divine status so that he could achieve this goal.

However, as time progressed, the evolutionary potential slowly percolated down through the layers of social class, eventually passing through the aristocracy and down to the mass of people, in what Perry refers to as a 'democratisation work of messianic visions'.[79] Whereas the image containing the evolutionary message had at first been confined to the personification of a divine king, remote and aloof from ordinary people, the concept of a messiah, which eventually evolved as the symbol of transcendence, was a model for everyone to emulate.

Perry's theory is that the course of acute schizophrenic imagery sequentially follows the developments of the Semitic/Judeo/ Christian religious traditions. These developments have been laid down, layer upon layer, in the collective unconscious so that the schizophrenic individual, who is working through this storehouse, encounters them in the order in which they were filed:

> It is my thesis that the visionary states we call psychosis recapitulate this entire history, as another instance of ontogeny repeating phylogeny. The renewal process attempts to evolve a new level of consciousness in the individual, and to accomplish this, induces an identification first with the mythology of sacral kingship, then with that of messianic democratisation, and finally reaches a vision of the potential spiritual consciousness for life in the world society of today.[80]

It is apparent that Perry's theoretical framework is seriously flawed. This is because it does not explain the nature of visionary states in people who do not have this Judeo/Christian background. A Chinese person with a Confucian background, for instance, is not likely to encounter this same sequence of archetypal material. Therefore, even if Perry's theory does correctly describe the pattern of psychotic experiences for people with Judeo/Christian backgrounds, it deals only with relatively superficial aspects of these experiences. It does not penetrate deeply enough to identify a denominator that is common to people of all religious and cultural backgrounds.

Perry's theoretical weakness is reminiscent of the problem with Laing's work, and probably originates with the same inadequacies in professional training. As with Laing, it is apparent that Perry recognised there were people undergoing spiritual/mystical emergencies who were mistakenly thought to have 'diseased' minds. He was prepared to listen carefully to what these people had to say about their inner experiences, sympathised with them, and was certainly better for them than any conventional drug-treating psychiatrist would have been. His patients were lucky to have him. But, as with Laing, he was trained in medicine and not in the appropriate body of knowledge associated with mysticism. Although his psychiatric training included a Jungian component, which apparently put him on the right track, it still proved to be an insufficient grounding on which to build a sound theoretical framework to properly explain what he observed.

Schizophrenia's Mystical Problem

Putting together a coherent account of the mystical problem associated with schizophrenia begins with the existential proposition that the consciousness of self presents all individual humans with a paradox. This paradox concerns the self's knowledge that because personal extinction is a foreseeable inevitability, and is unavoidable, the fear of it is therefore irrational. Yet despite the knowledge of this irrationality, the fear of death remains the foundation stone in the architecture of self-identity. The existential dilemma that confronts people who grow into an awareness of this problem concerns the difficulty in finding a purposeful form of self-expression in these circumstances.

The mystical quest is an attempt to transcend the self and to uncover a separate reality that is connected to a higher, deeper, or expanded level of consciousness. Everyone has the potential to reach this improved level of consciousness, which involves the replacement of the self's emotional dichotomy of fear-of-death/desire-for-life with a love/courage polarity focussed on transpersonal objectives. Mystical traditions, some of which have been in existence for more than two thousand years, teach their adherents a variety of techniques which are designed to induce this transition.

The transition phase itself involves a psychological crisis during which the person's mind is flooded with mythological images, putting it temporarily out of balance. The vast majority of people in modern industrial societies do not comprehend the meaning of mystical experience, and they mistakenly believe that people who display signs of this crisis are suffering from a mental disease and require urgent medical attention. This cultural belief in the existence of mental disease creates social conditions that are particularly dangerous for the many accidental mystics who stumble inadvertently into the mystical experience without protection or guidance from an organised discipline. These unfortunate people usually come to the attention of medical psychiatrists, who diagnose them with schizophrenia and routinely abort their mystical experience by the forced application of neuroleptic drugs.

Despite being handicapped with inappropriate training, a small number of psychiatrists have had the insight to see mystical experience rather than mental illness in the schizophrenic symptoms of their patients. Some of these psychiatrists, such as Laing and Perry, have realised that the crisis phase is only temporary, and that what the patients really need is a supportive and protective environment so they can complete the psychological transition.

When this psychological transition is successful, the benefits extend beyond the individual to the whole society. But these benefits are endangered by current psychiatric practices. Perry warns: 'If this way of viewing psychic turmoils is on target, then there is a grave danger in psychiatry's zeal to suppress them, and instead there is an urgent need to safeguard visionary experience for the benefit of the culture'.[81]

6

Shrinking Free Thought:
human rights and mystical experience

Psychiatrists violate fundamental human rights when they forcibly abort mystical experiences with drug treatments. The reason this is allowed to happen is frustratingly simple. Modern industrial societies are inherently biased against independent religious thought and belief. Our scientific age is willing to tolerate non-rational, religious thinking so long as it is contained within organised churches, but it will not abide the inflammatory visions of independent seers. This is particularly true of people with the temerity to suggest that they might have some kind of messianic mission to fulfil. Such people are thought to be a nuisance at best, and dangerous at worst.

Our culture feels the need to protect itself from these people, and has charged the psychiatric profession with the responsibility of identifying and neutralising them as quickly and efficiently as possible. In taking on this task, psychiatrists tacitly understand that the objective is really to silence such people, not to help them. That is why they are trained in the use of powerful drugs, and not in the knowledge of religion and mysticism.

However, this practice is not necessarily correct simply because it is culturally sanctioned. There are many practices and institutions in modern societies that are similarly supported by popular consensus which are demonstrably wrong—in the sense that they cause relative harm by retarding the societies that practise them, and also wrong in a more absolute moral sense. The scientific/military deployment of weapons of mass destruction is one example, and the market-driven destruction of the natural environment is another. Further examples that compare more closely are culturally based prejudices and sanctions against certain racial groups, against homosexuals, and against women. To put it bluntly, societies often don't know what is good for them. As a result, they sometimes develop practices and institutions that work against their collective interests.

Despite this pattern of self-inflicted cultural damage, there is another pattern whereby modern societies evolve their collective thinking and, with the passage of time, develop insights and correct their culturally based errors. Human rights have become an important tool in the development of this type of collective insight. In fact, it is largely through the educative efforts of human rights activists that various minority groups have been removed from culturally sanctioned blacklists, and recast as good and productive citizens. This brings us to a specific section within an international human rights covenant that was intended to protect the rights of differently minded people by asserting their universal right to the freedoms of thought and belief. The covenant is binding on all signatory nations.

Article 18

People diagnosed with schizophrenia have treatment forced upon them that aims to modify so-called delusions, hallucinations, and disordered thoughts. This intentional interference with mental functioning unequivocally abuses human rights, because the right of all individuals to have their own thoughts and to hold whatever beliefs they choose is protected under international law. Article 18 of the International Covenant on Civil and Political Rights (ICCPR) states:

1. Everyone shall have the right to freedom of thought, conscience and religion. This right shall include freedom to have or to adopt a religion or belief of his choice, and freedom, either individually or in community with others and in public or private, to manifest his religion or belief in worship, observance, practice and teaching.

2. No one shall be subject to coercion which would impair his freedom to have or to adopt a religion or belief of his choice.

3. Freedom to manifest one's religion or beliefs may be subject only to such limitations as are prescribed by law and are necessary to protect public safety, order, health, or morals or the fundamental rights and freedoms of others.[1]

The Article-18 rights that are most relevant to people who have undergone a mystical experience, and who are alleged to have schizophrenia, are the freedoms of thought, conscience, and belief; the freedom to manifest belief; and the protection against coercion which would impair freedom of belief. The only limitations that are allowed to be placed on these rights are in respect to the manifestation of beliefs. The protection of thoughts and beliefs is particularly relevant to people who have undergone mystical experience, because it is unusual varieties of thought and belief that characterise the residual phenomena of mystical experience.

Article 2 of the ICCPR specifies that the covenant protects the rights of all individuals 'without distinction of any kind'.[2] This means there is no scope for making exceptions for supposedly 'mentally ill' people. This point is pivotal for an Article-18 defence of mystical experience, because such a defence only becomes necessary after a person has been labelled mentally ill by medical psychiatrists.

The rights protected in Article 18 of the ICCPR are fundamental to the human experience. They were first specified in Article 18 of the Universal Declaration of Human Rights, and were restated as Article 1 of the more recently formulated United Nations Declaration on the Elimination of all Forms of Intolerance and of Discrimination Based on Religion or Belief.[3] Articles 18 of the ICCPR and the Universal Declaration, and Article 1 of the Declaration on Religion or Belief are almost identical. I have focussed my argument about human rights on Article 18 of ICCPR because covenants have higher standing in international law than declarations.

The Spirit of Article 18

The ideas behind the freedoms of thought, conscience, and belief, and the right to express beliefs, are as old as human society. Social organisation is inevitable for people who live in groups, and group members are usually required to conform with prescribed behavioural patterns and subscribe to commonly held beliefs. But these same people also have to face life as mortal individuals, and in this respect the knowledge of personal mortality imposes on individuals a consciousness that the self is unique and separate from the rest of the social group, and that it is often necessary to ignore the collective good in order to pursue personal needs.

John Stuart Mill sought to resolve the conflict between the good of the society and the good of the individual with a simple formula:

> The principle is that the sole end for which mankind are warranted, individually or collectively, in interfering with the liberty of action of any of their number is self-protection. That the only purpose for which power can be rightfully exercised over any member of a civilised community, against his will, is to prevent harm to others. His own good, either physical or moral, is not a sufficient warrant.[4]

Mill's utilitarian approach is based on the underlying moral principle that a person's action should be judged by evaluating the consequences of the action for all those who will be affected by it. Starting with the assumption that a fundamental benefit will accrue to individuals who exercise their right to act, the only justification for preventing such action is if greater harm can be expected to accrue to other people. Whether or not the performer of the action benefits should be of no concern to others.

The right of individuals to think freely and to discover their own beliefs is a principle that the European cultural tradition has defended against imposed conformity with particular ferocity since the Reformation. The words 'freethinking' and 'freethinker' did not begin to appear in English literature until the end of the seventeenth century, but there were people who described themselves as freethinkers as far back as the thirteenth century in Italy.[5] In the European Christian tradition, heretics have usually been severely punished, but at the same time there has also been a retrospective tendency to applaud heretics as 'heroes who were badgered by ignorant and vicious men'[6] and who often overcame great obstacles to bring new 'light' into the world.

One advocate of freedom in thought has argued that it is superstition that inhibits freethinking and that 'the mission of freethought is to relieve spiritual misery'.[7] The conquest of superstition is a widespread ideal in modern society, and the recognition of the role played by freethinking individuals in this quest is undoubtedly one of the reasons for the freedoms of thought, conscience, and belief having been enshrined in Article 18 as inviolable human rights.

The Technical Requirements of Article 18

The UN Centre for Human Rights compiles an annual report on action that the organisation has taken in regard to human rights. In a section that discusses resolutions formulated by the Commission on Human Rights, there is a cumulative record of how the commission has interpreted various human rights articles since its inception. Under the heading of 'Freedom of thought, conscience and religion or belief',[8] there is a record of the occasions when the commission has been called upon to interpret Article 18 and what it has resolved.

The discussions and resolutions recorded to date only concern matters of conscience and religion. There is a record of repeated discussions on the subject of conscientious objection to military service, particularly in relation to apartheid, and also on the religious rights of minorities. But the commission has not been called upon to make a ruling under Article 18 in regard to either mental health or psychiatric practice.

The key terms in Article 18—such as 'thought', 'conscience', and 'belief'—are straightforward. Individuals should be free to think their own thoughts and to hold whatever beliefs they choose without interference. One human rights analyst has argued that this right is inviolable because '[t]here are some aspects of person's lives that are so deeply personal and intrinsic, such as the right to freedom of thought ... that they are not subject to explicit balancing because there is no cumulative or collective interest that can justify an intrusion'.[9]

One interpretation by the Human Rights Committee of the United Nations seems particularly relevant to a possible defence against forced psychiatric treatment for schizophrenia:

> Article 18 protects theistic, non-theistic and atheistic beliefs, as well as the right not to profess any religion or beliefs. The terms belief and religion are to be broadly construed. Article 18 is not limited in its application to traditional religions or to religions and beliefs with institutional characteristics or practices analogous to those of traditional religions.[10]

A generalised UN interpretation of Article 18 emphasises the implied dichotomy of inner and outer. It says that 'no restriction of any kind may be imposed upon man's inner thoughts or moral conscience', but goes on to point out that external manifestations 'may be subject to legitimate limitations'.[11]

A conference of international jurists in 1984 made a detailed examination of the limitations allowed for in the ICCPR. The outcome of the conference was the Siracusa Principles,[12] which severely restrict the way in which limitations can be imposed. In relation to Article 18, for instance, the provision to limit the *manifestation* of beliefs could not be extended to limit the *holding* of beliefs. Nor would it be possible to place any limitations at all on a person's thoughts or conscience.

Article 18 allows for limitations to be placed on the manifestation of belief only when it is 'necessary to protect public safety, order, health, or morals or the fundamental rights and freedoms of others'. According to the Siracusa Principles, a 'necessary' act may only be undertaken 'in response to a pressing public need'.[13] The definitions of 'public safety' and 'public health' could probably be used as justifications for limiting the kinds of manifestations of belief likely to be made by a person who was thought to have schizophrenia. So would protection of the 'rights and freedoms of others'. But limitations on the grounds of public 'order' and 'morals' would probably not be allowed. For 'public order' to be invoked, 'the rules which ensure the functioning of society'[14] have to be endangered, and 'public morals' are generally recognised as being outside of the province of psychiatric practice.

According to the Siracusa Principles, mental health legislation does not violate human rights guaranteed under Article 18 when it empowers psychiatrists to limit a person's manifestations of belief, so long as those manifestations cause 'danger to the safety of persons, to their life or physical integrity, or serious damage to their property'.[15] Similarly, limitations are permitted to protect the rights of others. But other people's rights only have precedence if they are 'more fundamental' than the right to manifest a belief. Being more fundamental is indicated when a conflicting right is also specified in the ICCPR and has no limitations attached to it.[16] The limitation allowed on the grounds of protecting public health generally overlaps with public safety, but public health extends a little further and would probably include 'preventing disease or injury'[17] to the person who manifests the belief.

Despite the severe restrictions on the application of these limitations, their existence still generates some uncertainty about the level of protection that Article 18 can offer against the involuntary hospitalisation of people who are alleged to have schizophrenia. However, it seems certain that an outward manifestation of a false belief (delusion)—which takes the form of dangerous behaviour motivated by the false belief—is the only primary symptom of schizophrenia for which limitations, such as incarceration, can be legitimately imposed.

This means that it might sometimes be legitimate under the provisions of Article 18 to lock people up who manifest beliefs in a dangerous manner. But once they have been restrained they still retain inviolable rights to the freedoms of thought and conscience, and to *hold*, if not to manifest, whatever beliefs they like. If psychiatric practice on involuntary patients interferes with these rights, it unequivocally violates Article 18.

A Hypothetical Mental Patient

We can try to get a feeling for the human side of this problem by imagining the case of Kerry, a hypothetical mental patient. Kerry is a young person who has always felt a bit different from other people, perhaps because of a heightened feeling of vulnerability or self-consciousness. Kerry has long held a passion for poetry and eastern religions, and recently he/she began to find new meaning in favourite writings. After sitting up one night reading, he/she slipped into an altered state of consciousness involving visions and voices. When Kerry began to express unusual beliefs to the family over the next few days, together with fragmented quotations of poetry referring to 'slings and arrows of outrageous fortune' and taking 'arms against a sea of troubles', the family doctor was called in to make an examination. The doctor identified delusions, and thought Kerry was in need of care, treatment, and control. This led to Kerry's involuntary admission into a mental hospital.

DSM-IV defines delusions as false beliefs that are not 'ordinarily accepted by other members of the person's culture or subculture'.[18] This means that Kerry's family doctor, by virtue of being a medical practitioner, is presumed under the sanctions of typical mental health legislation to be a competent judge of ordinarily accepted beliefs, and is empowered to certify anyone who appears to hold beliefs that he or she thinks are culturally unacceptable.

It should be remembered that, after Kerry's incarceration in a hospital, there are still no laboratory tests available to confirm an underlying cause for the delusions identified by the family doctor. The hospital psychiatrists would therefore have to rely on monitoring Kerry's thoughts and beliefs, and their outward manifestations, to know whether his or her condition was improving or deteriorating. This means that treatment that is intended to 'improve' Kerry's condition will also be intended to coerce him or her to give up or change the 'false' beliefs that were the original symptoms of the illness. So long as Kerry's delusions remain in an unremitted state, it is likely that the treatment/coercion will continue.

This deduction allows us to establish a *prima facie* case that any involuntary psychiatric treatment given to a person alleged to have schizophrenia would violate Article 18 by subjecting the person 'to coercion which would impair his freedom to have or to adopt a religion or belief of his choice'.[19] A further case can be made that the standard neuroleptic drug treatment given to people who are alleged to have schizophrenia does not merely select delusions for modification, but also interferes with the person's freedom of thought by blocking the higher thinking centres of the brain.

Neuroleptic Treatment

Neuroleptic drugs are the treatment of first choice for schizophrenia.[20] (They are alternatively known as major tranquillisers and anti-psychotics.) The first commercially developed neuroleptic, chlorpromazine, was synthesised by French scientists in 1950 while they were attempting to develop an antihistamine.[21] Chlorpromazine was originally tried as an anaesthetic potentiator, but proved to be ineffectual. It was then used as an anti-emetic, but once again it was found to be not commercially useful until an experiment was carried out in 1953 on 'about 100 psychiatric patients and it was declared to be an effective antipsychotic'.[22] Thereafter it proved to be one of the most profitable drugs in pharmaceutical history.

This new drug was found to be highly sedating. One of the early French pioneers of its usage, a physician named Laborit, found it very useful in calming anxious surgery patients. He noted of his patients that, 'There is not any loss of consciousness, not any change in the patient's mentality, but a slight tendency to sleep and above all a disinterest [sic] in what goes on around him.'[23]

By targeting the dopamine neurotransmitter system of the brain, neuroleptics reduce the circulation of dopamine. Along with this reduction of dopamine, certain kinds of brain functions that depend on dopamine are also reduced. Some parts of the brain learn to compensate: 'Following neuroleptic blockade of A9 neurons, post-synaptic dopamine receptor targets in the striatum undergo a compensatory increase in both numbers of dopamine receptors and their sensitivity. This dopamine supersensitivity or hyper-reactivity in the striatum causes tardive dyskinesia.'[24]

Tardive dyskinesia is one of a number of serious side effects characterised by movement disorders that are associated with the use of neuroleptics. Once the dopamine supersensitivity has been established in this part of the brain, the movement disorders sometimes continue to get worse, and often remain permanently, even when treatment is discontinued. But it seems that other centres of the brain, which are also dependent on dopamine for proper functioning, and which regulate many of the higher emotional and mental activities, fail to make a similar compensatory adjustment by becoming supersensitive to dopamine. The result is that these higher mental centres close down, and this is why neuroleptic treatment has been referred to as a 'chemical lobotomy':

> Neuroleptics have their main impact by blunting the highest functions of the brain in the frontal lobes and the closely

connected basal ganglia. They can also impair the reticular activating or 'energising' system of the brain. These impairments result in relative degrees of apathy, indifference, emotional blandness, conformity, and submissiveness, as well as a reduction in all verbalisations, including complaints and protests. It is no exaggeration to call this effect a chemical lobotomy.[25]

In relation to the question of Article-18 rights, it is apparent that psychiatrists have prior knowledge that the thoughts and beliefs of their patients might be disrupted by neuroleptic treatment. However, there seems to be considerable divergence of opinion as to whether this disruption of thoughts will be beneficial to patients.

A recent text describes the psychiatric intention as benefiting the patient through 'Alterations in thought. Antipsychotic drugs improve reasoning, decrease ambivalence, and decrease delusions ... Antipsychotic drugs are effective in decreasing confusion and clouding ... hallucinations and illusions are reduced'.[26]

Some of these intended effects, such as the claim that the drugs 'improve reasoning', have to be treated with a certain amount of scepticism. 'Improved reasoning' is probably best interpreted as a euphemism for the fact that the patient's thinking has fallen more into line with the will of the psychiatrist administering the treatment.

But even if submission to the will of psychiatrists can be seen as leading to a beneficial outcome for the patient, neuroleptic treatment does not always go according to plan. For instance, the small print in an advertisement for the frequently prescribed neuroleptic Haldol [haloperidol is its generic name], warns of possible adverse reactions that are the opposite of those intended. Some of the possible effects are 'insomnia, restlessness, anxiety, euphoria, agitation, drowsiness, depression, lethargy, headache, confusion, vertigo, grand mal seizures, and exacerbation of psychotic symptoms including hallucinations and catatonic-like behaviour states which may be responsive to drug withdrawal'.[27] In addition to these possible reactions recognised by the manufacturer, researchers have also 'found in a controlled study that some patients have a marked increase in violence when treated with moderately high-dose haloperidol'.[28]

This paradoxical admission by a manufacturer that neuroleptics might exacerbate psychotic symptoms, rather than ameliorate them, does not weaken an Article-18 case against the drugs. On the contrary, regardless of whether a treatment diminishes or distorts a person's thinking processes, it still interferes with the person's right to freedom of thought and belief.

In a recent book, a British psychiatrist related how he had participated in an experiment that required him to take a 5 mg dose of haloperidol, which is a normal daily dose prescribed for adults with schizophrenia. The experiment was intended to test the effect of the drug on attention and concentration, and required him to sit in front of a computer screen and perform simple tasks:

> After an hour I felt terrible. The last thing I wanted to be doing was to be seated in front of that computer. Although I did not feel suicidal, I felt restless inside, as if I could not settle. On several occasions I had to get up and walk around. If I had not done so I don't know what would have happened. On two or three occasions I came close to putting my fist through the screen, because I was so intensely frustrated and bored with what was going on. This sensation was a real physical sensation located somewhere in the pit of my stomach. I felt irritated by everything that was going on at the time. The feeling persisted well into the next day, to the extent that I found it difficult to concentrate at work.[29]

Another psychiatrist who deliberately took a small dose of the commonly prescribed neuroleptic Thorazine [chlorpromazine], in order to find out what it was like, wrote a description of the experience: 'I felt overwhelmed by the blahs. I felt tired and lethargic, motivated to do nothing. My thinking was turned down from 78 to 16 rpms, my mouth got dry and I just didn't care all that much about anything'. He went on to describe the effects he had witnessed of neuroleptics on mental patients in hospitals:

> Thinking is slowed down—and at high enough doses 'dissolved'—so that so-called 'crazy' or 'delusional' thinking is prevented (along with other kinds of thinking—including creative thinking). Emotions are blunted, pushed down. The result is some degree of (often total) indifference and apathy. Sterile, zombie-like personalities result when indifference is combined with the drug's sedating effects. The sparkle, vitality and exuberance of an alive human being are cut off by these drugs.[30]

Surveys of patient attitudes towards neuroleptics have found that, almost universally, the people who take such drugs dislike them. Confirmation of this is to be found in the fact that, unlike the situation of most other mind-altering drugs, there is no black market for neuroleptics. One patient described the experience of enforced treatment with neuroleptics: 'They knock you out. They cause aches and pains all through your body. They make you apathetic. They stop the whole spiritual transformation process. It's like putting molasses in your brain. You can't even concentrate enough to read.'[31]

Another patient treated involuntarily with Thorazine said:

> The drugs caused me all kinds of problems. I couldn't see. I couldn't read my music or see across the room. I thought my eyes were going bad. The subjective feeling is actually one of disturbance. It's important for people to know that it's not a tranquillising effect at all. What you feel is a sense of inner turmoil. Viewed from the outside you might look less agitated because you're not going to make much noise or show your spirit. I had difficulty thinking. I remember once trying to make a list of books I needed from class and not being able to finish the list. I had difficulty moving my tongue which I really resent because I still have residual effects today.[32]

These testimonies make it clear that when people are alleged to have schizophrenia, and are given forced drug treatment, their Article-18 rights to the freedom of thought, conscience, and belief are violated. As if this isn't bad enough, there is also the likelihood of their incurring permanent brain damage as a side effect. When this possibility is combined with the argument that so-called treatment is in reality a 'chemical restraint', and is administered for the benefit of others rather than of the patient, it becomes apparent that psychiatric treatment for schizophrenia also harms a person's Article-12 right (as affirmed by the International Covenant on Economic, Social and Cultural Rights) 'to the enjoyment of the highest attainable standard of physical and mental health'.[33] The irony here is that Article 12 is supposed to provide the medical model with the basis for the 'right to treatment'. The 'right to treatment', in turn, provides the twisted logic that is supposed to justify psychiatric coercion.

From a human rights point of view, it is clear that forced psychiatric treatment of people undergoing a spiritual/mystical emergency is unequivocally wrong. However, these are not the only people whose human rights are abused by psychiatric labelling and forced treatment for schizophrenia. Many people experience this abuse when their real problems have more to do with their social relationships than with their minds.

7

Mental as Anything:
schizophrenic symptoms as manufactured artefacts

Many people whose minds function relatively normally are diagnosed with schizophrenia when they are neither undergoing a spiritual/mystical emergency nor displaying the classic symptoms of inner mental turmoil that indicate psychosis. Instead, they are effectively penalised for experiencing difficulties in their social relationships. In fact, so common is this type of false diagnosis that a substantial school of psychiatric criticism has developed which argues that everyone who is diagnosed as a schizophrenic can be fitted into this description, and that all 'mental illness' is a psychiatric myth.

However, the myth-of-mental-illness school neglects the problems of people who are diagnosed when they are undergoing genuine mystical emergencies, as described above. This neglect of the mystical problem in schizophrenia by some psychiatric critics is a serious but understandable error. It comes from having sufficient insight to see through the flaws in the medical model, but insufficient reflexivity or personal experience to overcome the cultural bias against mysticism. The result is that critics of the medical model are divided into two loosely assembled schools: one focuses on people abused for having mystical problems; the other focuses on people abused for having social problems.

Notwithstanding its failure to recognise a spiritual/mystical emergency, the latter school has very effectively criticised the institution of psychiatry with its argument that all mental illness is a myth. The basic premise of this argument is that there cannot be any disease of the mind because the mind is an abstract concept without any physical reality. The use of the term 'mental illness' to describe unusual patterns of thought and behaviour was originally clearly understood as being metaphorical. The subsequent application of a medical model to this metaphor, and the modern literal understanding of it, is therefore unsound. A 'sick' mind—like a 'sick' joke or a 'sick' society—cannot be treated medically, and would only be literally understood as a medical problem by a fool.

From this perspective, the only way that the symptoms of schizophrenia can be indicative of disease is if they are manifestations of a brain disease, not a mental disease. However, despite the many hypotheses that try to link schizophrenia with brain abnormalities, no firm pattern of schizophrenia-typical lesions has yet been detected in the brains of deceased schizophrenics. That is, there is no evidence for such a thing as a brain disease, let alone a mental disease, called 'schizophrenia'. This conclusion once prompted two US critics to state unequivocally: 'Schizophrenia is a moral verdict masquerading as a medical diagnosis'.[1]

The relatively large number of people supposedly displaying schizophrenic indicators does not threaten this position. On the one hand, critics argue that schizophrenic indicators fall within the range of natural psychological and behavioural experience, and that they have only been defined in pathological terms because they fall outside the boundaries of cultural tolerance. As such, there are social expectations that 'good citizens' will avoid these patterns of thought and behaviour. People who do not avoid them are subsequently identified as deviants because, in a metaphorical sense, they have 'sick' minds.

On the other hand, critics also argue that a provision by the medical profession of an otherwise non-existent category of human types called schizophrenics has required that individuals of this type be manufactured to fill it. To describe how this manufacturing process takes place, analogies are drawn between modern schizophrenics and medieval witches.[2] Just as it is now thought unlikely that people with magical powers and a compulsive desire to corrupt Christian citizens existed in late-medieval Europe, it is also thought unlikely that people manifest the extraordinary mental contortions and compulsive forms of dangerous behaviour attributed to modern schizophrenics.

What brings these types of people into existence is the human imagination. Belief in their existence is a kind of shared collective delusion which fulfils transitory cultural needs, and which can be initiated when the holders of knowledge-based authority categorically assert that such things are true. In other words, these culturally based delusions are initiated when transmission of the false belief proceeds from the top down.

The official process that led to the manufacture of late-medieval witches started with the publication of the *Malleus Maleficarum* in 1486. The *Maleficarum* was a precise diagnostic manual for witch-hunters, and it was published specifically to implement a papal bull empowering Inquisitors 'to proceed to the just correction, imprisonment, and punishment'[3] of heretics who corrupted the Catholic faith by conversing with devils. After its publication, 'there soon followed an epidemic of Witchcraft',[4] and people manifesting the malignant signs were discovered everywhere.

In the case of modern schizophrenics, the official declaration of their imagined existence cannot be so easily dated to a single publication. Kraepelin's and Bleuler's seminal works were part of an evolving definition of pathology to which many other researchers had contributed before them. To be valuable as scientific knowledge, the belief in schizophrenia must support continuing scientific research. Continuing research keeps the details of the concept shifting as new knowledge is negotiated into existence. This movement gives rise to the illusion that progress is being made and that break-throughs in scientific comprehension are imminent.

Needless to say, critics argue that this research is necessarily founded on false assumptions. If the indicators of schizophrenia are in reality quite natural forms of human expression which are only made abnormal by cultural restrictions, nothing more can be discovered about schizophrenics beyond what is already self-apparent: that is, that they are people who do not conform with unwritten codes of behaviour. On the other hand, if the supposed signs and symptoms are truly extraordinary (such as the ones that were supposed to identify witches), they exist in the minds of the observers of schizophrenia and not in the minds of the schizophrenics. If this is the case, we are confronted with a paradox: the minds that are routinely distorting reality are those that are researching into a non-existent disease by examining and deliberately modifying minds which would otherwise be quite normal. Once again, the persecution of witches by the Inquisition is a useful analogy.

Powerful as these arguments are, it is clear that they are only partially correct. For the most part, this type of critique has been developed by dissident mental health professionals—most notably, Thomas Szasz—and it reflects the already familiar weaknesses in the knowledge base of the psychiatric profession. Although these arguments are useful for introducing the dilemma of people who are diagnosed for having social problems, they only add to the confusion surrounding the mystical experience described in previous chapters. This line of psychiatric criticism developed by Szasz and his followers certainly applies to some schizophrenics, but not to those who undergo a spiritual/mystical emergency.

The people to whom these arguments do apply have the common denominator of a serious social problem without the added difficulty of a psychological crisis. In order to explain how a social problem can be mistaken for a mental disease, it is necessary to break down this class of people into three types.

The first type can be described as the cultural outsider. Schizophrenics of this type are, by definition, different from normal people, but only marginally so. Sometimes they might be aware of their difference, and deliberately cultivate it, and sometimes they might be surprised to discover that other people perceive them as abnormal. The invention of schizophrenia, and the use of forced medical treatments, are methods of dealing with people such as these who have wandered outside culturally defined boundaries.

The second type is the scapegoat. Here the person designated as schizophrenic is himself or herself quite normal, and would otherwise be content to live within cultural boundaries, but has the misfortune of belonging to a group that is under stress. The group might be a company, a neighbourhood, or even a nation, but most frequently it is a nuclear family.

The third type is the role-player who simulates the symptoms of schizophrenia. When this activity is initiated by the patient, it might be motivated by the desire to adopt the schizophrenic role as a career. When the role-playing is initiated by the diagnostician, it might involve the maintenance of professional norms. Either way, the result can be that the person who receives the diagnosis also receives a detailed script describing how to think and behave like a schizophrenic. A person who receives this script is thenceforth compelled by social expectations to rigidly adhere to it. This scripting of the schizophrenic role by diagnosis is often referred to as 'labelling'.[5]

The Cultural-Outsider Schizophrenic

Many psychiatric survivors claim to have had nothing wrong with their minds before encountering psychiatry. They say they were originally diagnosed with schizophrenia simply for being a little different to other people, or for being different from the way others expected them to be. These claims are usually made after long struggles to escape from the coercive grip of psychiatry—often lasting many years, sometimes decades—and are impossible to verify on an individual basis. However, it is fairly easy to demonstrate that this type of claim is likely to be true simply by analysing the diagnostic criteria for schizophrenia. If the guidelines direct clinicians to include this type of person, it is fair to assume that a substantial fraction of schizophrenics will be of this type.

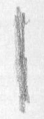

DSM-IV specifies the indicators for schizophrenia as being positive symptoms such as delusions, hallucinations, disorganised speech, and disorganised or catatonic behaviour; and/or negative symptoms such as affective flattening, alogia, and avolition.[6] These are the Criterion-A symptoms.[7] If any single 'bizarre' example of these symptoms, or any two examples if they are non-bizarre, correlate with a Criterion-B symptom—that is, a social/occupational dysfunction concerning matters such as work, interpersonal relations, or self-care—a diagnosis of schizophrenia can be made. It should be pointed out once again that there are no laboratory tests available to confirm a diagnosis, and nothing more needs to be done to make a definitive diagnosis than to follow the DSM-IV (or ICD-10)[8] guidelines.

Let us begin with delusions. In its Glossary of Technical Terms, DSM-IV describes a delusion as:

> A false belief based on incorrect inference about external reality that is firmly sustained despite what almost everyone else believes and despite what constitutes incontrovertible and obvious proof or evidence to the contrary. The belief is not one ordinarily accepted by other members of the person's culture or subculture (for example, it is not an article of religious faith).[9]

A delusion is said to have the additional pathology of 'bizarre' attached to it when it 'involves a phenomenon that the person's culture would regard as totally implausible'.[10]

Evidently there is no hard-and-fast division between bizarre and non-bizarre delusions, and what seems to differentiate a delusion from a false belief is a matter of cultural acceptance. This is a special psychiatric interpretation of the word 'delusion'. In normal lay usage a 'delusion' can be any kind of false belief, whether it is accepted by the person's culture or not.

There are two implications that can be drawn from this DSM-IV definition of delusion. Both concern the beliefs of the psychiatrists who have compiled the manual. The first is that culturally based beliefs can be false. The second is that false beliefs only become delusions, and therefore symptoms of schizophrenia, when they are culturally unacceptable.

If normal people and schizophrenics both have false beliefs, with the only difference between them being that normal peoples' beliefs are culturally acceptable and those of schizophrenics are culturally unacceptable, it is hard to avoid the conclusion that the use of delusions as a symptom can easily lead to the diagnosis of people who are simply cultural outsiders. The requirement to correlate delusions with a disturbance in social functioning (Criterion B) only strengthens this line of thinking.

The DSM-IV Glossary of Technical Terms defines a hallucination as a 'sensory perception that has the compelling sense of reality of a true perception but that occurs without external stimulation of the relevant sensory organ'.[11] But the manual warns that '[t]ransient hallucinatory experiences may occur in people without a mental disorder'. Hallucinations, in themselves, are thus not necessarily indicative of abnormality.

To be an indicator of schizophrenia, a hallucinatory experience should be beyond the range of normal experience. Certainly it should be more unusual than the common experience of a person who is distracted, or who is in a noisy environment, and imagines the voice of an accompanying person and asks, 'Did you say something?' When this happens there is usually no suspicion that it might be a symptom of mental disorder.

Exactly how different and unusual a hallucinatory experience has to be to qualify as a symptom of schizophrenia is not specified. But it is implied by the diagnostic criterion that the 'did you say something?' type of hallucination, although seemingly harmless to lay people, might be close to a schizophrenic marker. DSM-IV makes the point that some clinicians are only interested in hallucinations of external voices, and ignore those perceived as being inside the head. This clearly suggests that the 'did you say something?' kind of hallucination, being concerned with an imagined external source, is of the more serious kind.

In its diagnostic overview of schizophrenia, DSM-IV specifies that of all the types of hallucination possible, auditory hallucinations experienced as voices 'are by far the most common and characteristic of Schizophrenia'.[12] This is repeatedly confirmed in the psychiatric literature. So it seems that hearing imagined external voices is the most positive of the hallucinatory indicators for schizophrenia, even though this is a demonstrably common experience.

This lack of certainty about hallucinations means that the diagnostic emphasis has to be shifted onto the cross-referencing criterion of social/occupational dysfunction. Obviously, hallucinations by themselves might not properly distinguish a schizophrenic from a normal person. However, if a person is observed to hallucinate, and also to have a disturbance in his or her social functioning, the hallucinations might indicate schizophrenia. When the diagnostic criteria are interpreted this way, it seems that social functioning is exposed as a key determinant of schizophrenia. This gives support to the claim that sometimes schizophrenics are outsiders who have had the misfortune to wander into a diagnostic catchment-area.

The third symptom in the DSM-IV Criterion A for schizophrenia is disorganised speech. Examples given of such speech are 'derailment' or 'incoherence'. The manual makes it clear that disorganised speech is used as an indicator for an underlying disorganisation in the person's thinking, 'because in a clinical setting inferences about thought are based primarily on the individual's speech'.[13] For diagnostic purposes, the level of organisation apparent in a person's speech is assumed to represent his or her level of mental organisation as well.

However, in a further discussion about the varieties of disorganised speech to watch out for, the manual goes on to advise that, '[b]ecause mildly disorganised speech is common and nonspecific, the symptom must be severe enough to substantially impair effective communication'.[14] This means that the compilers of the manual recognise that normal people can have mildly disorganised thoughts, as is sometimes indicated by their speech, and that, in relation to this symptom, the threshold of mental illness is only crossed when a person's mind is so disorganised that the ability to communicate through speech is impaired.

But a diagnosis based on a judgement of ineffective communication combined with social/occupational dysfunction (Criterion B) seems to provide particularly strong evidence that schizophrenia can be culturally determined. A person who is diagnosed with schizophrenia in this way might lack sufficient interest in other people, or perhaps lack the social skills, to make themselves easily understood by others, and as a result have social/occupational difficulties. It is conceivable that the mental functioning of this person might otherwise be normal.

Nor does it follow that an impairment in communication necessarily indicates a short-coming in the person who is doing the speaking. In a clinical setting, the inability of the diagnostician to understand the patient should also be taken into account. The essential feature of this particular diagnostic tool is that the ability of the diagnostician to comprehend the speech of the patient is assumed to be a standard test of sanity. But this begs the question as to whether diagnosticians' minds are calibrated to make standard measurements in this regard; and, if they are, whether that standard is concerned with the measurement of mind or with cultural adaptation. If the latter is indeed the case, it offers strong support to the view of the outsider being typecast as a schizophrenic.

The fourth group of Criterion-A symptoms is 'grossly disorganised or catatonic behaviour'. The DSM-IV guidelines describe these symptoms as:

> Grossly disorganised behaviour (Criterion A4) may manifest itself in a variety of ways, ranging from childlike silliness to unpredictable agitation. Problems may be noted in any form of goal-directed behaviour, leading to difficulties in performing activities of daily living such as organising meals or maintaining hygiene. The person may appear markedly dishevelled, may dress in an unusual manner (for example, wearing multiple overcoats, scarves, and gloves on a hot day), or may display clearly inappropriate sexual behaviour (for

example, public masturbation) or unpredictable and untriggered agitation (for example, shouting or swearing).[15]

Whereas the instructions regarding the use of 'disorganised speech' specify that this symptom is only an external indicator of internal mental disorganisation, there is no similar instruction concerning 'grossly disorganised behaviour'. This means that disorganised behaviour is not meant to be read as an indicator of inner mental disorganisation. The types of disorganised behaviours listed above are merely some of the things that schizophrenics have been observed doing, and the behaviours do not directly reflect inner mental activity. This means that wearing multiple overcoats, or engaging in public masturbation, has the same kind of relationship to schizophrenia as the wearing of a hat has to baldness. Both bald and hirsute people might wear hats. But when a bald person wears one, baldness can serve as a convenient, though not necessarily correct, explanation for why the hat is worn.

Similarly, schizophrenia might serve as a convenient explanation for why a person might 'dress in an unusual manner', provided that the observer has already been informed that a person is indeed schizophrenic. But to use unusual dress as a diagnostic indicator of mental disorder seems as doubtful as assuming that any person wearing a hat is bald.

This symptom is transparently loaded with cultural bias. Even so, it is worth noting that although private masturbation is no longer considered to be either a cause or a symptom of madness, as it once was, public masturbation is clearly listed as an indicator of schizophrenia. What makes the difference here, apparently, is whether the setting of the behaviour, rather than the behaviour itself, is culturally acceptable.

Some of the examples of this symptom, such as wearing multiple overcoats in hot weather and public masturbation, only appear in the psychiatric literature as anecdotes, and have not been subjected to any kind of extensive scientific investigation. It is possible that these forms of behaviour might have more to do with homelessness than with mental disorder.

Negative Symptoms

The fifth and final group of symptoms in Criterion A are the negative symptoms such as affective flattening, alogia, and avolition. Positive symptoms are indicated by forms of deviant behavioural activity, and they are meant to disclose a commensurate level of inner mental deviance. Negative symptoms, on the other hand, are descriptions of behavioural inactivity, and are supposed to indicate a commensurate level of inner mental inactivity. If a person does not speak, or speaks as little as possible (alogia), it is assumed that there is insufficient thinking going on to generate communication.

The observed presence of both positive and negative symptoms for schizophrenia indicates that it is a mental disorder with an extraordinary variety of complications. A schizophrenic might be a person in a highly active delusional state, conversing incoherently with inner voices, wearing multiple overcoats and masturbating in public; or, alternatively, he or she could also be a person who says and feels and does, and presumably thinks, next to nothing. It is important to note at this point that the negative and positive symptoms have equal status as diagnostic criteria. This means that a person manifesting negative symptoms is not thought to be in remission, or in an inactive phase of the disease, but is at the time a full-blown schizophrenic and diagnosable.

Bearing in mind the diagnostic setting, which from the patient's point of view is a kind of interrogation session in which all power is transferred to the diagnostician,[16] it is worth considering the DSM-IV definition of alogia. This is one of the principal negative symptoms:

> **alogia** An impoverishment in thinking that is inferred from observing speech and language behaviour. There may be brief and concrete replies to questions and restrictions in the amount of

spontaneous speech (poverty of speech). Sometimes the speech is adequate in amount but conveys little information because it is overconcrete, over-abstract, repetitive, or stereotyped (poverty of content).[17]

'Concrete' is a key term, and it is used here to describe 'poverty' in both the quantity and quality of speech. In common usage, concrete means 'solid', 'firm', or 'serious'; is the opposite of 'light and airy'. In psychiatric literature, concrete is used variously to describe the opposite of metaphorical thinking and speech,[18] as well as to describe the opposite of abstract thinking and speech.[19] The inclusion of both extremes—over-concrete and over-abstract—in the above definition indicates that mentally healthy people stick to the middle ground.

Yet even though concreteness is viewed by psychiatric diagnosticians as indicative of schizophrenia in their patients, it is also viewed, strangely, as being a quality that therapists should develop in themselves for working with schizophrenics:

> The development of a therapeutic relationship is critically important in work with persons with schizophrenia (Frank & Gunderson, 1990; Lamb, 1982). Core skills of empathic attunement, warmth, genuineness, and concreteness were used to establish a supportive relationship (Anthony, 1980; Elson, 1986; Hepworth & Larsen, 1993).[20]

What can this contrariness mean? Why is concreteness associated with qualities such as 'empathic attunement, warmth, genuineness' when it is found in the therapists of schizophrenics, and with a pathological impoverishment of thinking when it is found in the schizophrenics themselves? Can there be anything wrong with concreteness if it is actually recommended as a therapeutic tool? Or, does a therapist who deliberately develops concreteness in speech for therapeutic purposes also run the risk of being diagnosed with schizophrenia?

Perhaps it could be seen as a demonstration of over-concrete thinking to question, in this way, the words used to describe schizophrenic symptoms. But it should be remembered that I am discussing a class of people who are diagnosed when their minds are functioning normally. They become schizophrenics simply because they can be fitted to the symptoms. For them, there is nothing more to schizophrenia than the supposed symptoms themselves. This means that the words which describe the symptoms are all-important, because from this perspective it is only a linguistic consensus amongst psychiatrists that brings this class of schizophrenics into existence.

Quite frequently, people are involuntary participants in the clinical procedures that lead to a diagnosis of schizophrenia. Psychiatrists are looked upon as interrogators who have been retained by a third party to ask probing questions about the person's private thoughts and beliefs, for the transparent purpose of acquiring damaging evidence. Under these circumstances, it might not be surprising if a perceptive and wary person seems concrete in their responses, and gives other evidence of DSM-IV negative symptoms such as 'brief, laconic, empty replies'.[21] In fact, when a diagnosis of schizophrenia is viewed as a label for a cultural outsider, the specification of negative symptoms such as these appear to create a 'Catch-22': anything that people say about themselves can be used against them; and if nothing of substance is said, that can be used, too.

Avolition is another of the negative symptoms:

> **avolition** An inability to initiate and persist in goal-directed activities. When severe enough to be considered pathological, avolition is pervasive and prevents the person from completing many different types of activities (for example, work, intellectual pursuits, self care).[22]

Consider a person who does not share with other people an appropriate level of culturally acquired goal-direction for specific activities such as formal education and career. This kind of person is often referred to as a 'loser', a 'drop-out', a 'bum', a 'hopeless case', or a 'never-do-well'. The specification of avolition as a symptom makes it apparent that 'schizophrenic' can also be added to this list of pejoratives.

In discussing the negative symptoms, DSM-IV warns: 'Although quite ubiquitous in Schizophrenia, negative symptoms are difficult to evaluate because they occur on a continuum with normality'. But this 'continuum with normality' is exactly what the outsider-as-schizophrenic case argues. Alogia might be no more than a disinclination for conversation, in situations where such a disinclination is culturally unacceptable. Similarly, avolition might be no more than a disinclination to participate in normal social intercourse. If these disinclinations are indeed on a continuum with normality, then—in relation to the negative symptoms at least—the outsider-as-schizophrenic case is very strong.

Criterion B is the second group of diagnostic indicators that are concerned with social or occupational dysfunction in the areas of interpersonal relations, work or education, or self-care. If Criterion-A symptoms have been identified, the diagnostician cross-checks to see whether there is any evidence of social or occupational dysfunction:

> Typically, functioning is clearly below that which had been achieved before the onset of symptoms. If the disturbance begins in childhood or adolescence, however, there may be failure to achieve what would have been expected for the individual rather than a deterioration in functioning. Comparing the individual with unaffected siblings may be helpful in making this determination. Educational progress is frequently disrupted, and the individual may be unable to finish school. Many individuals are unable to hold a job for sustained periods of time and are employed at a lower level than their parents ('downward drift'). The majority (60%–70%) of individuals with schizophrenia do not marry, and most have relatively limited social contacts.[23]

There seems to be some overlap here with avolition. A loss of interest in activities of social value, or a loss of interest in climbing the ladder of social status, or even failure to satisfy the status expectations of others, are all deemed to be indications of mental pathology. Ostensibly, Criterion-B indicators are primarily used as a cross-reference to evaluate the level of disability a person incurs from the presence of one or more Criterion-A symptoms. Unemployment, for instance, is only meant to be significant as a measure of the detrimental effect of a Criteria-A symptom such as delusions.

However, although Criterion-B indicators are supposedly only intended to give secondary confirmation of pathology, references can be found in the literature of mental health professionals arguing that '[i]mpairment in the ability to work is a defining characteristic of schizophrenia'.[24] Thomas Szasz has written emphatically about the way unemployment in young people can lead directly to a diagnosis of schizophrenia.[25]

It is quite apparent that people can be diagnosed, even though their thinking and behaviour might be on a continuum with that of normal people, simply because a psychiatrist observes personal attributes that are outside the boundary of cultural acceptance. There are numerous case studies in the literature of psychiatric survivors that confirm this contention. A particularly compelling story is told by Leonard Roy Frank. Frank is the author of a number of articles and books that argue against psychiatric coercion.

Frank recounts how he began a promising career in real estate sales in Florida and San Francisco. At a certain point, however, he decided to quit his job and take some time off to read books and follow an interest in philosophy. When his parents heard about his new life-style they went to visit him and, dismayed at his lack of interest in continuing his career in real estate, advised him to see a psychiatrist. When he refused, they signed the necessary papers to have him involuntarily committed to a mental hospital. He was diagnosed with paranoid schizophrenia and given 85 shock treatments. When he finally obtained his psychiatric records, twelve years later, he discovered that the symptoms which had been identified to justify his diagnosis and treatment included: 'not working, withdrawal, growing a beard, becoming a vegetarian, "bizarre behaviour", "negativism", "strong beliefs", "piercing eyes", and "religious preoccupations". The medical examiner's initial report said that I was living the "life of a beatnik—to a certain extent".'[26]

The Scapegoat Schizophrenic

Another way that a person can be diagnosed with schizophrenia is through belonging to an over-stressed group and being chosen as the group's scapegoat. Groups often focus negatively on individual members as a method of relieving stress. Indeed, psychotherapists routinely have to deal with the problem of schizophrenics being scapegoated by psychotherapy groups:

> the schizophrenic being the prime candidate in the group for the role of the scapegoat ... other members can deny their fears of intimacy and project them on to the scapegoat. The scapegoat acts as a safety valve that protects the group from the imagined dangers of closeness. Shifting attention away from the scapegoat can reduce his or her anxiety.[27]

The diagnostic criteria discussed in the previous section are largely irrelevant for understanding the scapegoat as a schizophrenic. Any alleged distinguishing indicators, such as delusions and hallucinations, are only artefacts of imagination manufactured by other members of the over-stressed group and/or the diagnostician.

The group from which the scapegoat schizophrenic has come before a diagnosis is made is most commonly a nuclear family; but other groups and organisations sometimes need scapegoats, too. Special conditions of collective stress are necessary to produce this type of schizophrenic, because 'the scapegoat selector—whether inquisitor or psychiatrist—does not work in a social vacuum. The persecution of a minority group is not imposed on a resistant population, but, on the contrary, grows out of bitter social conflicts.'[28]

In *The Manufacture of Madness*, Thomas Szasz undertakes the definitive analysis of the scapegoat as a schizophrenic. Psychiatric historians normally assert that witches who fell victim to the Inquisition were mentally ill people who were victimised on account of their mental illness. Szasz turns this conventional historical understanding on its head. He asserts that modern people diagnosed with mental illness are made scapegoats, in the same way as witches were in earlier times, by falsely labelling them with an imaginary form of deviance:

> the basic function of the medical theory of witchcraft—and, in my opinion, its basic immorality as well—lies in distracting from the persecutory practices of the institutional psychiatrists, and focussing it instead on the alleged disorders of the institutionalised mental patients.[29]

Szasz argues that the tendency for humans to be social and to always live in groups has a strong influence on shaping human nature. Membership of a group has a price: sometimes members are required to attack non-members as a means of further integrating themselves into the group, and also as a way of adding cohesion to the group itself. Group dynamics can also require that a member be selected for conversion into a non-member for the purpose of being sacrificed. When this happens, any members who do not participate in the scapegoating might themselves risk alienation and sacrifice.

The explanation for why this happens concerns the need for self-validation. By declaring an enemy, either internal or external, as invalid, and therefore bad, a person by implication declares himself or herself to be valid and good: 'Typically, we confirm our loyalty to our group by asserting the disloyalty of others (in or outside the group) to it; we thus purchase membership in the community by excluding others from it.'[30]

Contemporary people have acquired a habit of attributing subhuman status to classes of people who are selected for scapegoating. This attitude was applied to witches during the Inquisition and to Jews in Nazi Germany, and regularly happens to people who are ethnically or religiously affiliated with the enemy in times of war. Similarly, when family groups find the need to sacrifice a member, a convenient modern method is to declare that the person has a dysfunctional brain.

People who have been declared schizophrenics are usually the ones to supply a description of having been scapegoated into the role. Indeed, the dynamics of selecting and casting-out a scapegoat usually means that only victims of the group or outsiders are in a position to consciously observe the process. Of a number of such victim accounts, a particularly lucid story is told by John Modrow in *How To Become A Schizophrenic*.[31] Modrow recounts growing up in a family riddled with stress fractures inherited from previous generations. His mother was the daughter of Norwegian immigrants to the United States who, after her father died, had been forced to play the role of surrogate mother to her siblings while her own mother worked sixteen hours a day.

On Modrow's father's side of the family, his great-grandmother had died in an insane asylum, providing grounds for whispered expectations of a family curse that would surface once again. A story told to Modrow by his sister, who in turn had heard it from his mother shortly before she died, is critical to his story of selection as the family scapegoat. When he was very young, his mother and paternal grandmother were chatting in the kitchen while he was sitting outside in the sun, rocking back and forth, absorbed in thought. His mother, seeing him through the door, and thinking he looked cute, smiled and drew her mother-in-law's attention to him. The mother-in-law, however, misunderstood her meaning and angrily jumped to the defence of the child, accusing Modrow's mother of mocking him. The result, deduced by Modrow as an adult, was a life-long accusation levelled at Modrow by his mother that he would never let her love him.

After this incident, when Modrow was six, his mother decided that he was in need of a psychiatric examination. There was apparently a minor incident involving Modrow and a man in a wheelchair which triggered this unusual course of action, but the first psychiatrist was so unconcerned about it that he declined to make the examination. Six weeks later, Modrow's mother took him to be examined by a psychiatric team at the University of Washington. According to his mother, the psychiatrists told her: 'We don't know exactly what is wrong with your son, but whatever it is, it is very serious. We recommend that you have him committed immediately or else he will be completely psychotic within less than a year'.[32]

His mother did not follow the advice at the time, but the assumption that Modrow had a serious mental illness became incorporated into his family identity. Although by his own estimation there was nothing wrong with him, he was by degrees schooled into playing the role of the mad member of the family. Modrow's description is of a family with unusual levels of stress, and his supposed difference within this group allowed the other members of the family to contrast themselves with him and thereby assume normal roles. In this way, the family maintained outward signs of normality until Modrow was finally hospitalised for schizophrenia as an adolescent.

His stay in hospital was only brief, but it took him another three decades of introspection and family analysis to properly understand what had happened to him. Modrow says he wrote his book because he believes 'it is a fact beyond reasonable dispute that I had been victimised by a series of events—not by a disease. And I believe this can be demonstrated to be true of all people who have been labelled schizophrenic.'[33]

Families are not the only groups in need of scapegoats. Workplaces sometimes need them, too. For instance, there is a consistent pattern of scapegoating whistleblowers, who are usually somewhat out of the ordinary in that they are likely to have elevated levels of personal integrity and courage, combined with a naive faith in the prevalence of justice. If an organisation chooses to ignore a whistleblower's complaint, this combination of personality traits can easily lead the whistleblower into a situation of doggedly repeating assertions that something is wrong in the organisation. The whistleblower is then perfectly positioned to become a scapegoat for the organisation, to relieve the stress that might have been generated by the attempted revelation.

Employers commonly react by requiring a psychiatric examination of the whistleblower as a condition of continued employment, which often results in a diagnosis of mental illness.[34] This practice has even been documented in a recently released report by Australia's ombudsman's office. An investigation into the harassment of whistleblowers in the Australian Federal Police (AFP) found 'four relevant instances since 1992 where the AFP has arranged for officers to undergo inappropriate psychiatric assessments, either under duress, or without their knowledge or consent'.[35]

The support group Whistleblowers Australia is conducting a continuing survey of its members to discover how many have been treated in this way. It has found that many of them have received psychiatric diagnoses, ranging from non-specific conditions such as cognitive dysfunction to personality disorders and schizophrenia.[36]

At least one member of Whistleblowers Australia has lodged a complaint about her harassment with the World Psychiatric Association's Committee to Review the Abuse of Psychiatry. Shortly after receiving acknowledgment of the complaint from the secretary of the committee in Denmark, the complainant was asked to attend another psychiatric examination. The subsequent examination, presumably conducted under quality-control pressure from the peak body of the psychiatric profession, found she was in perfect mental health.

Schizophrenia as Role-Play

Social problems may be mistaken for mental illness when patterns of schizophrenic thought and behaviour are simulated. This can happen when the schizophrenic role is either deliberately chosen by the schizophrenic or imposed by other people. Analysts who argue that such roles are normally chosen by the schizophrenics themselves are inclined to see schizophrenics as predatory, exploitative types of people.[37] Conversely, those who prefer to see the schizophrenic role as an imposition tend to argue that schizophrenics are victims of labelling who, once diagnosed, are compelled by other people's expectations to behave in the prescribed manner of a schizophrenic.[38]

The evolution of Thomas Szasz's myth-of-mental-illness views has involved a passage through both the cultural-outsider-as-schizophrenic and the scapegoat-as-schizophrenic types. But more recently his attachment to libertarian philosophy has moved him into the schizophrenia-as-role-play camp. He shows a distinct lack of sympathy for people who willingly adopt the role of schizophrenic. In a recent article, descriptively entitled *Idleness and Lawlessness in the Therapeutic State*, he refers to schizophrenics as parasites. After establishing that modern society is divided between producers and parasites, he goes on to argue that people with 'real' illnesses who adopt the sick role are not idle and therefore not parasites. However, 'in contrast, most chronic mental patients—especially schizophrenics—are idle, economically dependent, and inclined (allegedly because of their illness) to lawlessness'.[39]

Szasz's view is that failure to make the necessary transitions in the process of maturation, from childhood through adolescence to adulthood, is what determines whether a person will become identified as a schizophrenic. If a person successfully passes through the first two stages, and establishes an adult identity by 'being useful to other people'[40]—that is, by having a productive occupation—the society will accept the person as being in mental health.

But '[i]f this process of maturation goes awry, the adolescent begins to envy his peers and to feel inferior to them'.[41] When this happens, the person might, in order to compensate, intentionally develop notions of self-importance, and perhaps begin to express unusual beliefs and mannerisms as marks of assumed distinction. According to Szasz, as such a person slides further away from a normal productive adult identity, family members, teachers, and friends tend to indulge the person and offer more leeway. The process of differentiation continues until the person gives some suggestion of potential violence. At this point, the person is likely to be brought into contact with a psychiatrist, who will give a diagnosis of schizophrenia. Henceforth the well-known symptoms of schizophrenia provide an easily followed identity-script to guide the person in his or her future career as a schizophrenic.

The assumption is that a person with parasitic tendencies will sometimes simulate schizophrenic symptoms as a way to gain access to the perquisites of mental patient-hood. These supposed perks include additional family attention, social welfare payments, and the right to be idle. This perception of exploitation is now so widespread that Szasz's myth-of-mental-illness arguments have even been raised by United States' policy analysts concerned about the growing welfare burden on taxpayers.[42]

Szasz's point of view is also shared by a significant proportion of the business community. Recent research has found that one-third of middle and senior-level business managers in Sydney and Melbourne believe that 'mental illnesses such as schizophrenia and manic depression are myths dreamed up by lazy workers' as excuses 'used to escape work or gain personal rewards'.[43]

The simulation of madness for personal advantage or disguise is not a new idea. It must have been well understood in late-sixteenth-century England, for instance, because characters in a number of Shakespeare's plays feign madness in order to disguise either their identities or their intentions. Hamlet feigns madness to put his enemies off guard. In *King Lear*, Edgar adopts the persona of the madman, Poor Tom. When he fears for his life, he flees into the countryside. But before he goes he tells the audience about the disguise he will adopt to avoid detection—and also to help him earn a living:

> My face I'll grime with filth,
> Blanket my loins, elf all my hair in knots,

> And with the presented nakedness outface
> The winds and persecutions of the sky.
> The country gives me proof and precedent
> Of Bedlam beggars, who with roaring voices,
> Strike in their numb'd and mortified bare arms
> Pins, wooden pricks, nails, sprigs of rosemary;
> And with this horrible object, from low farms,
> Poor pelting villages, sheep-cotes, and mills,
> Sometime with lunatic bans, sometime with prayers,
> Enforce their charity. Poor Turlygood! poor Tom!
> That's something yet: Edgar I nothing am.[44]

Curiously, DSM-IV now has a diagnostic label for people who fabricate madness in the way that Edgar does. In fact, there are two different disorders to choose from. If Edgar were detected in the act of feigning madness by a modern psychiatrist, he might be diagnosed with 'Malingering'—but only if the diagnostician thought that 'enforcement of charity' was Edgar's motivation. Malingering is used to describe a person who is perceived to intentionally produce false or exaggerated psychological or physical symptoms because he or she is 'motivated by external incentives such as avoiding military duty, avoiding work, obtaining financial compensation, evading criminal prosecution, or obtaining drugs'.[45]

The alternative diagnosis for feigners of madness is 'Factitious Disorder—With Predominantly Psychological Signs and Symptoms'. This label is used when there is the same intentional feigning 'of psychological (often psychotic) symptoms that are suggestive of a mental disorder' and 'the motivation for the behaviour is to assume the sick role'.[46] But unlike Malingering, people with Factitious Disorder are not motivated by external incentives such as economic gain. Factitious Disorder is also known as Munchausen Syndrome.[47]

The existence of these disease categories in DSM-IV confirms the claim that schizophrenia can be simulated, and is therefore sometimes a psychiatric myth. But it also reveals a somewhat bizarre divergence of opinion between medical psychiatry and the psychiatric-myth school. What DSM-IV is claiming is that mentally healthy people who pretend to be mentally ill are, by virtue of their pretence, mentally ill. Psychiatrists believe that the pretence is itself a form of mental illness. This sort of twisted logic offers a free kick to the myth-of-mental-illness sceptics.

The paradoxical situation that arises from the medicalisation of play-acting is further compounded by the inclusion of a variant of Factitious Disorder, called Factitious Disorder By Proxy (FDBP), in an appendix of DSM-IV.[48] FDBP is one of a number of mental disorders that are already recognised by large sections of the psychiatric profession, but which have yet to achieve consensual endorsement. In DSM-IV's Appendix B, descriptions are given of these disorders, and further research into them is recommended. The essential feature of FDBP

> is the deliberate production of physical or psychological signs or symptoms in another person who is under the individual's care ... The motivation for the perpetrator's behaviour is presumed to be a psychological need to assume the sick role by proxy ... The perpetrator induces or simulates the illness or disease process in the victim and then presents the victim for medical care while disclaiming any knowledge of the actual etiology of the problem.[49]

To a psychiatric sceptic, FDBP might appear at first glance to provide the simplest of all explanations for the cause of schizophrenia. That is, schizophrenic symptoms are fabricated by relatives and psychiatrists who are suffering from FDBP, and who are adopting the sick role by proxy. However, FDBP presents sceptics of the myth-of-mental-illness school with a conundrum: if all mental illness is a myth, so is FDBP.

But even if Malingering and the Factitious Disorders present problems of usage by the psychiatric-myth school, their inclusion in DSM-IV confirms that mainstream psychiatry recognises that schizophrenia is sometimes only role-playing. The problem is that nobody seems to know how many schizophrenics are either role-playing themselves, or are the victims of role-playing by relatives and psychiatrists.

Tests have shown fairly conclusively that people without a diagnosis of schizophrenia can fabricate the symptoms on request so well that psychiatrists are willing to diagnose them with schizophrenia. The authors of one of these studies concluded that all that is required for normal people to successfully simulate schizophrenia is that they have some prior knowledge of the symptoms.[50] Another survey found that when normal people were coached in the methods of detecting schizophrenic simulation one-third of them could feign schizophrenia without detection.[51]

However, an accurate knowledge of either the symptoms of schizophrenia or methods for detecting simulators might not be necessary for pretenders in real-life situations outside the laboratory. The much-cited Rosenhan experiment found that a high level of accuracy is not required in the simulation of symptoms, and that practising mental health professionals are unlikely to expose pretenders.[52]

In an experiment conducted in the early 1970s, David Rosenhan enlisted eight volunteers to act as pseudo-patients. Over a period of time, the pseudo-patients presented themselves at twelve psychiatric hospitals and complained of hearing voices saying the words 'empty', 'hollow', and 'thud'. These words had been chosen because their existential connotations suggested the emptiness of life and because they had never appeared in psychiatric literature as being symptoms of mental illness.

No other symptoms were fabricated. On each occasion, the pseudo-patients were admitted to the hospitals, and on all but one occasion they were diagnosed as having schizophrenia. After the initial interview the volunteers did not mention the voices again, and acted their normal sane selves. The agreement they had made with the co-ordinator of the experiment was that they would each have to gain their own release without any outside assistance. This had to be done by convincing the hospital staff that they were sane.

The length of hospitalisation ranged from seven to 52 days, with an average of nineteen days. All those originally diagnosed as having schizophrenia were released with the diagnosis of 'schizophrenia in remission'.

One conclusion made by the co-ordinator of the experiment was that, '[p]sychiatric diagnoses ... are in the minds of the observers and are not valid summaries of the characteristics displayed by the observed'.[53] Rosenhan's principal contention was that mental hospitals could not tell the sane from the insane.

Rosenhan was a psychologist, and when his study was first published in the journal *Science* there was widespread protest from psychiatrists. The next issue of the journal contained fifteen letters in response, only one of which was favourable. When a symposium discussing his experiment was subsequently published in the *Journal of Abnormal Psychology*, all of the five psychologists who contributed articles were critical of Rosenhan.[54]

Most of the criticism concerned either the ethics or the methodology of the experiment. The ethical problems mostly focussed on the deliberate intent to deceive hospital staff that was inherent in the design of the experiment. Only one commentator, Thomas Scheff, writing at a later date, seems to have raised a further ethical question concerning the considerable risks that were taken by the pseudo-patients in subjecting themselves to an average nineteen days' incarceration and psychiatric treatments.[55]

One of the major criticisms of Rosenhan's methodology was the lack of controls. Indeed, one of the contributors to the symposium argued that the experiment was of little value because no controls had been used. It was proposed that, had there been a control group that was unaware of the purpose of the experiment, its members might have tried a lot harder to get out of hospital than did Rosenhan's pseudo-patients.[56]

Despite these criticisms, Rosenhan's findings still had a considerable impact on the psychiatric profession in the United States by temporarily undermining confidence in the validity of psychiatric diagnoses. Kirk and Kutchins relate how Rosenhan's work particularly affected Robert Spitzer, who was one of the principal architects of the DSM revision that became DSM-III: 'He obviously took Rosenhan's work very seriously; it constituted a frontal assault on psychiatric diagnosis.'[57]

Spitzer challenged Rosenhan in an article entitled 'On pseudoscience in science, logic in remission, and psychiatric diagnosis: a critique of Rosenhan's "On being sane in insane places"'. In this article, Spitzer offered the simplistic argument that, 'A correct interpretation of [Rosenhan's] own data contradicts his own conclusions. In the setting of a psychiatric hospital psychiatrists are remarkably able to distinguish the "sane" from the "insane"'. Spitzer argued that being released from hospital with 'schizophrenia in remission' was tantamount to being found sane.[58]

Although Spitzer claimed a successful refutation, Rosenhan's study is still 'often discussed in introductory college courses in psychology and sociology'[59] to illustrate problems with psychiatric diagnosis. It has also been recommended in legal literature for use as a courtroom reference to refute the certainty of psychiatric assessments: 'Plaintiffs' experts should be asked to admit that psychiatrists can be fooled and that malingering is difficult to detect. In this connection, defence counsel should use the famous Rosenhan study'.[60] Despite many criticisms, Rosenhan's experiment has survived as a landmark demonstration of how easy it is to simulate symptoms that lead to a diagnosis of schizophrenia.

Another elaborate experiment has demonstrated the converse of Rosenhan's findings. That is, in order to comply with falsely conceived professional standards, psychiatric and psychological diagnosticians sometimes imagine the symptoms of mental illness in people who are behaving normally. Maurice Temerlin of the University of Okalahoma demonstrated this when he presented a man in perfect mental health for diagnosis by various groups of psychiatrists, psychologists, and psychology students. Before these diagnosticians were allowed to observe the man, they were supplied with a fabricated suggestion by an expert in the field that the man was mentally disordered.[61]

To set up his experiment, Temerlin had a professional actor trained to portray a mentally healthy man:

> he was happy and effective in his work; he established a warm, gracious and satisfying relationship with the interviewer; he was self-confident and secure, but without being arrogant, competitive, or grandiose. He was identified with the parent of the same sex, was happily married and in love with his wife, and consistently enjoyed sexual intercourse. He felt that sex was fun, unrelated to anxiety, social-role conflict, or status striving. This was built into his role because mental patients allegedly are sexually anhedonic.[62]

The actor's role also required him to be agnostic and uninterested in extrasensory perception or occult phenomena. This was to avoid subjects often associated with schizophrenia. He also had a gentle, self-mocking sense of humour to combat the normal perception that mental patients are humourless people who have no insight into themselves. The actor's script required him to deny that he had ever experienced hallucinations, delusions, or any other phenomena associated with psychosis.

To cap it off, a happy childhood was created for him, together with mild anxieties about current political affairs, in order to demonstrate social concern and the absence of self-obsession. His domestic life was happy, punctuated only by occasional disagreements with his wife about church-going and infrequent musings about whether he was raising his children correctly.

The experiment required a recording to be made of Temerlin interviewing the actor as if he were a prospective patient. In order to account for the clinical setting, so that sickness would not automatically be assumed by the audience, the script described the actor as 'a successful and productive physical scientist and mathematician (a profession as far away from psychiatry as possible) who had read a book on psychotherapy and wanted to talk about it'.[63]

The actor himself was not told the purpose of the experiment.

After the recording was made, three clinical psychologists evaluated the interview to ensure that the actor had indeed portrayed a man in perfect mental health. Temerlin then recruited 25 practising psychologists, 25 psychiatrists, and 45 graduate students enrolled in doctoral programmes in clinical psychology.

The purpose of the experiment was to test whether diagnosticians could be influenced in their clinical judgement by a false statement given by a 'prestige confederate'. Before the psychologists and psychology students heard the interview, they were told by a well-known psychologist who had gained many professional honours that the patient on the taped interview they were about to listen to was 'a very interesting man because he looks neurotic, but actually is quite psychotic'. Similarly, the 25 psychiatrists were told that 'two board-certified psychiatrists, one also a psychoanalyst, had found the recording interesting because the patient looked neurotic but actually was quite psychotic'.[64]

Control groups were also tested. One control group was asked to diagnose the actor without any prior prestige suggestion at all. Another group made diagnoses after hearing a prestige suggestion that the actor was mentally healthy. The results were quite extraordinary. As can be seen in the following table, the psychiatrists were particularly vulnerable to being misled by the 'prestige suggestion'.

Diagnosing by suggestion

	Psychosis	Neurosis	Mental Health
Professional & student groups			
Psychiatrists (25)	15	10	0
Clinical Psychologists (25)	7	15	3
Psychology Students (45)	5	35	5
Control groups			
No prestige suggestion (21)	0	9	12
Suggestion of mental health (20)	0	0	20

Adapted from: Maurice K. Temerlin, 'Suggestion Effects in Psychiatric Diagnosis', in Thomas J. Scheff, *Labelling Madness*, Prentice-Hall, Englewood Cliffs N.J., 1975, p. 50.

Schizophrenia was the most common form of psychosis diagnosed, and the results in many ways speak for themselves. After analysing the data, Temerlin concluded that professional identity was the relevant variable and that there was no relationship in diagnostic outcomes with either length of training or experience. What is apparent is that the psychiatrists in particular were inclined to adopt a professional role-play after the appropriate script was supplied to them by a prestige confederate whose opinion could be assumed to represent professional standards.

In attempting to explain why the psychiatrists were more easily led into diagnosing a healthy person as psychotic, Temerlin observed that: 'Psychiatrists are, first and foremost, physicians. It is characteristic of physicians in diagnostically uncertain situations to follow the implicit rule "when in doubt, diagnose illness", because it is a less dangerous error than diagnosing health when illness is in fact present.' This point was punctuated by a statement from one psychiatrist who, after learning about his error, defended a diagnosis of psychosis by arguing: 'Of course he looked healthy, but hell, most people are a little neurotic, and who can accept appearance at face value anyway?'[65]

There is scope to speculate about the role of patient fees in this apparent willingness by psychiatrists to diagnose mental illness in healthy people. DSM-IV identifies Malingering as a diagnosis for use when patients fabricate symptoms for personal gain. But, unlike Factitious Disorder, the manual does not supply a proxy complement of Malingering that could be used when mental health professionals fabricate symptoms for their personal gain. It is not surprising that Malingering By Proxy fails to even make it into Appendix B, as an area recommended for further research. But this omission leaves the way open for cynics to argue that the compilers of DSM-IV might have insufficient insight into the real cause of at least some cases of supposed schizophrenia.

There is little likelihood a method can be developed that will eliminate role-playing as a factor in schizophrenia. Most mental diseases share the same conceptual weakness of not having laboratory tests to confirm diagnoses. With schizophrenia, this problem is compounded. As presently conceived, schizophrenia is a condition in which the mind plays tricks on itself. This means that once a person is diagnosed, and becomes known as a 'schizophrenic', psychiatrists and relatives expect the person to make improbable claims about mental functions. An attempted confession of role-playing, or a claim to have been a victim of other peoples' role-playing, simply provides evidence that a person lacks insight into his or her diseased mental state. This means that once a diagnosis has been given on the basis of role-playing it is unlikely to be overturned. As Rosenhan's pseudo-patients found, a verdict of 'schizophrenia in remission' is the best that can be expected.

A notable exception is the New Zealand writer Janet Frame. Frame has given a detailed account in her autobiography of how she came to be diagnosed with schizophrenia and incarcerated in the back ward of a mental hospital. It seems that, as a painfully shy young woman, she became infatuated with a former psychology lecturer who had taken an interest in what he called her 'loneliness of the inner soul'.

To attract, and maintain, the attention of the young psychologist, Frame simulated the symptoms of schizophrenia:

> I built up a formidable schizophrenic repertoire: I'd lie on the couch while the young handsome John Forrest, glistening with newly-applied Freud, took note of what I said and did, and suddenly I'd put on a glazed look in my eye, as if I were in a dream, and begin to relate a fantasy as if I experienced it as a reality. I'd describe it in detail while John Forrest listened, impressed, serious. Usually I incorporated in the fantasy details of my reading on schizophrenia.[66]

The unexpected penalty for this 'game, half in earnest, to win the attention of a likeable young man',[67] was involuntary commitment for eight years in an infamous mental hospital. Here she received more than 200 electro-shock treatments, and was on a short list for psychosurgery, when a book she had written many years before unexpectedly won a major literary prize. This amazing stroke of good fortune allowed a new hospital psychiatrist to accept 'me as I appeared to him and not as he learned about me from my "history" or reports of me'.[68] As a result she was rapidly rehabilitated and released. But her subsequent confession of role-playing as being the original cause of her troubles is probably only credible because she is now regarded as New Zealand's best-known living author. Without a prominent post-schizophrenia career to demonstrate her sanity, it is unlikely that Janet Frame's version of events would be believable.

8

Punishing the Patient:
human rights and psychiatric coercion

When psychiatrists diagnose people with schizophrenia they are not usually interested in making distinctions between types of schizophrenics along the lines discussed in this book. Most schizophrenics, therefore, are treated in much the same way after diagnosis. They are usually hospitalised for observation, and treated with neuroleptic drugs. If the diagnosed person disagrees with this procedure, legal sanctions are invoked and it is conducted by force. The person is usually held in this captive situation until a demonstration of 'insight' is made. This is an acknowledgment by the patient that the diagnosis is correct and that a mental disease is indeed present. The patient is also expected to demonstrate a willingness to continue drug treatment after release from hospital.

The seemingly unreasonable treatment of people diagnosed with schizophrenia can only be partly explained by the psychiatric belief in an underlying disease. It takes an understanding of the stressful conditions imposed on psychiatrists by the existence of the insanity plea to complete the explanation.

Background to the Insanity Plea

There is a long-standing tradition in most legal systems that allows two kinds of excuses to be used as a justification for breaking the law. The first is the argument that the illegal act was committed in ignorance: for example, someone who had shot another person might claim it was an accident because he or she didn't know the gun was loaded; or one person might admit to poisoning another after cooking a meal, and claim that he or she didn't know that rat poison was kept in the jar marked 'food colouring'. The excusing of children from legal culpability is derived from this area, and when a child is found to have committed a serious offence it is assumed that he or she didn't know any better.

The second kind of excuse occurs when the perpetrator can claim that he or she was compelled to act in a particular way. Self-defence and extreme provocation come into this category. Acts committed under duress, as well as behaviour that is motivated by extremes of emotion, might also be excused on the grounds of compulsion.

There is a long history of excusing people who are deemed to be insane at the time of their having committed a crime, on one or the other, or both, of these grounds. Roman law of the later Empire period excused insane people because an analogy was drawn between them and children. Ancient Hebraic law 'recognised that deaf-mutes, idiots and minors were not responsible for their actions' and '[a]ncient Mohammedan law applied punishment only to individuals who have attained their majority, and who are in full possession of their faculties'.[1]

In modern times, countries with legal systems derived from British law have developed a test for insanity which excuses legal culpability when the person, at the time of committing the crime, is believed to be unaware of the difference between good and evil. The legal precedent which established this test is known as the M'Naghten case.[2]

In England in 1843, Daniel M'Naghten assassinated Edward Drummond, the private secretary of the prime minister. M'Naghten claimed to believe that a number of people, including the prime minister, were persecuting him in various ways. At his trial M'Naghten successfully defended his actions on the grounds of insanity; but after the trial many people still believed he might have been feigning his madness. As a result, the judges in the case were asked to appear before the House of Lords to explain the test of insanity that they had applied to M'Naghten. The answer that they supplied has since become the basis for a test of criminal insanity:

> To establish a defence on the grounds of insanity, it must be conclusively proved that, at the time of the committing of the act, the party accused was labouring under such a defect of reason, from the disease of the mind, as not to know the nature and quality of the act he was doing; or if he did know it, that he did not know what he was doing was wrong. (*Regina v. M'Naghten*, 10 Clark and F. 200, 8 Eng. Rep. 718 (1843)).[3]

The so-called M'Naghten test soon became established in English-speaking countries as the principal test of legal insanity, but it also came under persistent criticism because it was thought to be too narrow in its definition. This was because it only covered the traditional defence of ignorance. It did not provide a defence for a person who was aware of the nature of his or her act and, aware that it was wrong, was nevertheless compelled by mad impulses to act in ways that were contrary to the law.

In the United States, this controversy finally produced a definition by the American Law Institute that incorporated both defences:

> a person is not responsible for criminal conduct if at the time of such conduct as a result of mental disease or defect he lacks substantial capacity either to appreciate the criminality of his conduct or to conform his conduct to the requirements of the law.[4]

A more recent trend is to define 'mental illness' in mental health legislation so that the interpretation of the condition is a legal matter as well as a medical matter. The terminology of criminal insanity is replaced with 'mental illness'. A person who at the time an offence was committed is deemed to have been mentally ill, according to the legal definition of mental illness, is thus not to be held responsible for criminal acts.

Under most pieces of modern mental health legislation, a medical practitioner who encounters a person manifesting positive symptoms of schizophrenia, and who believes him or her to be dangerous, disruptive, or likely to deteriorate, is legally authorised to have the person incarcerated in a mental hospital. This is where the existence of the insanity plea is important as a background motivator for the medical impositions that are placed on the patient.

Ostensibly, the doctor is free to choose to have the person incarcerated or not, according to the best interests of the patient. But in many respects a doctor involved in psychiatric matters is simply an agent of social control. As such, the doctor is required to consider the social and legal consequences of allowing the person with schizophrenic symptoms to remain free. Having diagnosed the person as schizophrenic, and therefore as being mentally ill in a legal sense, the doctor has in effect provided the person with a legal excuse to get away with murder, or any other crime, in the future.

From the criminal justice perspective, therefore, the production of a diagnosis of serious mental illness without a subsequent imposition of control has to be seen as a sign of professional irresponsibility. The precautionary control of people who could possibly invoke an insanity plea is a necessary social-control task that goes with the job of being a doctor.

A recent case in the United States is a good illustration of this principle in action. On 10 October 1998 the *New York Times* published an amazing-but-true front-page story under the headline: 'Killer Sues His Therapist and Wins $500,000'.[5]

Wendell Williamson was a law student at the University of North Carolina. After he disrupted a class by claiming that he had telepathic powers, he was directed to attend a consultation with Myron B. Liptzin, the head of student psychiatric services. Liptzin diagnosed Williamson with delusional disorder grandiose, and prescribed neuroleptic medication. After eight consultations, Liptzin informed Williamson that, since he was soon to retire, Williamson should find another psychiatrist. Williamson did not follow Liptzin's advice, and instead of finding another psychiatrist simply stopped taking his medication.

Eight months after his last contact with Liptzin, Williamson shot and killed two men in the street without provocation. He was diagnosed with paranoid schizophrenia, and at his trial was found not guilty on the grounds of insanity. At a subsequent trial he was awarded $500,000 in damages against Liptzin, his former psychiatrist. The jury believed that Liptzin had not correctly perceived the seriousness of Williamson's disorder, and had not imposed the necessary control measures. A newspaper report said Williamson claimed that:

> the verdict in the civil case showed that he and the people he killed were all victims of Dr. Liptzin's failure. 'The murders would not have happened if Dr. Liptzin had done his job properly.' Williamson testified at trial of his suit last month, telling the jurors that Dr. Liptzin 'had more control over the situation than I did.'[6]

Williamson's success with this unlikely argument is an unequivocal message to psychiatrists that the justice system expects them to impose precautionary control measures on anyone they encounter who is likely to commit a crime and might escape criminal liability with an insanity plea. This type of message is particularly disturbing for critics of medical psychiatry, because it reinforces the expectations of an authoritarian imposition of the medical model. Thomas Szasz and Jeffrey Schaler are leading critics of medical psychiatry, and they both responded within a few days of the Williamson story with letters to the editor:

> That killers can successfully blame their therapists for their actions (front page, Oct. 10) is the consequence of the fiction of

mental illness and the junk science of psychiatry that it supports. Although lawyers, psychiatrists and society conspire in the twin charades of civil commitment and the insanity defence, the main culprits are the mental health professionals. If they believed in personal responsibility rather than in mental illness—and rejected the practices of depriving innocent people of liberty and excusing guilty people of crimes—we would be spared the spectacle of criminals' being acquitted of crimes and collecting damages as if they were the victims of untreated diseases.

   THOMAS SZASZ, M.D. Syracuse, Oct. 10, 1998
The writer is professor emeritus of psychiatry at SUNY Health Science Center.[7]

Why did a jury hold a psychiatrist, Myron B. Liptzin, accountable for Wendell Williamson's murderous acts (front page, Oct. 10)? Because psychiatrists invented and perpetuate the myth of mental illness. As long as people believe in mental illness as a cause for behaviour, those who receive such a 'diagnosis' will be exculpated—and someone else will be culpable.

   Since psychiatrists removed the blame, it is only fitting that they should be saddled with it.

   JEFFREY A. SCHALER, Silver Spring, Md., Oct. 10, 1998
The writer is an adjunct professor of justice, law and society at American University.[8]

Despite the numerous doubtful applications of the insanity plea such as Williamson's, the concept is deeply entrenched in legal custom, and most people still agree that it should be available. But its continued existence is presenting acute problems for civil liberties. In the modern context, any positive effect it might have for human rights is disproportionately counter-balanced by the negative effect of large numbers of innocent people being made victims of precautionary psychiatric controls.

Some comparative figures might be useful to illustrate this point. In New South Wales in 1996, for instance, ten people who were tried for criminal offences were found not guilty by reason of mental illness. A further three people were found mentally unfit for trial. These thirteen people who escaped criminal liability in that year can be compared with 7,601 involuntary admissions to mental hospitals, 2,095 community treatment orders, and 167 community counselling orders—totalling 9,863 involuntary impositions in the same legal jurisdiction in the same year.[9]

All these impositions required as justification medical opinions that the people involved were at risk of causing serious physical harm to themselves or others. But what was the real risk? For every case where a person successfully evaded criminal liability on the grounds of mental illness there were some 760 occasions on which people had their human rights violated as a precautionary measure.

Relevant Human Rights

Deprivation of liberty and forced treatment are the two most serious human rights problems that arise for the socially alienated class of schizophrenics. Article 9 of the International Covenant on Civil and Political Rights (ICCPR) guarantees that:

> Everyone has the right to liberty and security of person. No one shall be subjected to arbitrary arrest or detention. No one shall be deprived of his liberty except on such grounds and in accordance with procedure as are established by law.[10]

The key word here is 'arbitrary'. If correct procedures are followed and there is good reason to arrest a person, because he or she has broken a law, the person no longer has a right to liberty. But, on most occasions, schizophrenics are involuntarily hospitalised as a precautionary measure. Is this arbitrary? Assuming that there is no disease underlying the symptoms, and that medical treatment is therefore unnecessary, the answer hangs on whether the people selected are still in need of control because they are dangerous to themselves or to other people.

A great deal of research has been undertaken to determine whether people with the symptoms of schizophrenia and other mental disorders are more dangerous than other people. The results of this research vary from 'not at all' to 'marginally more dangerous'. Some classes of people, such as young men between the ages of fifteen and 25, and men consuming alcohol, are statistically far more dangerous to other people than schizophrenics. However, it is unthinkable that all young men, and all alcohol drinkers, should be incarcerated as a precautionary measure. This often raises the rhetorical question of why it is thought to be just to incarcerate a statistically less dangerous group, such as people with the symptoms of schizophrenia, on the grounds of their supposed dangerousness.

The same holds for the supposedly high suicide-rate of schizophrenics. A far higher suicide-rate prevails amongst people who have already attempted to kill themselves, particularly when there is a background of childhood sexual abuse. This is a group on whom no precautionary incarceration is imposed. Nor is there any institutionalised intervention in the lives of people who pursue dangerous sports, such as mountain climbing and car racing. On the contrary, such people are encouraged because they inspire normal people with their willingness to take risks.

There is an interesting statistic that relates to the practice of incarcerating schizophrenics to protect them from themselves. It seems that schizophrenics undergo a particularly high risk of suicide shortly after they are released from hospital.[11] This can be interpreted in a number of different ways. On the one hand, it could be argued that hospitalisation protects a person from suicidal impulses, and that those who suicide after release should have been kept in longer. On the other hand, it can also be argued that it is the treatment, or the humiliation of the incarceration experience, that causes people to suicide as soon they get a chance.

The possibility that hospitalisation and the accompanying neuroleptic drug treatment might induce suicidal or violent reactions is very disturbing. Neuroleptic-induced akathisia is a side-effect of standard drug treatment for schizophrenia: 'The individual is virtually tortured from inside his or her own body as feelings of irritability and anxiety compel the person into constant motion, sometimes to the point of continuous suffering'.[12] DSM-IV is unequivocal about the risks of suicide and violence associated with neuroleptic medication:

> Akathisia may be associated with dysphoria, irritability, aggression, or suicide attempts. Worsening of psychotic symptoms or behavioural dysfunction may lead to an increase in neuroleptic medication dose, which may exacerbate the problem. Akathisia can develop very rapidly after initiating or increasing neuroleptic medication. The development of akathisia appears to be dose dependent and to be more frequently associated with particular neuroleptic medications. Acute akathisia tends to persist for as long as neuroleptic medications are continued, although the intensity may fluctuate over time. The reported prevalence of akathisia among individuals receiving neuroleptic medication has varied widely (20%–75%).[13]

DSM-IV is not a polemic written by critics of medical psychiatry. As explained in previous chapters, it is an officially recognised manual, and is perhaps the most important contemporary document supporting the medical view of mental disorders. Its statement immediately above—in effect, that up to 75 per cent of the people given drug treatment for schizophrenia are put at increased risk of suicide—is a consensus opinion of the psychiatric profession. In the face of this admission, it seems bizarre that the same profession regularly claims that there is a need to incarcerate schizophrenics to ensure that they are given this treatment to *protect* them from suicide.

Torture and Cruel Treatment

Another article of human rights law that is of particular interest to critics of medical psychiatry is Article 7 of the ICCPR:

> No one shall be subjected to torture or to cruel, inhuman or degrading treatment or punishment. In particular, no one shall be subjected without his free consent to medical or scientific experimentation.[14]

The linkage in Article 7 between torture and unreasonable forms of punishment, on the one hand, and medical experimentation on the other, is noteworthy. For sceptics, all medical treatment for mental illnesses is, and must be, experimental. Further, since it is implausible that any illness underlies the symptoms of schizophrenia, the rationale for applying medical treatment can only be explained in terms of punishment. That is, individuals are punished for allowing their thoughts, beliefs, and behaviour to cross a threshold of social tolerance.

Concerns about torture and unreasonable forms of punishment are so fundamental to human rights that a special United Nations convention is dedicated to their elimination, which is supplementary to Article 7. The Convention against Torture and Other Cruel, Inhuman or Degrading Treatment or Punishment conveniently supplies a definition of torture as:

> any act by which severe pain or suffering, whether physical or mental, is intentionally inflicted on a person for such purposes as obtaining from him or a third person information or a confession, punishing him for an act he or a third person has committed or is suspected of having committed, or intimidating or coercing him or a third person, or for any reason based on discrimination of any kind, when such pain or suffering is inflicted by or at the instigation of or with the consent or acquiescence of a public official or other person acting in an official capacity. It does not include pain or suffering arising only from, inherent in or incidental to lawful sanctions.[15]

The exclusion described in the last sentence is concerned with the application of prescribed punishments for specific breaches of the law. In some countries, for instance, whipping is still used as a punishment for certain criminal offences, and the intention of the convention is to exclude such 'lawful sanctions' from the definition of torture. However, if medical treatment for schizophrenia can be shown to fit the former part of the definition of torture, it is unlikely that it would be excluded merely because it has lawful sanction under mental health legislation. It can be assumed that the lawful sanction for the application of medical treatment for schizophrenia is only given on the assumption that it will benefit the patient—not that it will deliberately cause pain and suffering.

An argument can be easily made that medical treatment for schizophrenia fits the above definition of torture because it causes severe physical and mental suffering; it is intentionally inflicted on a person for the purpose of obtaining a confession in the form of a demonstration of 'insight'; it intimidates and coerces the person to change his or her pattern of thinking and belief; and, in the case of involuntary treatment, the mental suffering is inflicted by a government-employed psychiatrist acting in an official capacity.

It is not difficult to establish that schizophrenia treatment causes physical and mental suffering in those who receive it. Medical treatments for madness, from the fifteenth century onwards, have almost always done so. Noteworthy were 'stone operations—that is, pretending to remove stones from incisions made in the heads of patients thought to be mad'.[16] This European practice, which flourished between the fifteenth and seventeenth centuries, is thought to be the origin of the description of mad people as having 'rocks in their heads'.

A seventeenth-century English medical textbook on madness relates 'that the observations that sword wounds penetrating the skull sometimes produced a cure for insanity led to operations to let out the "fuliginous humours" by boring the skull'.[17] The nineteenth century saw the widespread use of treatments such as prolonged exposure in cold water, shock therapy by suddenly opening a trap-door and dropping a patient into cold water, and a rotating swing device in which the patient's head was strapped into a position in which the centrifugal force pushed more blood into the brain.

There have also been various kinds of infection therapies whereby pustules and running sores have been deliberately induced on the scalp so that they could be incised to let 'the black vapours escape'.[18] Early in the twentieth century, fever therapies were used by infecting psychiatric patients with tuberculin, typhoid, and malaria. The exponents of all these improbable treatments claimed success at the time that they were applying them. If it is true that such applications can indeed eliminate the symptoms of schizophrenia, it is simply a demonstration that torture and punishment can persuade people to change their minds and behaviour.

It was not until well into the twentieth century, with the advent of more sophisticated medical treatments such as insulin coma treatment in the late 1920s, and in the 1930s metrazol convulsive treatment, psychosurgery, and electro-convulsive treatment (ECT), that schizophrenic patients were introduced to modern medical practices.

Insulin and metrazol have long ago been phased out as schizophrenia treatments, but the record of their usage is relevant to the current discussion on torture. Early psychiatric pioneers of these treatments were often candid in their opinions about the usefulness of insulin and metrazol in 'fear therapy':

> No reasonable explanation of the action of hypoglycaemic (insulin) shock or of epileptic fits in the cure of schizophrenia is forthcoming, and I would suggest as a possibility that as with the surprise bath and the swinging bed, the 'modus operandi' may be the bringing of the patient into touch with reality through the strong stimulation of the emotion of fear, (and) that the intense apprehension felt by the patient after an injection of cardiazol (metrazol), and so feared by the patient, may be akin to the apprehension of the patient threatened with the swinging bed. The exponents of the latter pointed out that fear of repetition was an important element in success.[19]

During insulin treatment a person experienced a range of symptoms, beginning with clouding of consciousness and progressing to wild excitement, involuntary gasping and sucking, protrusion of the tongue, snarling, grimacing, twitching, convulsions, spasms, and deep coma. It is reported to have been a very unpleasant experience.

A point from the above observation that needs to be emphasised is the 'bringing of the patient into touch with reality through the strong stimulation of the emotion of fear'. The reality presented to the patient was that if he or she was not prepared to cease manifesting schizophrenic symptoms, and make the required adjustments of thinking and belief, the patient would be made to suffer more insulin or metrazol treatments. This is a fairly concise description of torture, and the objective of torture—that is, compliance. One psychiatrist summed it up this way:

> The patient is mentally sick, his behaviour is irrational; this 'displeases' the physician and, therefore, the patient is treated with injections of insulin which make him quite sick. In this extremely miserable condition he seeks help from anyone who can give it. Who can give help to a sick person, if not the physician who is constantly on the ward, near the patient, and watches over him as over a sick child?[20]

Don Weitz is a psychiatric survivor and an anti-psychiatry activist based in Toronto, Canada. He is co-editor of a book, *Shrink Resistant: the struggle against psychiatry in Canada*. He also produces an anti-psychiatry radio programme called Shrinkrap and is the co-founder of a Toronto-based organisation called People Against Coercive Treatment (PACT). A perception that the forced insulin treatment he received as a young man was a deliberate form of torture motivates his continuing campaign against psychiatric coercion:

> I was once tortured for six weeks 46 years ago—it happened in December 1951 and January 1952. I was forcibly subjected to a

series of over 50 sub-coma insulin shocks which psychiatrist Douglas Sharpe prescribed as a treatment for 'schizophrenia'. I never believed I was 'schizophrenic' or 'mentally ill'—just a very confused college student struggling to find himself, a common identity crisis. I was an involuntary psychiatric patient in McLean Hospital (a teaching-research facility affiliated with Harvard Medical School and Massachusetts General Hospital).

Psychiatrist Douglas Sharpe prescribed a series of insulin shock treatments for me because I was openly angry and defiant. Here's a telling excerpt by Dr. Sharpe in my medical records: 'The patient was finally placed on sub-coma insulin and after a month of sub-coma insulin three times a day he showed tremendous improvement ... There was no longer the outbursts of anger ... He spends most of his time trying to figure out what the effect of insulin has on him ... '

The shock treatments terrorised and debilitated me. I once went into a coma and thought I was dying—a 'side effect' Dr. Sharpe and other psychiatrists never warned me about. When I frequently complained to Dr. Sharpe about the maddening hunger, profuse sweating and convulsions I was forced to experience everyday on insulin-shock and that it was torture, he dismissed my complaints and calmly replied, 'I'm not torturing you. These complaints are just part of your problem.' The usual blame-the-victim game. I was finally released in 1953 only after I promised to conform to the psychiatrists' stereotype of a middle-class young student—study and go back to college.

It took me almost 20 years to understand my forced psychiatric incarceration and forced treatment in political terms, 20 years to realise that I was a political prisoner of psychiatry—locked up against my will, tortured, no right to a hearing or trial before losing my freedom, no right to appeal.[21]

Like insulin treatment, ECT has also earned a reputation as a 'fear therapy'. Sylvia Plath described a personal experience of ECT in *The Bell Jar*:

'Don't worry,' the nurse grinned down at me. 'Their first time everybody's scared to death.'

I tried to smile, but my skin had gone stiff, like parchment.

Doctor Gordon was fitting two metal plates on either side of my head. He buckled them into place with a strap that dented my forehead, and gave me a wire to bite.

I shut my eyes.

There was a brief silence, like an indrawn breath. Then something bent down, and took hold of me and shook me like the end of the world. Whee-ee-ee-ee-ee, it shrilled, through an air crackling with blue light, and with each flash a great jolt drubbed me till I thought my bones would break and the sap fly out of me like a split plant. I wondered what terrible thing it was that I had done.[22]

Unlike insulin and metrazol, ECT is still widely used as a psychiatric treatment, although these days patients are anaesthetised first. Even so, fear of the experience has been well documented. One group of researchers exploring the role of fear in ECT elicited comments from patients who had undergone it:

Reaction ranged from strong denial of fear, such as 'I'm glad to take it,' to fear of total mental destruction or death, such as 'Shock will destroy my mind,' 'My heart will stop,' 'I will die.' Many subjects expressed fears of being electrocuted, such as one who said, 'It's like being burned to a crisp.' Often the subject revealed under questioning a high degree of fear after first denying any fear, such as a depressed subject who admitted 'I'm scared to death every time. I never know if I'm going to come out of it or not.' A very psychotic subject described ECT as 'like crossing a river.'[23]

In the past ECT was, for a time, the main treatment for schizophrenia. More recently it has been largely reserved for so-called drug-resistant cases of severe depression. However, ECT is still recommended for treating acute symptoms of schizophrenia 'in certain patients who are in severe states of withdrawal (catatonia) or who present with significant affective symptoms such as uncontrolled mania'.[24]

The medical profession often seems to have a blind spot in its collective conscience concerning the difference between treatment and torture when electric shocks are involved. When electric shock is applied to the genitals it is unequivocally 'torture'. However, when a person is imprisoned in a mental hospital, and subjected to toxic chemicals and electric shocks to the head, it is called 'treatment'.

A recent report to Amnesty International on the use of electric torture does not have the same trouble making the distinction between treatment and torture when ECT is involved. The report identifies ECT machines as being one of two electrical devices that are specifically suited and routinely used for torture: 'the story of human torture cannot be conducted without the study of the torture of the insane ... This is quite clearly illustrated in the story of the development of the ECT machine ... '[25]

Psychosurgery is another psychiatric treatment that was widely used for schizophrenia in the past, but which contemporary psychiatrists now reserve for other mental illnesses such as depression and obsessive-compulsive disorder.[26] Psychosurgery is a form of psychiatric treatment which ordinary people have little trouble understanding. Its conception is not much more sophisticated than an operation to cut a rotten spot out of an apple. It relies on crudely conceived brain-mapping which purports to locate specific forms of deviant mental activity in certain areas of the brain. The basic principle is that unwanted mental activity can be surgically removed. The effects of psychosurgery are irreversible.

Psychosurgery has been 'practised in most countries with the necessary technical skills', but it boomed in the United States in the late 1940s and early 1950s, shortly before the widespread adoption of anti-psychotic drugs. In Britain between 1942 and 1954, 10,365 people were given leucotomy operations, two-thirds of them being performed on schizophrenics.[27] At this time insulin and metrazol were passing out of favour for schizophrenia treatment, and mental hospitals were over-crowded with war veterans from World War II.

The popularisation of psychosurgery in the United States was largely attributable to a neuropsychiatrist called Walter Freeman and a neurosurgeon called James Watts, who jointly developed new techniques. In 1946 they performed the first operation using a new, all-purpose technique called 'transorbital lobotomy': 'The only instrument needed was a simple penetrating and cutting tool, which was forced through the bony orbit over the eye to enter the region of the frontal lobes'.[28]

This instrument, which Freeman referred to as resembling 'an ice-pick',[29] was called a leucotome, and, being a blunt instrument in both literal and metaphorical senses, was driven into the frontal lobe area with the aid of a mallet. Once in place it was rotated 'so that the cutting edge would destroy fibres at the base of the frontal lobes'.[30] Estimates for the number of first-wave lobotomy operations performed in the United States using this method range up to 50,000.[31] One of the main reasons for this popularisation was that:

> transorbital lobotomies were relatively easy to perform and electroconvulsive shock was frequently used in place of anaesthesia, the surgery was commonly performed by psychiatrists without the involvement of neurosurgeons, anaesthetists, and surgical amphitheatres. In some instances, the operation was performed as an office procedure and the patient was taken home by the family a few hours after the operation.[32]

However, the family took home a very different person to the one they had taken in:

> Typically the patient tends to become more inert, and shows less zest and intensity of emotion. His spontaneous activity tends to be reduced, and he becomes less capable of creative productivity, which is independent of the intelligence level ... With these

changes in initiative and control of behaviour, our patients resemble those with frontal lobe lesions.[33]

An extensive study undertaken by P. MacDonald Tow in 1955 of *Personality Changes Following Frontal Leucotomy* found very significant changes in intellectual functions, including 'impairment of the powers of abstraction and synthesis; of perception of relations and differences; of the ability to deal with complex situations, planning and thinking out of the next action and its consequences; and appreciation of one's own mistakes ... There is also impairment of the power of sustained attention and of the capacity for fine discrimination; and a dulled appreciation of the subject's own level of success or failure'.[34]

Tow also examined journals written by patients before and after their psychosurgery. The post-surgery journals were particularly good indicators of the effects of the operation, and showed that patients had deeply felt concerns about loss of creativity and self-awareness; in particular, they frequently had 'a terrible fear of being harmed and controlled by scientific and psychiatric technology'.[35] Breggin describes having made similar observations in post-psychosurgery patients: 'I have observed a florid paranoid schizophrenic with terror of being controlled by psychiatric technology following amygdalotomy'.[36]

There is little doubt that psychosurgery, and chemical and electrical shock treatments, and the variety of crude treatments used in earlier centuries, can all be easily construed as forms of punishment and neatly fitted into the United Nations definition of torture. However, if the past history of medical treatment for schizophrenia is so clearly a tale of punishment and torture, can the same be said of the current forms of drug treatment?

Neuroleptics and the Right to Liberty

As discussed in previous chapters, a group of drugs called neuroleptics, formerly known as major tranquillisers and antipsychotics, is the contemporary psychiatric treatment of first choice for schizophrenia. It is not difficult to demonstrate that forced treatment with neuroleptics violates both the right to liberty and the right to protection from torture.

An involuntary patient usually undergoes a loss of liberty in two different ways. The incarceration process physically removes the person from the community. The forced treatment with neuroleptic medication effectively restricts brain activity, and thereby restrains the person's ability to be physically and mentally active. Neuroleptic drugging is so efficient that earlier methods of physical restraint such as straitjackets are now rarely needed. In fact, neuroleptic treatment itself is sometimes referred to as a 'chemical straitjacket'.

So efficient is this straitjacket that incarcerated people, although they may be considered still in need of control, are now often released under community treatment orders which ensure that their minds and bodies remain under restraint after release from hospital. In the United States, this process is called outpatients' commitment, and states are progressively passing legislation to enable it. People are subjected to a legally binding order under which mobile treatment teams have access to their homes in order to inject them with long-acting neuroleptics at the required intervals. There is usually a prescribed maximum period for which an order is effective, but successive orders can be made for an indefinite period.

Neuroleptic treatment applied in this way cannot possibly have a therapeutic benefit if there is no underlying illness on which to apply the therapy. The justification in such cases could only be that the treatment is administered for social-control reasons. The people who are thereby controlled have their right to liberty violated because the process by which their mental functions are restrained with forced drugging is arbitrary.

The same drugs which are given to schizophrenics as therapy to supposedly rebalance their brain chemistry are used in many different institutional settings purely as restraining devices to control the behaviour of non-psychotic people. When they are used on non-psychotic people there is no pretence of a therapeutic purpose. This suggests that the only effective use of neuroleptics is for chemical restraint.

Neuroleptics are used widely for treating agitation in elderly people, and there are varying opinions within the psychiatric profession about the correctness of this procedure. While one text protests that 'the use of antipsychotic drugs to control disturbed behaviour in elderly patients with dementia is a widespread practice that should be deplored' and that 'antipsychotic drugs should not be used in the routine treatment of non-psychotic patients,'[37] other texts and professional papers canvass a very different point of view.

The influential *Synopsis of Psychiatry* recommends that '[i]n addition to treating overt signs of psychosis, such as hallucinations and delusions, antipsychotics have also been used to deal effectively with violent, agitated, and abusive geriatric patients'.[38] This view is supported by another text which says that neuroleptics are in 'widespread use for the control of behavioural complications' in nursing homes and hostel settings where from 20 to 70 per cent of institutionalised patients with dementia are receiving the drugs.[39] (Dementia is not regarded as a psychosis but is a symptom of brain damage/brain atrophy arising from a variety of causes.)

Studies of neuroleptic use in nursing homes have found that informed consent is often not sought in advance but is usually 'presumed', and that treatment continues unless it becomes apparent that the patient no longer acquiesces.[40] Studies have also found that the neuroleptic drugging has a detrimental effect and hastens the decline of elderly people. One recent study found that the intellectual capabilities of elderly people receiving neuroleptics were only half those of untreated elderly people.[41] Another study implicated neuroleptics in an increased incidence of injurious falls in nursing homes.[42]

In its 1995 federal Budget submission, the Australian Council on the Ageing recommended that Commonwealth funds be allocated to specifically address a number of matters raised by the Inquiry into Human Rights and Mental Illness. One of these matters was referred to as 'the use of chemical restraint in residential care for older people'.[43] The human rights inquiry had been told that old people with dementia 'get zonked out with medication or tied to their chairs'[44] in some nursing homes as a matter of course, and that 'elderly patients are routinely sedated as a management technique—rather than for therapeutic purposes'.[45]

But there is no equivocation when it comes to prescribing neuroleptic drugs for mentally retarded people: 'Treatment of behavioural disturbances in the mentally retarded has tended to rely heavily on medication resulting in up to 50% of retarded people in institutions and community residences being on psychotropic drugs'.[46] (Neuroleptics are a sub-set of the psychotropic group.) A second textbook confirms the 50 per cent figure as being normal, and enthusiastically recommends the neuroleptics Mellaril and Haldol as being 'useful in reducing unwanted behaviour, such as self-stimulation, aggression, and motor activity'.[47]

Neuroleptics are also routinely used by psychiatrists to treat children and adolescents who have had complaints laid against them for being disruptive. High strength neuroleptics such as Haldol, for instance, are routinely prescribed for conduct disorder.[48] Conduct disorder is specific to children and adolescents, and is essentially a tendency towards disobedience. Conduct disorder is considered a non-psychotic condition and so, unlike the dopamine hypothesis for schizophrenia, there is no attempt at formulating an underlying therapeutic rationale for using neuroleptic medication to control it. This has left drug treatment for conduct disorder open to severe criticism. A recent study of children and adolescents receiving neuroleptics in New York found that one-third of them had developed symptoms of Parkinsonism, and one-eighth had developed tardive dyskinesia, as a result.[49]

When neuroleptic drugs are openly used in these ways to control troublesome behavioural patterns, without any pretence of a therapeutic purpose, it is obvious there is no truth in claims that they have a therapeutic effect on schizophrenics. It is apparent that the drugs are administered to schizophrenics for the same reason as they are given to disruptive non-psychotic people in institutions—primarily to control their behaviour. This means that all involuntary dosing with these drugs is a restriction of personal liberty and therefore a violation of Article 9 of the International Covenant on Civil and Political Rights.

Neuroleptics: Treatment or Torture?

When medical psychiatrists in Western democracies use neuroleptics on their own patients, they claim it is a relatively safe, necessary, and effective therapy. However, when the same mainstream psychiatric professionals observed Soviet psychiatrists using the same drugs on people diagnosed with schizophrenia during the last decades of the communist era, they proclaimed that the drugs were being used as a form of punishment and torture. This was despite evidence that Soviet psychiatrists approached the concept of mental illness in almost identical ways to those of Western psychiatrists. An investigator of Soviet psychiatry at the end of the communist era found that:

> The dopamine hypothesis of schizophrenia and amine hypothesis of depression are widely quoted. There is a more intense approach to treatment in the early stages of an illness, and the range of drugs used is similar to that in the West. Interestingly, clozapine [an atypical neuroleptic] was used in the Soviet Union long before it became available in Western countries.[50]

The World Psychiatric Association (WPA), the professional body representing psychiatrists at an international level, was very prominent in the early 1980s in a campaign of condemnation of Soviet psychiatry. There was a widespread perception in the West that Soviet psychiatrists were using neuroleptics as a form of torture on dissidents who had been diagnosed with schizophrenia.

Leonid Plyushch, a Russian scientist and political dissident of the 1970s who eventually fled to the United States, told how he had been drugged in a Soviet psychoprison on small doses of the neuroleptic Haldol: 'I was horrified to see how I deteriorated intellectually, morally and emotionally from day to day. My interest in political problems quickly disappeared, then my interest in scientific problems, and then my interest in my wife and children.'[51] Haldol is not a Soviet invention. It is manufactured in the United States by McNeil Pharmaceuticals. In 1995, Haldol had 24 per cent of the neuroleptic market in the United States.[52]

The professional body representing Soviet psychiatrists resigned from the WPA under pressure in 1983, and in 1989 a *Time* article warned about the dangers of allowing Soviet psychiatrists to rejoin the WPA. The article canvassed the opinion that psychiatric methods remained essentially unchanged in the Soviet Union, and reviewed some of the abuses of the past. At its supposed worst, Soviet psychiatry was dominated by Dr Andrei Snezhnevsky, the director of the Institute of Psychiatry of the USSR Academy of Medical Sciences. Snezhnevsky, who had died in 1987, had been the leading figure in Soviet psychiatry since the early 1950s, and his influence was still felt. It was Snezhnevsky who

> broadened the definition of schizophrenia by adding the category 'sluggish schizophrenia.' He defined the disorder as a slow-developing illness without the hallucinations that are a classic element in the Western definition of many schizophrenias. Instead, the 'symptoms' could be nearly all forms of behaviour—unsociability, mild pessimism, stubbornness—that deviated from the social or political ideal.[53]

This description of schizophrenia could easily be derived from the current DSM-IV diagnostic criteria, in which 'hallucinations' are only one of five possible Criterion-A symptoms and are not an essential feature of schizophrenia. Evidence of 'unsociability, mild pessimism, stubbornness, that deviated from the social ideal', could easily trigger a diagnosis of schizophrenia using DSM-IV guidelines. 'Disorganised behaviour' (Criterion A4) combined with negative symptoms such as 'affective flattening' (Criterion A5) and 'social dysfunction' (Criterion B) would probably be sufficient. If a person was troublesome to their family or a social nuisance in a Western country, there is little doubt that the Soviet criteria could be used for at least a tentative schizophrenia label such as 'schizophreniform disorder' (DSM-IV) or 'simple schizophrenia' (ICD-10).

The same *Time* article described the Soviet dissidents being tortured/punished by being 'hospitalised for years under prison-like conditions and put on powerful drugs that turned them into zombies'.[54] But the powerful drugs that violated human rights by turning Soviet dissidents into zombies are the same neuroleptics used on similar types of people by Western psychiatrists.

Another indignant description of Soviet psychiatry describes sluggish schizophrenia again: 'One manifestation of this novel ailment was "stubbornness and inflexibility of convictions"; the usual treatment consisted of megadoses of powerful tranquillisers such as Thorazine for "prophylactic" purposes'.[55] Once again, 'inflexibility of convictions' is just another way of describing 'delusions with lack of insight', which is a common feature of the diagnosis of schizophrenia in the West. 'Prophylactic purposes' is called 'maintenance treatment' by Western psychiatrists and, as with Haldol in the earlier description, the drug used to supposedly 'punish' Soviet dissidents, Thorazine, is routinely applied to schizophrenics by Western psychiatrists. Thorazine is the brand, and chlorpromazine the generic name, of a commonly used neuroleptic that had 12 per cent of the market for neuroleptics in the United States in 1995.[56] In Britain, this drug is known as Largactil.

Thomas Szasz argues that the spectacle of the Western psychiatric profession loudly condemning Soviet psychiatrists for their abuse of professional standards was largely an exercise in hypocrisy. Szasz maintains that it is psychiatric power that is the problem from which psychiatric abuse arises, and that psychiatric power is just as prevalent in democratic societies as it was in the

Soviet Union: 'Psychiatric abuse, such as we usually associate with practices in the former Soviet Union, is related not to the misuse of psychiatric diagnoses, but to the political power intrinsic to the social role of the psychiatrist in totalitarian and democratic societies alike'.[57] If one accepts the argument that neuroleptic treatment was a form of torture when it was used by Soviet psychiatrists, there is little reason to have a different opinion about its current usage by Western psychiatrists.

Lawrence Stevens, a lawyer in the United States who represents victims of psychiatric injustice, goes beyond the punishment/torture model for forced treatment with neuroleptics. He compares the practice to rape:

> In both cases, the victim's pants are pulled down. In both cases, a tube is inserted into the victim's body against her (or his) will. In the case of sexual rape, the tube is a penis. In the case of what could be called psychiatric rape, the tube is a hypodermic needle. In both cases, a fluid is injected into the victim's body against her or his will.[58]

Descriptions given by patients of the treatment they have received sometimes gives confirmation of Stevens's assertion, despite his hyperbole. One woman patient, who had read a number of books about psychiatric theories of schizophrenia before her incarceration, had the temerity to demand of the hospital staff that they test her dopamine levels before giving her neuroleptic medication, in order to confirm that she did indeed have a chemical imbalance in her brain:

> When I was demanding testing at Shellharbour [a psychiatric hospital in New South Wales], I refused to lay on the bed for an injection unless they tested my levels first. The hospital brought in the hospital security men who forced me around to the TV room via a back corridor. They held me down and forced the injection on me.[59]

This same former patient goes on to describe how neuroleptics affect patient behaviour by the same 'fear therapy' principle as earlier forms of treatment:

> When the side effects of the drugs started taking effect I told staff that the side effects were totally unacceptable and that the drugs were toxic. Worse, they were forcing untested drugs on untested patients. The psychiatrist 'treating' me was furious. She said in response that I wasn't allowed to leave the ward with the other patients. I was therefore effectively put in isolation on the ward. I had to endure the side effects etc in silence because there is always ECT down the corridor. Staff then naively believed that I had calmed down because of the drugs. One psychiatric nurse said 'Look how much better you are now'. This woman honestly believed that I had calmed down because of biological intervention. I hadn't changed my attitudes or feelings one skerrick. It was just that I was too terrified to say anything because this woman 'treating' me was vicious. She meant business. I gave up the fight out of fear of an increased risk of brain damage from increased doses over a longer period of time.[60]

The fear of 'ECT down the corridor' is a particularly noteworthy element in the fear therapy that was applied to this patient. She further clarified the therapeutic principle: 'Because biopsychiatrists dehumanise and depersonalise schizophrenics they can't comprehend the fact that we respond rapidly to abuse like anyone else. If someone puts the fear of God into you, you shut up. Because of the silence they think the patient has calmed down and recovered because of biological intervention'.[61]

The history of treatment for schizophrenia reveals a long tradition of applying torture and cruel punishment as forms of 'fear therapy'. In the past, psychiatrists have candidly described the principle of fear therapy as giving patients a choice between better behaviour or more pain. Contemporary treatment in the form of neuroleptic medication, while still clearly retaining the same fear-therapy principle, also restricts a person's liberty by acting as a chemical straitjacket. In this way, neuroleptic medication appears to violate human rights that protect against the loss of liberty, as well as human rights that protect against torture and cruel punishment.

This is bad enough, but the situation is now worsening. Not content with the 1-2 per cent of the population traditionally caught in the diagnostic dragnet, the psychiatric profession is now engaged in a project to expand the numbers. In what appears to be a strategy largely developed by the pharmaceutical industry, psychiatrists are now embarked on a preventive medicine campaign to detect and treat schizophrenics who are still in a supposed pre-psychotic stage. Given that it is unlikely there is any disease to prevent—and that the implementation of a preventive medicine campaign is therefore far more likely to increase rather than reduce the number of people who receive a diagnosis—the reasoning behind this campaign is doubtful. However, it is not difficult to guess at the outcomes, whether intended or not: there will be an extension of psychiatric precautionary-control measures, together with an expansion of the market for a new generation of atypical neuroleptics.

9

Early Psychosis:
expanding the market for preventive medicine

Various countries are now implementing detection and intervention programmes that extend the definition of schizophrenia to include a 'pre-psychotic' phase. As a consequence, neuroleptic medication is being prescribed in the belief that it can prevent the development of psychosis in people who are thought to be 'at-risk'.[1] The pre-psychotic signs of schizophrenia are usually referred to as 'early psychosis' or as 'prodromal symptoms'.[2] These pre-psychotic symptoms, however, are only tentative, and researchers themselves sometimes describe them as being 'putative'.[3]

Promoters of the concept see pre-psychosis detection and intervention as a form of preventive medicine. They argue that if the incidence of schizophrenia can be reduced by early identification and treatment, as is the case for some somatic diseases, community benefits—such as cost savings and avoidance of personal trauma and family disruption—will follow.[4]

Early-Psychosis Detection and Intervention

Early-psychosis detection and intervention programmes generally aim to reduce the duration of untreated psychosis (DUP). The DUP is a hypothetical period preceding first treatment for schizophrenia during which symptoms and signs of an impending psychological or social crisis are present. Medical psychiatrists argue that the DUP for most people who develop psychosis is much longer than it should be, often lasting for years.[5]

It has been claimed that 'the cost of treatment for patients with a DUP greater than 6 months is twice the cost of those with a DUP less than 6 months'. Some argue that brain damage occurs during the DUP, and that the longer it continues the less chance a person has of ultimate recovery: 'most of the neurobiological damage is already accomplished by the time it is possible to make a valid DSM-IV diagnosis', and 'applying existing schizophrenia treatment as soon as possible in the course of the disorder may slow or stop deterioration'.[6] But apart from the equivocal evidence of initial pilot studies,[7] no substantial findings support these contentions.

Nevertheless, despite the weak theoretical base, it has been claimed that a programme of early detection and intervention which was trialled at Buckingham in the United Kingdom in the mid-1980s resulted in the incidence of schizophrenia in the community being measurably reduced.[8] These findings have not been replicated. This is not surprising, as the Buckingham Project's 'diagnostic thresholds for functional psychotic disorders' appear to have been uniquely flexible, and a considerable number of cases 'with symptom patterns suggesting an early phase of a florid schizophrenic episode'[9] were not counted. This diagnostic flexibility is the most likely explanation for the supposedly 'successful' outcome of the project.

Yet the claimed success of the Buckingham Project has been the basis for a growing body of literature and the initiation of early-psychosis projects in other parts of the world. The promoters of these programmes now face the task of reaching consensus on three points: an inventory of easily recognisable pre-psychotic symptoms; the design of a community-based catchment system that funnels at-risk people into a clinical setting; and an appropriate pre-psychosis treatment programme.

Research in Australia

Australia has become a particularly active site for this type of research, and in 1996 a National Early Psychosis Project (NEPP) was launched as 'a collaborative endeavour between the Commonwealth, State and Territory governments of Australia to develop and promote a national model of best practice for early intervention in psychosis'. This model of best practice is now embodied in the recently published *Australian Clinical Guidelines for Early Psychosis*. These guidelines extend the definition of psychosis to include 'the period described as the prodrome'.[10]

The most advanced early-psychosis programme in Australia, consistently cited as a model, is run by the Early Psychosis Prevention and Intervention Centre (EPPIC) in Melbourne, Victoria. EPPIC assumed a leadership role in Australia after winning the government tender to establish the NEPP. Much of the policy development embodied in the clinical guidelines has come out of EPPIC research programmes.

A major problem for psychiatrists researching into a supposed prodromal phase of schizophrenia is a lack of consensus about prepsychotic symptoms. The EPPIC team had at first intended to adopt the nine prodromal symptoms supplied in DSM-III-R.[11] However, when EPPIC conducted a community survey of Australian high school students to determine the prevalence of these symptoms in the general population of adolescents, they found that 'nearly half the sample (49.2%) had two or more symptoms and hence met the criteria for DSM-III-R schizophrenia prodrome'. This remarkably high figure caused the researchers to adjust the threshold for diagnosis by reducing the number of possible symptoms from nine to four. After testing the restricted criteria on ordinary high school students, they found that only '10 to 15 percent of the sample met the criteria for schizophrenia prodrome'.[12] As I will show, this was an under-estimate.

Satisfied that the modified criteria could be used to correctly identify their target group, the EPPIC researchers went on to implement 'a specialised outpatient service to monitor and care for young people thought to be at high risk for psychosis'.[13] The new clinic was called Personal Assistance and Crisis Evaluation (PACE).

Initially, the PACE clinic targeted young people between sixteen and 30 years of age. These were divided into three groups. In Group 1 were people who met the complete DSM-III-R criteria for schizophrenia prodrome and who also had a first- or second-degree relative with a history of a DSM-III-R psychotic disorder or schizotypal personality disorder. In Group 2 were people who had one or more of the four DSM-III-R positive-only criteria for schizophrenia prodrome: markedly peculiar behaviour; digressive, vague, overelaborate, or metaphorical speech; odd or bizarre ideation, or magical thinking; and unusual perceptual experiences. In Group 3 were 'young people with a history of fleeting psychotic experiences that spontaneously resolved (called brief limited intermittent psychotic symptoms, or BLIPS) within 1 week'.[14]

To detect these types of people in the community and to channel them into the PACE clinic, a public education campaign was launched, aimed particularly at general practitioners and other specialised professionals—such as school counsellors, teachers, and youth workers—who frequently come in contact with young people. Treatment involved psychosocial therapy or neuroleptic medication, sometimes both. Of the patients treated, '[t]he most frequently occurring DSM-III-R prodromal symptoms were magical thinking, perceptual disturbance, and impaired role function, present in 67.7, 54.8, and 54.8 percent of the subjects, respectively'.[15]

The fact that nearly 70 per cent of these young people were treated for 'magical thinking' is quite extraordinary. According to a description in DSM-IV's glossary of technical terms, magical thinking is not a particularly debilitating symptom. It is:

> The erroneous belief that one's thoughts, words, or actions will cause or prevent a specific outcome in some way that defies commonly understood laws of cause and effect. Magical thinking may be part of normal child development.[16]

The logic of schizophrenia prevention is that although some of the prodromal symptoms might not be serious handicaps in themselves they are, all the same, signs of approaching psychosis. However, members of the EPPIC team had previously discovered in other research that 51 per cent of normal Australian sixteen-year-olds experience magical thinking.[17] The fact that magical thinking was one of the symptoms used to identify these supposedly pre-psychotic young people, and that it did not have to be combined with other symptoms, means that the selection criteria were still targeting over 50 per cent of the population. Having already rejected the possibility that half of all Australian teenagers are afflicted with the prodrome for schizophrenia, why did the EPPIC team not realise that magical thinking is simply a part of normal adolescent psychology?

By 1996 the EPPIC researchers were ready to claim success for the initial PACE programme, and asserted that 'it is possible to identify and follow possibly prodromal individuals in the community'.[18] But they were concerned that many of the patients monitored during the course of the programme did not make the transition to full psychosis. The transition rate to psychosis presents an interesting problem of interpretation. On the one hand, if most of the young people fail to cross the threshold into psychosis, it can be claimed that the preventive treatment was successful. On the other hand, it might also indicate that the prodromal indicators were not accurate, and that many of the patients had been given a false positive diagnosis.

Inventing the Diagnostic Criteria

The EPPIC researchers decided to interpret the low transition-rate of their patients as indicating that a substantial fraction were false positives.[19] They promptly began a new prospective study of at-risk individuals using updated diagnostic criteria. The same sixteen-to-30 years age group was targeted, with the same division of the subjects into three groups. This time, however, the DSM-III-R prodromal symptoms were replaced with DSM-IV symptoms for Schizotypal Personality Disorder. This switch to using the symptoms of a personality disorder, which psychiatrists think of as a milder form of deviance than a psychosis, was necessary because the newer, fourth revision of the DSM had dropped the prodromal symptoms of schizophrenia from its specifications.

DSM-IV specifies nine symptoms for Schizotypal Personality Disorder:

(1) ideas of reference;
(2) odd beliefs or magical thinking;
(3) unusual perceptual experiences;
(4) odd thinking and speech;
(5) suspiciousness or paranoid ideation;
(6) inappropriate or constricted affect;
(7) behaviour or appearance that is odd, eccentric, or peculiar;
(8) lack of close friends or confidantes other than first-degree relatives; and
(9) excessive social anxiety.

A diagnosis normally requires the presence of five or more of these symptoms. But the researchers at the PACE clinic decided that only one symptom would be sufficient to indicate the presence of the schizophrenia prodrome. This assumption was in defiance of the DSM-IV view that 'Schizotypal Personality Disorder has a relatively stable course, with only a small proportion of individuals going on to develop Schizophrenia or another Psychotic Disorder'.[20] If this is true about people who meet the normal diagnostic criteria for Schizotypal Personality Disorder by having five or more symptoms, what is to be assumed about the real risk of psychosis for people who met the PACE diagnostic criteria by only having one symptom? It should be noted that magical thinking is once again on the list, so we know that over 50 per cent of the adolescent popluation would be identified by this method.

Defying expectations, the PACE research found that 48 per cent of the people inducted into the programme using the diluted schizotypal indicators became psychotic within twelve months. The transition rate to psychosis at six months was 40 per cent. But these results still raised ethical questions about treatment of the non-psychotic majority: 'because over 50% of cases do not develop psychosis within twelve months routine treatment of this group would result in many young people being subject to unnecessary treatment and labelling'.[21]

These claims of having calculated a precise rate of transition into psychosis suggest that the threshold of psychosis is a well-defined boundary, and that non-psychotic people can be easily distinguished from psychotic people. But this is not the case. In a recent publication, the EPPIC researchers admitted that psychosis has no precise definition, and that '[t]he point of onset is difficult to define prospectively and has to be defined arbitrarily'.[22]

When the point of psychotic onset is determined retrospectively, which is the usual way of making a determination, it can be simply pegged to the point in time at which a psychiatrist judged that a person's behaviour required urgent psychiatric treatment. But psychiatric treatment was given to the people in the PACE study while they were still in an acknowledged 'pre-psychotic' state. This blurred the distinction, and made it impossible to tell with any certainty when the psychotic threshold had been crossed.

The whole purpose of the research was to follow the progress of supposedly pre-psychotic patients and determine whether they crossed the threshold into psychosis. But because the threshold is an arbitrarily defined boundary, as the researchers admitted, the significance of their findings must be called into question. If the criteria for determining psychosis is arbitrary then, arguably, the researchers were at-risk of producing results that suited their purpose. These doubts are compounded by the apparent lack of control groups in the design of the research.

It should be noted here that a serious gap exists in the material published about the efficacy of pre-psychotic treatment programmes. No convincing evidence has been provided to support claims that a particular type of prophylactic treatment can help to prevent psychosis. Nor is there evidence that a lack of treatment will lead to psychosis. It is quite possible, from the anecdotal evidence provided so far, that attempts to apply prophylactic treatments might actually exacerbate symptoms, rather than ameliorate them, and thereby induce psychosis.

Australian Clinical Guidelines

Although heavily influenced in its developmental stage by the EPPIC researchers, the *Australian Clinical Guidelines for Early Psychosis* do not recommend the use of the schizotypal symptoms. Instead, a newly contrived sixteen-item list of 'Prodromal Symptoms and Signs' of psychosis is provided:

> Suspiciousness; Depression; Anxiety; Tension; Irritability; Mood swings; Anger; Sleep disturbances.
> Appetite changes; Loss of energy or motivation; Memory or concentration difficulties; Perception that things around them have changed; Belief that thoughts have speeded up or slowed down; Deterioration in work or study; Withdrawal and loss of interest in socialising; Emerging unusual beliefs.[23]

The authors of the clinical guidelines acknowledge that 'these signs and symptoms are not usually indicative of a developing psychosis'. This is apparently said to prevent over-zealous usage and to minimise the alarm that might arise in normal people who encounter this list and reflect on themselves. The clinical guidelines advise that these signs are only meant to be used as symptoms of impending psychosis when 'they occur in individuals who have been identified as "at-risk" of psychosis'.

A separate list of indicators identifies those who are at-risk. The idea is to first narrow down the field before applying the prodromal signs and symptoms. The narrowed field primarily focuses on adolescents and young people. But there is a fairly extraordinary mixture of further risk factors that range from the relatively specific 'Family history of psychotic disorder' to the equivocal 'Season of birth', to the thoroughly non-specific 'Life events' and 'Subjective/functional change in the person'.[24] In actuality, these risk factors fit almost any young person who is a bit worrisome to parents, school teachers, or other authority figures.

Apart from supplying its own lists of symptoms and risk factors, the clinical guidelines also advise that '[i]nformation currently available to promote awareness and identification of symptoms is captured in the pamphlet "Something is Not Quite Right" (SANE Australia)'.[25] SANE Australia is a business name of Schizophrenia Australia Foundation, which generally purports to represent the interests of relatives of schizophrenic people, but is also funded by drug companies. (See Chapter 4.)

The SANE pamphlet is directed at parents, teachers, employers, and workmates of 'difficult' people. Two checklists of symptoms are supplied to assist in recognising the severity of the underlying mental illness that might be giving rise to the difficulties. Boxes are provided beside each symptom so that observers can tick off a person's faults. Checklist 1 is:

> Behaviour which is considered **normal** although difficult. *Difficult behaviour at home, school or in the workplace.* People may be—
>
> | | | |
> |---|---|---|
> | rude | irritable | over-sensitive |
> | lazy | rebellious | weepy |
> | argumentative | over-emotional | withdrawn |
> | thoughtless | shy [26] | |

Observers are warned that these behaviours may not be cause for alarm but, if they persist or are too disruptive, advice should be sought from a GP, a school or workplace counsellor, a Citizens Advice Bureau or a mental health centre.

Checklist 2 is a list of 18 behaviours which are said to be definitely abnormal and which require an urgent medical assessment:

- withdraw completely from family, friends and workmates.
- be afraid to leave the house (particularly in daylight hours).
- sleep or eat poorly. Sleep by day and stay awake at night, often pacing around.
- be extremely preoccupied with a particular theme, for example, death, politics, or religion.
- uncharacteristically neglect household or personal or parental responsibilities, or personal hygiene or appearance.
- deteriorate in performance at school or work, or leave jobs.
- have difficulty concentrating, following conversation or remembering things.
- talk about or write things which do not really make sense.
- panic, be extremely anxious or markedly depressed, or suicidal.
- lose variation in mood, be *flat*. Lack emotional expression, for example, humour, friendliness.
- have marked changes in mood, for example from quiet to excited or agitated.
- have inappropriate emotional responses, for example, giggling on hearing sad news.
- hear voices that no-one else can hear.
- believe, without reason, that others are plotting against, spying on, or following them and have extreme fear of, or anger at, those people.
- believe they are being harmed, or influenced to do things against their will—by television, radio, aliens or the devil, for example.
- believe they have special powers, for example—that they are important religious leaders, politicians or scientists when this is not the case.
- believe their thoughts are being interfered with or that they can influence the thoughts of others.
- spend extravagant and unrealistic sums of money.[27]

The SANE pamphlet advises that if the person demonstrates 'outright resistance to the idea of visiting the doctor, consult with the doctor yourself to work out a plan over time. It may be possible and appropriate for the doctor to assess the person at home'.[28] In a situation such as this, where a person is reluctant to submit to a medical assessment, it is likely that a doctor would see the complaining friends or relatives—rather than the person to be assessed—as the real clients. This introduces a great deal of scope for bias in the doctor's assessment, which necessarily relies on subjective reports from the complainants. Summary detention in a mental hospital, or coercion to participate in a pre-psychosis treatment programme, are likely outcomes for a person who is the target of these types of complaints.

The SANE checklists of symptoms have been given elevated status by their endorsement in the clinical guidelines. The official recognition now makes them part of the consensus understanding of pre-psychotic schizophrenia. The SANE programme of using non-medical people as front-line diagnosticians, and encouraging them to identify and report people who are irritating/offensive/disturbing, must give some pause for thought. There is great potential for this system to be exploited by people motivated by personal grudges, or people who might want to punish others for holding opinions or beliefs with which they disagree. The possibility of using pre-psychotic intervention for social control is particularly evident in the fourth symptom of the above list: 'be extremely preoccupied with a particular theme, for example, death, politics, or religion'.

The aptly named 'Something is Not Quite Right' pamphlet is distributed by SANE with a note on its letterhead which announces that the pharmaceutical company Pfizer is one of the organisation's sponsors. (Pfizer makes a new atypical neuroleptic called ziprasidone.)

Drug Company Influence

Some of the risk factors listed in the clinical guidelines are based on theories about the cause of schizophrenia that remain unconfirmed. One of these, 'Season of birth', is a theory of very doubtful merit. It is based on observations that records in a few countries indicate a slightly higher birth-rate for schizophrenics in the late winter/early spring months.[29] Researchers in other countries have not been able to confirm the link,[30] and its use as a diagnostic indicator is highly questionable. The supposed risk season only lasts a few months and, although the rate of schizophrenia in some countries might be slightly higher amongst people born in these months, most of the people who go on to develop the condition later in life are still born outside this period. Similarly, the vast majority of people who are born within this period are obviously not at any risk at all of developing schizophrenia.

These anomalies indicate a certain level of imprecision by the compilers of the clinical guidelines. Indeed, both the list of 'risk factors' and the list of 'symptoms and signs' were not originally devised for the clinical guidelines, but were adopted without comment from a publication called the *Early Psychosis Training Pack*.[31] Although the principal authors of the training pack were the director and assistant director of EPPIC, the document was produced by Gardiner-Caldwell Communications, a British public relations company which specialises in pharmaceutical marketing. The training pack was funded by an 'educational grant' from the pharmaceutical company Janssen-Cilag, which manufactures risperidone, an atypical neuroleptic used for treating schizophrenia.

It may be worth noting that while the clinical guidelines were being prepared, Gardiner-Caldwell was publishing a web-based journal entitled *Influenza Bulletin*[32] for an organisation called the European Scientific Working-Group on Influenza (ESWI). ESWI received funding from a number of pharmaceutical companies, including Solvay Pharma and SmithKline Beecham, both of whom manufacture influenza vaccines. Gardiner-Caldwell appears to have developed a public relations specialty that provides promotional assistance for medical researchers and which, at the same time, also helps to expand the potential markets for their pharmaceutical sponsors. The *Early Psychosis Training Pack* should be considered in this light, which raises questions as to why the clinical guidelines for early psychosis 'best practice' in Australia use material from the training pack without explanation.

A popular theory among schizophrenia researchers about the season of birth postulates a link between influenza infection of mothers in the second trimester of pregnancy and schizophrenia in offspring. A review of the evidence shows this hypothesis to be doubtful.[33] Still, some psychiatric researchers have called for an influenza-vaccination programme for all women of child-bearing age to prevent mental disorders.[34] It is interesting to speculate whether public relations activity on behalf of influenza-vaccine manufacturers might have helped to position season-of-birth as a leading risk-factor for schizophrenia. The stage is now set for interested parties to argue that influenza vaccination of child-bearing-age women is a necessary part of future 'best practice' for preventing schizophrenia.

This type of public relations activity on behalf of drug companies does seem to play a role in other early-psychosis research. Most often, the public relations work is undertaken on behalf of companies that manufacture the newer neuroleptics. For example, a community education programme supporting a new two-step programme for early intervention in first-episode psychosis at the London Health Sciences Centre in London, Ontario is sponsored by Zeneca.[35] It involves teaching doctors, parents, school teachers, college teachers, and guidance counsellors how to identify the signs and symptoms of early psychosis in young people, and where to direct them for psychiatric intervention. Zeneca manufacture quetiapine, an atypical neuroleptic.

The Western Psychiatric Institute and Clinic (WPIC) in Pittsburg, Pennsylvania, is running a Program for Assessment and Care in Early Schizophrenia (PACES).[36] To facilitate this research, WPIC educates primary health care suppliers and educational professionals in their catchment area about the early signs of psychosis. Part of the research in conjunction with this programme aims to test the efficacy of three new atypical neuroleptics, with funding provided by the manufacturers of the drugs—Janssen-Cilag, Eli Lilly, and Pfizer.

A recently established programme in the United States aims to increase the awareness of schizophrenia by emphasising the importance of early intervention and detection. 'The SOS programme—known in full as "SOS—Signs of Schizophrenia: What To Look For, What To Do"—was set up by the National Mental Health Association in conjunction with Janssen Pharmaceutica in the USA'.[37]

In Australia, EPPIC's preventive-treatment centre for young people, PACE, also receives drug company funding from Janssen-Cilag.[38] This may have paid off handsomely for the company. The EPPIC researchers have established a leadership role in early-psychosis research and treatment in Australia, as was apparent in the organisation of NEPP and the clinical guidelines that emerged from the project. It may not be coincidental that a half page of the clinical guidelines is dedicated to dosage recommendations for using Janssen-Cilag's risperidone in first-episode psychosis.[39] The clinical guidelines do not extend these dosage recommendations to include other schizophrenia drugs, and the recommendations for risperidone give the appearance of an official endorsement of the drug.

Drug company involvement is particularly evident in the organisation of early-psychosis conferences. For instance, the Second International Conference on Early Psychosis—'Future Possible'—held in New York in March/April 2000, was sponsored by Pfizer, Lilly, Janssen-Cilag, and AstraZeneca (all manufacturers of new atypical neuroleptics). A similar conference, sponsored by Pfizer, Lilly, Janssen-Cilag, and Novartis, was hosted by EPPIC at the Hobart Casino, Tasmania, in September 1998. The foyer of the Hobart conference venue was given a carnival atmosphere by the presence of stalls set up by the drug companies. During intervals between conference sessions, barkers from the drug company stalls competed with one another for the attention of conference delegates, with public relations teams distributing literature, coffee, and various gifts such as pens, tea-towels, writing pads, and rubber balls. Sponge-rubber brains from Eli Lilly were very popular.

In the final plenary session of the Hobart conference, I asked a question of the assembled delegates: 'why are early-psychosis programmes taking off now—and why is it happening in Australia—when there does not seem to have been a breakthrough in knowledge about the cause of schizophrenia and Australia does not normally lead the world in mental health initiatives?' The delegates became animated as they questioned one another for the answer, but none was provided.

There seems to be only one plausible answer to this question: early-psychosis research and intervention programmes are driven by funding and lobbying from the pharmaceutical companies that have recently launched atypical neuroleptics onto the market. The objective of these pharmaceutical companies is to expand the market for their new drugs. The size of the existing market for palliative treatment of the psychotic and post-psychotic stages of schizophrenia is limited by diagnostic conventions. But the size of the market for prophylactic treatment of pre-psychotic schizophrenia is open-ended. Australia figures prominently in this strategy because it is being used as a testing ground for the idea of preventive medicine for schizophrenia. This is in preparation for the introduction of full-scale preventive medicine campaigns in the much larger drug markets of North America and Europe.

Atypical Neuroleptics as Prophylactic Treatment

Prophylactic treatment with atypical neuroleptic drugs of people who have not manifested a psychological crisis carries an enormous burden of ethical responsibility. This is because of the severe risks of drug-induced diseases incurred by taking neuroleptics. There is an extraordinary range of these drug-induced diseases, and sometimes the manufacturers' warnings in advertisements published in psychiatric journals run to two pages of extremely small type.

The more serious adverse reactions, such as agranulocytosis[40] and neuroleptic malignant syndrome,[41] may cause sudden death. The manufacturers also warn that laboratory evidence indicates that the new drugs are carcinogens[42] and mutagens.[43] Despite the claims from some quarters that tardive dyskinesia is not a problem with atypicals, most of the drug companies warn that their drugs do cause the disease. An advertisement for Risperdal [risperidone] clearly warns about this risk.[44]

The manufacturers also warn about the possibility of adverse mental and behavioural reactions. Many of these psychiatric reactions are the very disorders that treatment with the drugs is intended to prevent. An advertisement published by Zeneca Pharmaceuticals, for instance, after warning about an extraordinary variety of ways that their new atypical quetiapine [Seroquel] can induce ill-health, identifies 'Other Adverse Events Observed During the Pre-Marketing Evaluation of Seroquel'. These include:

> abnormal dreams, dyskinesia, thinking abnormal, tardive dyskinesia, vertigo, involuntary movements, confusion, amnesia, psychosis, hallucinations, hyperkinesia, libido increased, urinary retention, incoordination, paranoid reaction, abnormal gait, myoclonus, delusions, manic reaction, apathy, ataxia, depersonalisation, stupor, bruxism, catatonic reaction, hemiplegia.[45]

A Clozaril [clozapine] advertisement also warns about the risk of a variety of drug-induced negative and positive symptoms, such as loss of speech, amentia, delusions/hallucinations, and paranoia.[46] If treatment with atypical neuroleptics can sometimes induce psychosis, hallucinations, and delusions (as is frankly admitted by the manufacturers), questions must arise about the application of these drugs as prophylactics against psychosis. In the long term, will prophylactic treatment actually increase the incidence of psychosis? This question does not seem to have been considered in the psychiatric literature.

Another question to be addressed concerns how to interpret the significance of the transition to psychosis by a person who has been receiving prophylactic drug treatment. Given the nature of traditional thinking in the field, such an event will probably be taken to indicate accuracy in the diagnosis of prodromal symptoms, but ineffectiveness in the prophylactic treatment. This interpretation might encourage the prescription of increased doses of prophylactic drug treatment for other patients. But if it is clear that psychosis can be induced by the drugs themselves, as the manufacturers warn, such an event could simply indicate an adverse drug reaction. This interpretation would be a warning that other patients should be taken off their prophylactic medication altogether, rather than have their dosage increased. Once again, these lines of discussion do not arise in the literature.

Perhaps the most insidious of the ethical burdens for the promoters of the prophylactic use of atypicals comes from the growing body of evidence that withdrawal from some of these drugs can sometimes cause a psychotic reaction. Withdrawal reactions from typical neuroleptics have long been documented. It is now becoming apparent that the brain chemistry of some people treated with atypicals is changed in a way that makes them dependent on continued treatment. When atypical neuroleptic treatment is withdrawn they experience an immediate psychotic reaction that can only be rectified by recommencement of treatment.[47]

The ethical burden for psychiatrists treating the 'prodrome' of schizophrenia will include resisting the temptation to interpret psychosis induced by atypical withdrawal as evidence that the person was correctly diagnosed initially. Psychiatrists will be tempted to argue that it was the prophylactic treatment that, up to the point of withdrawal, prevented the person from entering psychosis. In this way, the original diagnosis and prophylactic treatment could easily be vindicated—when in fact they might both be at fault.

Is Preventive Medicine for Schizophrenia Valid?

It is hard to tell what the PACE research really indicates without being in possession of details of symptoms, treatment, and transition to psychosis for individual patients. The most benign interpretation would be that about 50 per cent of their patients had false positive diagnoses, and were therefore treated without the normal level of evidence for mental illness. However, it is entirely possible that all or most of their patients had false diagnoses, and that any transitions to psychosis were only adverse reactions to treatment.

Despite the honourable intentions of many of the researchers in this field, problems with symptomatology and treatment make it unlikely that pre-psychosis detection and intervention programmes will ever deliver the kind of unequivocal social and community health advantages that are generally expected from preventive medicine campaigns. This means that the extension of the definition of schizophrenia into a prodromal phase is unlikely to further enhance the plausibility of the medical model of schizophrenia.

In fact, it is quite likely that, in the long run, pre-psychotic programmes will damage the credibility of the medical model. When psychiatrists openly refer to pre-psychotic indicators as being 'putative', and then proceed to intervene in the lives of people who are thought to manifest them by treating them with the same potent neuroleptics that are used on supposedly full-blown schizophrenia, the argument that schizophrenia is just a psychiatric myth looks ever more persuasive.

This point is further emphasised by the commercial opportunism demonstrated by pharmaceutical companies in this area. A preventive medicine campaign based on the type of prodromal symptoms and risk factors specified in the *Australian Clinical Guidelines for Early Psychosis* potentially defines a whole generation of young people as being at-risk and in need of treatment. If pharmaceutical marketing strategies are eventually exposed as the primary motivating force behind the concept, it will make it a lot easier to argue that the whole medical model for schizophrenia is a psychiatric myth invented to serve special interests.

There are several fundamental knowledge gaps in the pre-psychosis concept that need to be explored. Firstly, no firm consensus exists about what psychosis is. DSM-IV introduces the spectrum of psychotic disorders by stating: 'The term *psychosis* has historically received a number of different definitions, none of which has achieved universal acceptance'.[48] The manual goes on to discuss various narrower and broader definitions of psychosis.

Is it a narrower or a broader form of psychosis that is to be prevented with pre-psychotic treatment? This question is not discussed by pre-psychosis researchers. But how can pre-psychotic detection criteria even be considered until a consensus is reached about how to define the psychosis that is to be prevented? If a broader definition of psychosis is agreed upon, this will inevitably mean that a broader range of pre-psychotic symptoms are required to predict it. The opposite is true for a narrower definition.

Closely associated with this is the problem of establishing a baseline for the lifetime prevalence of psychosis in the general community. Once again, this issue does not arise in the pre-psychosis literature. But if a baseline of prevalence has not been calculated before pre-psychotic detection and treatment begins, it will be impossible to determine whether pre-psychotic treatment reduces or increases the rate of psychosis in the general community.

Another closely related unresolved problem is imprecision in determining the threshold of psychosis. This is particularly important when people are being given pre-psychotic treatment. Without a precise definition of the threshold, it is impossible to compare the efficacy of preventive treatments. This problem has been discussed in the literature, and the EPPIC researchers have admitted that they are forced to make determinations of psychosis 'arbitrarily'.

A serious deficit in the concept of pre-psychotic detection is the failure to compare the prevalence rate of supposed pre-psychotic indicators with the prevalence rate for psychosis. (The prevalence rate is the percentage of the general community who exhibit the symptoms.) If the two rates do not correspond fairly closely, the pre-psychotic indicators are unlikely to be accurate. A common assumption is that psychotic disorders have a lifetime prevalence of about 2 to 3 per cent.[49] For argument's sake, let us choose the higher figure and use it to test the prodromal symptoms used by the EPPIC researchers.

The EPPIC researchers experimented with a couple of different sets of prodromal symptoms to select the people who they thought were pre-psychotic. Both of these sets used 'magical thinking' as a symptom; each time it was used, magical thinking alone could indicate a pre-psychotic condition. This means that the prevalence rate of magical thinking in the general community represents the minimum prevalence rates for people selected by these sets of early-warning symptoms. In other words, since we know that 51 per cent of adolescents experience magical thinking, we also know that EPPIC's pre-psychotic indicators identify at least 51 per cent of the general population of young people.

If we compare the 50 per cent prevalence rate for the pre-psychotic selection criteria with the 3 per cent prevalence rate for psychosis, we can begin to see the scale of the problem that will emerge with wide-scale implementation of pre-psychotic treatment programmes. Something like 50 per cent of young people could be targeted and treated, when only 3 per cent are at-risk. As well, it is not even certain that the selection criteria identify the 3 per cent who are actually at-risk. Perhaps the 50 per cent target group is composed wholly of people who, if left alone, would never experience psychosis.

But the outcome of the PACE research tells an even worse story. It was claimed that 40 per cent of the patients selected by these means became psychotic after six months of treatment, and 48 per cent became psychotic within twelve months. Assuming the 50 per cent prevalence rate for the selection criteria, this means that, if this program were adopted on a large scale, the rate of psychosis in the general community would be increased, by the application of six months' prophylactic treatment, from the baseline of 3 per cent to something like 20 per cent. And the longer the treatment is given, the higher the psychosis rate goes. A full year of prophylactic treatment would raise the prevalence rate of psychosis from 3 per cent to about 25 per cent.

A Very Suspicious Concept

The pseudo-authoritativeness characterising much of the literature in the early-psychosis field regularly demonstrates a lack of reflection on the part of researchers about the superficial nature of their claims. A good example of this can be found in the *Early Psychosis Training Pack*. Under the heading of 'How to achieve early recognition—triggers for considering psychosis or pre-psychosis', the training pack advises doctors dealing with adolescents and young people to be sure of '[m]aintaining a high index of suspicion—signs to look out for'.[50] This advice is followed by the 16-item list of 'Signs and Symptoms' adopted by the *Australian Clinical Guidelines for Early Psychosis* and reprinted on page 231 in this chapter. The first item on this list is 'suspiciousness'. This juxtapositioning of the idea of suspicion, first as an efficiency measure for diagnosticians and then as a sign of pathology in patients, begs the question: is it credible for psychiatrists to claim that 'suspiciousness' in young people is a sign of serious mental illness when the same psychiatrists argue that clinicians should cultivate an attitude of suspicion in themselves as an efficiency measure?

There is a certain degree of irony here, where suspicion is encouraged to uncover suspicion, which apparently escapes the authors of the training pack. But the contrariness raises an important question as to whether suspiciousness and the other putative signs and symptoms are correctly judged to be indications of an underlying serious mental illness. The authors seem to be claiming that suspicion is a worthy quality when it is used as a tool of efficiency by a person with authority, but it becomes a sign of pathology when it is found in a person of low status, or in a person who is challenging authority.

The EPPIC researchers have cited a 1938 article by D. Ewen Cameron as their original source of authority for believing that 'suspiciousness may predict subsequent psychosis'.[51] This is itself a decidedly suspicious source. Cameron is the Canadian psychiatrist who gained notoriety in the 1980s after it was revealed that he had undertaken cruel and unethical experiments on his patients during the 1950s and 1960s with funding from the CIA.[52]

Using a deep sleep technique combined with multiple daily assaults of ECT, Cameron attempted to cure schizophrenia by erasing all memory of self from his patients' minds. The CIA was apparently interested in utilising these techniques in espionage work. In 1988 the CIA acknowledged complicity in Cameron's work, when they arranged to pay $750,000 in compensation to some of the victims.[53] Cameron's exploits were the subject of a 1979 book by John Marks entitled *The Search for the Manchurian Candidate*.[54]

Cameron is perhaps the most widely discredited psychiatrist of all time, and contemporary psychiatric researchers who cite him as a source of authority for their own work demonstrate, at the very least, a deficiency of judgement. Nevertheless the Cameron-inspired symptomatology has been incorporated into the *Australian Clinical Guidelines for Early Psychosis*, in which suspiciousness is given as the leading symptom of pre-psychotic schizophrenia.[55] The linking of Cameron's name with a government-sponsored preventive medicine campaign for schizophrenia is a fairly extraordinary development.

But the deficiency of judgement regarding Cameron extends beyond merely adopting his suggestion about the use of suspiciousness as a symptom. Proponents of early psychosis repeatedly cite Cameron as the originator of the whole concept of early detection and intervention programmes for schizophrenia.[56] Patrick McGorry, the director of EPPIC, even quoted an extract of Cameron's article to lead his introductory essay to a June 1998 early-psychosis supplement he edited of the *British Journal of Psychiatry*:

> Very early schizophrenia still constitutes a relatively unexplored territory. Entry into this territory calls for new ideas on the social problems involved in bringing the early schizophrenic promptly under treatment, or where the treatment should be carried out and in what it should consist. D. Ewen Cameron (1938)[57]

In his 1938 article, Cameron wrote enthusiastically about the effectiveness of 'the newer therapeutic techniques used in schizophrenia'. But apparently unnoticed by McGorry, in its original publication form, Cameron's article was immediately followed with a commentary by the leading authority on schizophrenia at the time, Harry Stack Sullivan. Unlike McGorry, and obviously without foreknowledge of Cameron's future notoriety, Sullivan demonstrated disgust with Cameron's proposal, and issued a strong rebuttal:

> I would be very deeply disturbed if, as is implied by the last speaker [Cameron], people who show signs of personality disorders, early mental disorder of an indeterminate kind, were to be rushed through treatment with insulin, metrazol and camphor on the chance that they might otherwise have developed schizophrenia. I privately have a suspicion that might have a distinctly unfavourable effect on the general intelligence level and so on of the community.
>
> What does it mean that a person will have schizophrenia which can be detected by the intelligent layman months to years before the schizophrenia appears? In seven and half years of exclusive preoccupation with the schizophrenia problem I was unable to put my finger on anything sufficiently simple and obvious to service this purpose.[58]

Sullivan's scorn in 1938 apparently helped to knock out the idea of schizophrenia prevention for almost 60 years. But what are we to make of its recent resurrection? If it is now feasible to use the latest form of pharmacological shock—atypical neuroleptics—

perhaps it is only because there is no longer any figure in the psychiatric profession, such as Sullivan, with both a high-enough stature and a sufficiently developed social conscience to mount the necessary protest.

Subjective opinions about people, across generations, involving concepts such as 'odd beliefs or magical thinking', 'odd thinking', and 'odd appearance' are never going to lend themselves to genuine scientific research. Indeed, it would be decidedly odd if psychiatric researchers actually believed that they would. So what is going on with pre-psychotic research? Is it just well-meaning but misguided? Breggin and Cohen, for their part, have explained the anomalous nature of much psychiatric research this way: 'The sad truth is that, in the field of psychiatry, it is impossible to "trust in research". Nearly all the research in this field is paid for by drug companies and conducted by people who "deliver" in the best way possible for those companies'.[59]

Conclusion

The concept of a pre-psychotic phase of schizophrenia clearly demonstrates that psychiatrists view the symptoms of schizophrenia as being on a continuum with normal human thinking and behavioural patterns. This means that people who travel down the road towards a diagnosis of schizophrenia are likely to begin their journey within the realm of normality. The diagnosis only occurs at the point in the journey where the attention of a psychiatrist is drawn to them and observations are made that they have travelled too far from normal. This point of psychiatric interception need not be the same for everyone. There is no definitive feature on the landscape that clearly marks the boundary between normal behaviour and schizophrenic symptoms.

To illustrate the continuum from normality to schizophrenia, an analogy can be drawn with a road. Imagine a road that leads from an urban setting of tower buildings (downtown Normal), through suburbs (outer Normal), through a mixed landscape on the city fringe of suburban houses and vegetable farms (early psychosis), to pastures interspersed with bushland (schizophrenic symptoms of social/occupational dysfunction) and, eventually, by degrees, into pristine wilderness (florid psychosis). Some people go all the way down the road to the wilderness before they are intercepted psychiatrically; others only get as far as the pastures and bushland. The new plan of preventive medicine is to catch young people on the outskirts of Normal, even before they leave town.

There is a bigger picture. Globalism is a new phenomenon that is beginning to deeply affect the lives of most people on the planet. Satellite broadcasting is penetrating into remote corners of the globe, and television images have initiated most of humanity into the mass culture of consumerism. The great diversity in human cultures that once guided tribes, nations, and religious groupings in their varied approaches to life has been largely melted down into a homogenous global mind-set focussed on worship of the shopping mall and the products on sale there.

It is not at all clear what sort of brave new world we are currently constructing for ourselves, but it is likely to contain at least two features that are relevant to the problems discussed in this book. The first is that an idealised market-based approach to life is not a culture to which all humanity can happily adapt. This means that an impulse towards human diversity will continue to manifest itself at the individual level. The second is that the psychiatric profession and the pharmaceutical industry are together being positioned to play an ever-more important role in controlling the minds and behaviour of people who find it difficult to adapt to this new global culture.

In the last decades of the Soviet Union, when the communist authorities found it necessary to use psychiatry to control dissidents who could not or would not conform with their own particular brand of cultural ideology, a diagnosis of schizophrenia was found to be the most convenient method. This was because schizophrenia effectively labels non-conformists as having a serious mental disease that makes them irredeemably abnormal and potentially dangerous. Once this much is accepted about people it is relatively easy to add the corollary that it is necessary to force powerful drugs on them and imprison them in a state of permanent semi-stupor, perhaps for the rest of their lives.

To understand how Soviet psychiatrists came to be used for social control it isn't necessary to assume that their professional ethics were corrupted. They were only doing what psychiatrists do everywhere: they were identifying and 'alienating' individuals who could not be fitted into the social fabric. To do this they simply followed normal diagnostic procedures. And, as I have demonstrated, the diagnostic criteria for schizophrenia can be easily made to fit people who have the kinds of social and occupational problems that you would expect of the average misfit or dissident.

The use of psychiatry for social control is caused not so much by a deficiency in the professional ethics of psychiatrists as by the prevailing cultural attitude towards dissidence and social maladaptation. If a society does not respect the rights of social misfits, it is a fairly normal response to complement the criminal justice system with psychiatric measures as a means of controlling them. In the Soviet Union there was very little tolerance for such people. The current trend to develop early detection and intervention programmes for budding social misfits, as detailed in the preceding chapter, indicates that our own Western democracies are developing similar levels of intolerance.

I realise that many people might agree with this argument, and yet still have misgivings about my overall position. They might share my view that the diagnostic methods used for schizophrenia cast too wide a net, and that it is apparent some people are diagnosed with the condition when they only have social problems. They might also agree that measures need to be taken to ensure that diagnoses of schizophrenia are not used either for social control or for the commercial benefit of drug companies seeking captive markets. But they might go on to argue that these concerns do not negate the fact that there is still a problem to solve with 'real' schizophrenics. 'Real' schizophrenics, they might say, are people who do have a serious mental disease and do need medical treatment.

'Real' schizophrenics, or perhaps the belief in 'real' schizophrenics, is indeed still the central problem. If a lay person who believed in the concept of 'real' schizophrenia were asked to describe a sufferer of the condition, the answer would probably be—to use the analogy given above—that such a person has travelled all the way down the road to the psychotic wilderness at the end. An account might be given of a relative or friend who had been observed in full psychotic flight. It might involve a sketch of a person hallucinating, deluded, talking to voices, unpredictable, and generally being irritating, embarrassing, and frightening company. The portrayal would be of a person whose behaviour had no apparent relationship to normality. This image would be proffered as prima facie evidence that 'real' schizophrenia does exist, and that an underlying disease of some kind is the only plausible explanation of the cause.

If a psychiatrist were listening to such a conversation he or she might take the opportunity to affirm this point of view. The psychiatrist might go on to say that 'real' schizophrenics are not just recognisable in this florid state at the end of the road but, to experts with psychiatric training, they are also detectable in much earlier states of deterioration. And, at this point, we might all begin to realise that the argument had gone full circle, and that the psychiatrist was asking us not to worry our lay minds about highly specialised tasks such as diagnosing schizophrenia. The implication would be that we should simply accept the status quo and trust in the judgement of experts.

But experts—all types of professional experts—simply represent the interests of their clients. One of the paradoxes in the relationship between psychiatrists and schizophrenics is that schizophrenics are rarely seen as the clients of the psychiatrists who attend to them. Far more often, a psychiatrist's client is the State, and/or the schizophrenic's relatives. This means that when schizophrenics are in conflict with family or authorities, which is usually what brings them to the attention of psychiatrists, their psychiatrist will be representing the interests of their opponents. This raises the question as to whether the disease model used to explain schizophrenia might be a professional service supplied by psychiatrists to ease the minds of their clients.

Relatives, friends, and authorities are usually desperate for some kind of professional advice when they form a perception that a person who has not broken the law needs to be controlled. They might be uncertain about the best method of achieving their goal, and might also feel anxious about the breach of trust and the violation of civil liberties involved. It is not hard to see that the most compelling way in which a psychiatrist can relieve these doubts is by explaining that the behaviour in need of control is caused by a disease. The schizophrenic is then controlled with powerful drugs, the psychiatrist has provided a professional service, the clients' problems of guilt and confusion have been solved, and everyone can carry on as normal—everyone, that is, except the person diagnosed with schizophrenia. And the only reason the schizophrenic can't be normal is because he or she has apparently developed an incurable disease. But, at least, everyone can be comforted in the belief that the best possible medical treatment has been made available.

However, what relatives, friends, and authorities are not told is that there is no scientific evidence to support the psychiatric explanation that the person in need of control has a diseased mind. Instead, the medical explanation of schizophrenic symptoms is based on four unproven, interdependent assumptions:

- The nosological (classification) assumption that the wide variety of schizophrenic symptoms all point to a discrete, underlying 'mental disease';
- The aetiological (causal) assumption that the underlying cause of the symptoms is accessible to scientific investigation and will eventually be revealed;
- The diagnostic assumption that psychiatrists can use schizophrenic symptoms to accurately and uniformly detect the presence of this unknown underlying disease in individual patients, without the aid of laboratory tests; and
- The treatment assumption that neuroleptic drugs are an appropriate way of treating the symptoms, even though the cause remains unknown.

When they are examined in detail, all of these assumptions are doubtful. To begin with, schizophrenia does not fit the conventional notions of 'disease'. Indeed, an analysis of its history reveals that it was brought into existence through a long process of compromise and professional consensus-building amongst psychiatrists. This consensus-building was so successful that schizophrenia has managed to exist in the minds of psychiatrists for more than one hundred years without any scientific verification. The 'disease' interpretation of schizophrenic symptoms is still an unconfirmed hypothesis that relies on faith rather than hard scientific evidence to support it.

This faith is enough to maintain the medical consensus, but it is still only considered an interim measure by psychiatrists. The quest for scientific evidence about the cause has been something of a holy grail for psychiatric researchers over the past century, and a virtual army is currently engaged on the search. But they are pursuing so many widely divergent threads of inquiry that, of necessity, most of them have to be dead-ends. Not only that, but the methods these researchers are forced to use are decidedly unscientific.

Research into the cause essentially involves taking groups of schizophrenics and looking for a common denominator that makes them different from normal people. This means, apart from anything else, that the legitimacy of the research is reliant on the accuracy of the schizophrenia diagnoses of the subjects used in the research. If the diagnoses are inaccurate, and the subjects are not all of the same type, no common denominator can be found. Similarly, the value of the research also depends on schizophrenic subjects being otherwise healthy. If they have other mental/brain diseases, as well as schizophrenia, the search for the cause of schizophrenia will be confounded.

A good reason to be sceptical about the scientific basis of this aetiological research is the inability of researchers to find groups of schizophrenic subjects that meet these requirements. The diagnostic methods used to detect schizophrenia, with no support from laboratory tests, mean that there is no certainty that all the members of a group are of the same type. Different psychiatrists at different places and different times might have decided that each member of a group has schizophrenic symptoms. But the diagnostic methods used will have been varied, highly personalised, and subjective. The symptoms identified will not necessarily be the same ones, and the degree of severity of the symptoms might vary considerably. On top of this, all the members of a schizophrenic cohort assembled for research purposes will have, of necessity, varying degrees of disturbance in their brain chemistry as a result of the neuroleptic medication used to treat their schizophrenia.

These inevitable circumstances mean that the only common denominators amongst any research group of schizophrenics are likely to be a shared stigma of having been branded as mental patients and a common history of having been treated with neuroleptic drugs. Yet despite the unsuitability of schizophrenic subjects for use in scientific research, investigations into the cause of schizophrenia cannot proceed without them. This is because their living, human forms are the only evidence that schizophrenia exists. As a result, all the claims of 'promising' leads that come out of this type of research—such as divergent patterns in brain waves and malformations in brain architecture—are scientifically very doubtful, at best. In most cases, these results are much better explained as artefacts of the neuroleptic drugs used for treating schizophrenia, rather than as indications of the underlying cause of schizophrenia itself.

This problem of confusing schizophrenia with the effects of schizophrenia treatment extends beyond aetiological research. Normally, schizophrenics are promptly medicated upon first diagnosis. This means that psychiatrists generally have a very narrow window of opportunity through which to observe the symptoms of never-medicated schizophrenics. Most psychiatric knowledge about the nature of schizophrenia and the behaviour of schizophrenics is derived from observing medicated schizophrenics.

Once applied, neuroleptic drugs quickly suppress the diverse and bizarre schizophrenic symptoms for which the person was diagnosed, and then replace them with the relatively homogeneous and medically comprehensible symptoms of neuroleptic intoxication and neuroleptic-induced movement disorders. These drug-induced disorders are true medical problems, and they provide the common denominators of pathology which help to persuade psychiatrists that they are treating a discrete disease entity. The drug-induced movement disorders also help to convince relatives and friends that the person is indeed seriously ill.

Very few contemporary psychiatrists attempt to treat newly diagnosed schizophrenics without drugs. Those who do, such as John Weir Perry, interpret the cause of the symptoms very differently from their drug-treating colleagues. They tend to find that 'real' schizophrenics—that is, people who are deluded and hallucinating and in the midst of a florid psychosis—are not diseased, but are undergoing a spiritual/mystical emergency. Perry found that when he gave these people the right sort of supportive environment they would recover completely, without medical treatment, in about six weeks.

This brings me to the point of this book, which is to provide the basis for a simple argument: involuntary medical treatment for people with schizophrenic symptoms is wrong. It is wrong factually, because there is no scientific evidence to confirm the existence of an underlying mental disease in need of treatment; it is wrong ethically, because it violates basic human rights; and it is wrong spiritually, because it robs people of their vision of life's meaning.

Stating this wrong is not particularly difficult; righting it is another matter, of enormous proportions. It isn't simply a matter of stating the 'truth'. Anyone who has taken up one side or the other of a religious debate knows that it is not possible to prove conclusively to a committed believer that something does not exist. This is particularly so when a belief is as deeply embedded in the culture as the medical explanation for schizophrenic symptoms.

Not only is the cultural belief deeply embedded, but it is constantly reinforced with skilfully directed public-relations campaigning. Vested interests such as drug companies have very good reasons to ensure that it remains deeply embedded. The worldwide market for schizophrenia drugs is now a multi-billion dollar industry.

The ethical aspect of this wrong also involves deeply embedded attitudes. Although it is fairly simple to show that involuntary treatment for schizophrenia violates basic human rights, it is far more difficult to interest human rights watchdog groups in the problem. From my own experience, I have found that presenting human rights organisations with sound arguments for why they should take action against psychiatric coercion can even do more harm than good.

This was evident recently, for instance, when I attempted to raise the issue of psychiatric coercion with the Australian Human Rights and Equal Opportunity Commission. At the time, the Commission was preparing legislative recommendations to protect the freedom of religion and belief in Australia, and was seeking advice from interested parties. Despite (or because of) my extensive submission, the problem of psychiatric coercion was ignored in the Commission's recommendations. Even worse, to ensure that lawmakers would not allow human rights to interfere with continued psychiatric coercion, a definition of 'belief' was provided which specifically excludes from protection any 'beliefs which are caused by mental illness'.[1] It seems to me that my submission might have simply alerted the Commission to a perceived need to recommend protection against the very type of human rights challenge I had urged them to make.

When I questioned the recommendation with a high-ranking official, a carefully prepared response was given. I was told that the Human Rights Commission believed in the existence of mental illness, and believed that mentally ill people have two kinds of belief: those which are manifestations of mental illness, and which are not protected by articles of human rights law; and those which are not manifestations of mental illness, and which are protected by Article 18 of the ICCPR. The Human Rights Commission is apparently willing to allow psychiatrists to determine whether particular beliefs are protected or not, depending on whether they are deemed to be manifestations of mental illness. When I explained that psychiatric drug treatment did not selectively target the supposed symptoms of mental illness, leaving other thoughts and beliefs unaffected, the official had no prepared response.

It seems to me that human rights organisations in the Western democracies have become so accustomed to associating human rights problems with non-democratic political systems that they are incapable of directing their vigilance to their own backyards. As a consequence, they tend to give knee-jerk support to all the cultural values of the democratic societies from which they arose. This means turning a blind eye to the use of psychiatric coercion for social control. For the time being, therefore, the human rights arguments that have been presented in this book are most useful as rhetorical tools in public debate, rather than as legal devices to be used in law courts. Although they can be used to clearly establish the moral ascendancy of people who want to refuse forced psychiatric treatment, they do not provide—under prevailing social conditions—the means for legal redress.

The third and final aspect of the wrong that is intrinsic to involuntary treatment, and which is at the heart of this book, is the spiritual aspect. This is the wrong that is caused when a person is thwarted in an attempt to grasp some personal insight about the meaning of his or her life. The mass culture guiding the direction of the new world order largely locates the meaning of human existence in the commercial marketplace. Life is a struggle to work, and to buy, and to sell. We have families so we can rear children to do the same. Underneath the cacophony of lifestyles and choices that are endlessly available, there is little that is culturally valued that does not point in the direction of the marketplace and consumerism.

Anyone who even begins to think about the possibility of there being a deeper or alternative meaning to life is going to look a little weird to those who conform. Almost by definition, someone who believes that he or she has found some alternative meaning, through internal revelation, is mentally disordered. Perhaps a way of making sense of the road out of Normal, and of how it relates to a diagnosis of schizophrenia, is to look at it this way: a person on the outskirts of Normal, with pre-psychotic symptoms, is a young person with an inclination to look for an alternative meaning in life; someone intercepted halfway down the road, who has become socially alienated, is one who is actively seeking an alternative meaning; and someone in the midst of a florid psychosis, in the wilderness at the end of the road, is a person who thinks he or she has found an alternative meaning, through some kind of direct revelation.

This analogy will probably raise the question of 'real' schizophrenia once again in the minds of some readers. Anyone who has spent any time with a person in the midst of this type of 'revelation' at the end of the road, and who knows how extreme it can be, might find the analogy naive. This is particularly so if readers have witnessed a young person seeming to fall into psychosis quite suddenly, without any prior indication of having embarked on a spiritual quest. The quest for meaning in life might sound like a noble and worthwhile pursuit, to which everybody should have a right of access. But, to unprepared observers, florid psychosis usually appears to be a thoroughly degrading experience; and to suggest that it has redeeming qualities might seem absurd. Yet this is exactly what John Weir Perry found to be the case in regard to his patients at Diabasis. Joseph Campbell, the mythologist, also saw merit in the experience of psychosis. From his angle, this was the same mystical experience that mythological heroes undergo.

The problem for young people in our contemporary society, who stumble into it accidentally, is that they are untrained and unprepared for its rigours. This is why it degrades them. It is not so much the nature of the experience that is degrading, but the fact that people enter it without tutoring and support from experts who understand it. This is the very problem that both Laing and Perry sought to redress by setting up refuges for schizophrenics, staffed with spiritual guides who had themselves successfully negotiated the experience.

It might be that Perry exaggerated his success in using this method. Perhaps, in truth, a substantial fraction of people who enter into a spiritual/mystical emergency do not have whatever it takes to successfully emerge on the other side. Perhaps, despite the lack of scientific evidence, there is even a type of schizophrenic who has an incurable underlying disease of the mind or brain, after the fashion hypothesised by psychiatrists, who cannot possibly benefit from the assistance of spiritual guides. But, even if these possibilities are true, I am still convinced that most of the people who are diagnosed with schizophrenia, when they are floridly psychotic, do not have a disease but are in fact undergoing a spiritual/mystical emergency. Further, I am convinced that, under the right conditions, they can emerge from this psychological crisis with a deeper understanding about the meaning of their lives.

This finally brings me to the point at which I can try to describe the type of reform that I think should be undertaken in order to correct the brutality and ignorance that currently dominates the treatment of people diagnosed with schizophrenia.

The first reform necessary is to alter the diagnostic criteria so that only people who are in an acute psychological crisis—what I have been describing as florid psychosis—may be called schizophrenic. These are the people who have gone all the way to the end of the road out of Normal, and have become lost in the wilderness. People who are observed at other stages of the road, who only have social and occupational problems, should not be diagnosed with schizophrenia. Changes must be made to the diagnostic criteria so that these types of people are specifically excluded. It is a misuse of psychiatric power to justify intercepting them by claiming that they are at risk of becoming psychotic.

This is not to deny that some of them may well continue down the road to psychosis. But which ones? All car drivers are at risk of motor accidents, too. Should they all be dragged out of their cars to prevent some of them having accidents? Why should it be assumed that a person is heading for a psychological crisis simply because he or she wants to explore beyond the city limits of Normal? Pre-psychotic preventive medicine programmes for schizophrenia should be stopped dead in their tracks. They have the potential to do enormous harm to human individuality and diversity.

The second reform is concerned with the mental health system that handles people who have become floridly psychotic. When a person becomes psychotic for the first time, it is usual for them to pass fairly rapidly through a catchment system that ends in a psychiatric ward. Here the person is observed and diagnosed, and drug treatment is commenced. If the person is undergoing a spiritual/mystical emergency, the drugs begin to interfere with the continuity of the experience—as they are intended to do—and the person loses contact with the source of inner revelation. Most of the people who go through this drug-induced psychic abortion will never get the opportunity to properly reconnect with their true inner world again. If, at a later time, they once again become psychotic, their natural brain chemistry will have been altered by drugs, their self-identities will have been debased by labelling with mental disease and, as a result, their inner experiences will be clouded with doubt, confusion, and impurities.

What I have in mind to correct this problem is the addition of an extra filter to the standard procedures that are currently followed. People who develop the symptoms of florid psychosis already pass through one very important filter under the current standard practices. This is the medical filter at the point of diagnosis. One of the problems that complicates the handling of psychotic people is the existence of a number of disorders that are clearly medical in nature, with symptoms that overlap those of schizophrenia. Diagnostic conventions require psychiatrists to consider a variety of alternative complaints to ensure that a candidate-for-diagnosis does not have one of these. Under the heading of Differential Diagnosis, DSM-IV offers the following advice to diagnosticians:

> A wide variety of general medical conditions can present with psychotic symptoms. **Psychotic Disorder Due to a General Medical Condition, delirium,** or **dementia** is diagnosed when there is evidence from the history, physical examination, or laboratory tests that indicates that the delusions or hallucinations are the direct physiological consequence of a general medical condition (for example, Cushing's syndrome, brain tumor). **Substance-Induced Psychotic Disorder, Substance-Induced**

Delirium, and **Substance-Induced Persisting Dementia** are distinguished from Schizophrenia by the fact that a substance (for example, a drug of abuse, a medication, or exposure to a toxin) is judged to be etiologically related to the delusions or hallucinations. Many different types of **Substance-Related Disorders** may produce symptoms similar to those of Schizophrenia (for example, sustained amphetamine or cocaine use may produce delusions or hallucinations; phencyclidine may produce a mixture of positive and negative symptoms).[2]

I am proposing that the current practice of first-stop medical assessment of psychotic people should be retained. The objective of this medical assessment is to filter out people whose psychosis is caused by known diseases so they can be given the appropriate medical attention. The change of policy I am proposing comes after schizophrenia is diagnosed. At this point, instead of commencing neuroleptic drug treatment, the person should be referred on to a residential facility modelled along the lines of John Weir Perry's Diabasis.

This drug-free residential facility would act as a second filter so that people undergoing a spiritual/mystical emergency could be distinguished from a hypothetical residue of 'real' schizophrenics. Here, people in the midst of psychological crisis would be given every opportunity and support to help them through what would be assumed to be (until proven otherwise) a spiritual/mystical emergency. The advice and attention of non-psychiatrists, who had themselves been through the experience, would be an important component. These arrangements need not exclude psychiatric supervision. Indeed, psychiatric supervision would probably be necessary if such a facility were to be seen as a filter attached to the mainstream mental-health catchment system.

If there were people who clearly could not benefit from this type of supportive treatment, they would form a separate group. Assessments of the members of this group would have to be made to ensure that their continuing problems were not caused by limitations in the facility, and in difficulties conforming to its rules and restrictions. Perhaps within such a hypothetical residual group the elusive 'real' schizophrenic, with the underlying disease, might at last be recognisable.

But the question of how to properly define this hypothetical residual group, and how to best treat them, is not something that can be sensibly guessed at here. If this second filter of a spiritual/mystical emergency refuge were to be added to the current mental health model, the one thing that is certain is that most of the people who develop florid psychoses would emerge from their psychological crisis in much better shape. As a result, there would be enormous social benefits from the creative input of those who had recovered, as well as long-term cost savings on disability pensions and government-subsidised medication.

The main obstacles that can be envisaged to running a trial of an extra filter such as this are only the obvious ones—the vested interests that stand to lose. These are the transnational drug companies, the biomedically oriented elements of the psychiatric profession, and those people and institutions that are already committed to a brave new world order of mass conformity.

Endnotes

Introduction
1. Peter Macdonald, 'Mental Health Support and Counselling Services'.

Chapter One
1. Anthony Browne, Health Editor, 'Doctors could soon prescribe behaviour-controlling chemicals to pre-teens against their parents' wishes'.
2. John R. Clayer et al., 'Prevalence of psychiatric disorders in rural South Australia', pp. 124–8.
3. Ronald Leifer, 'The Medical Model as the Ideology of the Therapeutic State', pp. 247–58.
4. Gareth Williams and Jennie Popay, 'Lay Knowledge and the Privilege of Experience', p. 118.
5. Stuart A. Kirk and Herb Kutchins, *The Selling of DSM: The Rhetoric of Science in Psychiatry*, pp. 4–5.
6. G. L. Klerman, 'The Advantages of DSM III', p. 539.
7. L. J. Davis, 'Diagnostic and Statistical Manual of Mental Disorders, 4th ed.', *Harper's Magazine*, p. 61.
8. American Psychiatric Association, *Diagnostic and Statistical Manual of Mental Disorders*, fourth edition, (DSM IV), pp. 646–7.
9. Michele T. Pathe and Paul E. Mullen, 'The Dangerousness of the DSM-III-R', p. 48.
10. Kirk and Kutchins, *op. cit.*, p. 60.
11. *Ibid.*, pp. 8–9.
12. Schizophrenia Information Centre, 'Schizophrenia: the early signs'.
13. Andrew T. Russell, 'The Clinical Presentation of Childhood-Onset Schizophrenia', *Schizophrenia Bulletin*, pp. 631–46.
14. *Ibid.*, p. 631.
15. *Ibid.*, p. 632.
16. Robert Wright, 'The Biology of Violence', pp. 68–77.
17. Human Rights and Equal Opportunity Commission, *Human Rights and Mental Illness*, p. 855.
18. Kathleen McKenna et al., pp. 636–45.
19. American Psychiatric Association, *op. cit.*, pp. 85–6.
20. Harold I. Kaplan and Benjamin J. Sadock, *Synopsis of Psychiatry: behavioural sciences, clinical psychology*, pp. 798–9.

21 Human Rights and Equal Opportunity Commission, *op. cit*, p. 857.
22 Richard Warner, *Recovery From Schizophrenia*, pp. 35, 132.
23 Thomas Szasz, *Cruel Compassion: psychiatric control of society's unwanted*, p. 145.
24 American Psychiatric Association, *op. cit.*, p. 7.
25 *Ibid.*, pp. 277–8.
26 World Health Organisation, *The ICD-10 Classification of Mental Disorders and Behavioral Disorders: Clinical Descriptions and Diagnostic Guidelines*, p. 95.
27 Philip E. T. Lewis and Paul Koshy, "Youth employment, unemployment and school participation', p. 42.
28 Human Rights and Equal Opportunity Commission, *op. cit.*, p. 846.
29 Mental Health Review Tribunal, *Annual Report,* pp. 13, 17, 20.
30 *Ibid.,* p. 20.
31 Mental Health Review Tribunal, *Annual Report*, 1992, p. 91.
32 *Ibid.*, 1995, p. 58.
33 *Ibid.*, 1998, p. 70.
34 *Ibid.*, 1994, p. 41.
35 *Ibid.*, 1995, p. 28.
36 *Ibid.*, 1998, p. 47.
37 *Ibid.*, 1995, p. 20.
38 Reuter Information Service, *Drugmakers look for home-runs with schizophrenia drugs.*
39 Arthur Kleinman and Alex Cohen, 'Psychiatry's Global Challenge', *Scientific American*, March 1997.
40 Robert Jay Lifton, *The Nazi Doctors: medical killing and the psychology of genocide,* p. 46.
41 *Ibid.,* pp. 34, 134–44.
42 United Nations, 'International Covenant on Economic, Social and Cultural Rights', Article 12 (1), p. 16.
43 J. K. Wing, 'Psychiatry in the Soviet Union', p. 435.
44 David Cohen, *Soviet Psychiatry: politics and mental health in the USSR today*, pp. 24, 44.
45 A. L. Halpern, 'Current Dilemmas in the Aftermath of the US Delegation's Inspection of the Soviet Psychiatric Hospitals', p. 11.
46 C. Shaw, 'The World Psychiatric Association and Soviet Psychiatry', p. 50.
47 K. W. M. Fulford, A. Y. U. Smirnov and E. Snow, 'Concepts of Disease and the Abuse of Psychiatry in the USSR', pp. 801–810.
48 Yo Kubota, 'The Institutional Response', p. 115.
49 United Nations, 'Principles for the Protection of Persons with Mental Illness and for the Improvement of Mental Health Care', pp. 989–1005.
50 *Ibid.*, Principle 11, pp. 994–995.
51 New South Wales Parliament, *NSW Mental Health Act 1990, Reprinted as in force at 17 October,* Section 9, p. 5.
52 United Nations, 'Principles for the Protection of Persons with Mental Illness

and for the Improvement of Mental Health Care', Principle 16, p. 1000.
53   *Ibid.*, Principle 4, p. 992.
54   Brian Burdekin, Federal Human Rights Commissioner, opening address to Sydney hearings, National Inquiry into Human Rights and Mental Illness, 17 June 1991, personal observation.
55   Human Rights and Equal Opportunity Commission, *op. cit.*, p. 5.
56   Leonard Roy Frank, 'An Interview with Bruce Ennis', in Sherry Hirsch, Joe Adams, Leonard Frank, Wade Hudson and David Richman (eds), *Madness Network News Reader*, p. 165.
57   Human Rights and Equal Opportunity Commission, *op. cit.*, p. 13.

Chapter Two

1   German E. Berrios, *The History of Mental Symptoms*, p. 85.
2   Arnulphe d'Aumont, 1754, quoted in Berrios, *ibid.*
3   Vincenzo Chiarugi, quoted in Berrios, *ibid.*, p. 86.
4   Thomas Hobbes, quoted in Berrios, *ibid.*, pp. 86–87.
5   John Locke, quoted in Berrios, *ibid.*, p. 88.
6   David Hartley, quoted in Berrios, *ibid.*, pp. 88–89.
7   Jean Francois Dufor, quoted in Berrios, *ibid.*, p. 35.
8   Berrios, *ibid.*, p. 35.
9   E. Esquirol, quoted in Berrios, *ibid.*, p. 37.
10 *Ibid.*
11 *Ibid.*
12 *Ibid.*, pp. 37–8.
13 J. Baillarger, quoted in Berrios, *ibid.*, p. 39.
14 C. F. Michéa, quoted in Berrios, *ibid.*
15 Berrios, *ibid.*, p. 40.
16 Berrios, *ibid.*, p. 72.
17 *Ibid.*
18 Richard Warner, *Recovery From Schizophrenia*, p. 10.
19 Nancy C. Andreasen et al., 'Regional brain abnormalities in schizophrenia measured with magnetic resonance imaging', pp. 1763–70.
20 Warner, *op. cit.*, p. 14.
21 Eugen Bleuler, *Dementia Praecox or the Group of Schizophrenias*, pp. 13, 14.
22 *Ibid.*, p. 13.
23 *Ibid.*, p. 15.
24 *Ibid.*, p. 22.
25 R. D. Laing, *The Politics of Experience*.
26 Fred R. Volkmar, 'Childhood and adolescent psychosis: a review of the past 10 years', pp. 843–52.
27 Loren J. Chapman and Jean P. Chapman, *Disordered Thought in Schizophrenia*, p. 208.
28 Donald W. Black et al., 'Schizophrenia, Schizophreniform Disorder, and Delusional (Paranoid) Disorders', p. 358.
29 World Health Organisation, *The ICD-10 Classification of Mental Disorders*

      and Behavioral Disorders: Clinical Descriptions and Diagnostic Guidelines.
30   American Psychiatric Association, *Diagnostic and Statistical Manual of Mental Disorders.*
31   *Ibid.*, p. xxi.
32   *Ibid.*, p. 273.
33   *Ibid.*, p. 770.
34   *Ibid.*, p. 274.
35   World Health Organisation, *op. cit.*, p. 86.
36   *Ibid.*
37   *Ibid.*, p. 87.
38   American Psychiatric Association, *op. cit.*, p. 275.
39   *Ibid.*
40   *Ibid.*
41   *Ibid.*, p. 276.
42   *Ibid.*
43   *Ibid.*
44   *Ibid.*
45   *Ibid.*, p. 277.
46   *Ibid.*, pp. 285–6.
47   *Ibid.*, p. 284.
48   *Ibid.*, p. 765.
49   *Ibid.*, p. 297.
50   *Ibid.*
51   'Delusions' is one of five symptoms specified in the NSW Mental Health Act which, if identified by a medical practitioner, can lead to involuntary incarceration and treatment. See New South Wales Parliament, *Mental Health Act 1990.*
52   American Psychiatric Association, *op. cit.*, p. 765.
53   *Ibid.*, p. 297.
54   Jenny J. van Drimmelen-Krabbe et al., 'Homosexuality in the International Classification of Diseases: a clarification', p. 1660.
55   Lawrie Reznek, *The Nature of Disease*, p. 98.
56   *Ibid.*, p. 100.
57   Jacqueline Messite and Steven D. Stellman, 'Accuracy of death certificate completion: the need for formalized physician training', pp. 794–7.
58   Reznek, *op. cit.*, p. 208.
59   Royal College of Psychiatrists, 'Stereotypical attitudes towards Christian names and gender may influence diagnosis'.

Chapter Three

1   Norman L. Keltner, 'Schizophrenia and Other Psychoses', in Norman L. Keltner et al., (eds.), *Psychiatric Nursing*, p. 367.
2   Harold I. Kaplan and Benjamin J. Sadock, *Synopsis of Psychiatry*, p. 639.
3   David Richman, 'Pursuing Psychiatric Pill Pushers', p. 113. (For a more extensive description of the effects of neuroleptics, see Chapter 6.)

4 American Psychiatric Association, *Diagnostic and Statistical Manual of Mental Disorders (DSM)*, Fourth Edition, pp. 735–51.
5 *Ibid.*, p. 743.
6 *Ibid.*, p. 745.
7 *Ibid.*, pp. 747–9.
8 *Ibid.*, p. 748.
9 Moisey Wolf et al., 'Clozapine Treatment in Russia: A Review of Clinical Research', p. 256.
10 Peter Breggin, *Toxic Psychiatry*, p. 106.
11 Keltner et al., *op. cit.*, p. 245.
12 M. Weatherall, 'An end to the search for new drugs', p. 387.
13 Breggin, *op. cit.*, p. 447.
14 Sandoz has since merged with Ciba-Geigy and the new conglomerate is named Novartis.
15 Keltner et al., *op. cit.*, pp. 245–6.
16 Kaplan and Sadock, *op. cit.*, p. 648.
17 Breggin, *op. cit.*, p. 105.
18 Wolf et al., *op. cit.*, pp. 256, 258.
19 T. M. Shiovitz et al., 'Cholinergic rebound and rapid onset psychosis following abrupt clozapine withdrawal', pp. 591–5.
20 Daniel R. Weinberger, 'From neuropathology to neurodevelopment', pp. 552–8.
21 R. Sandyk et al., 'Atrophy of the Cerebellar Vermis: relevance to the symptoms of schizophrenia', pp. 205–12.
22 Nancy C. Andreasen et al., 'Regional brain abnormalities in schizophrenia measured with magnetic resonance imaging', pp. 1763–70.
23 B. Bower, 'Brain Anatomy Yields Schizophrenia Clues', p. 182.
24 *Ibid.*
25 D. B. Double, 'Understanding Schizophrenia'.
26 Thomas Szasz, *Schizophrenia: The Sacred Symbol of Psychiatry*, p. 7.
27 R. L. O'Reilly, 'Viruses and Schizophrenia', pp. 222–8.
28 E. F. Torrey, 'Viral-Anatomical Explanation of Schizophrenia', pp. 15–18.
29 M. A. Coggiano et al., 'The Continued Search for Evidence of Retroviral Infection in Schizophrenic Patients', pp. 243–7.
30 J. A. Richt et al., 'Failure to detect Borna disease virus infection in peripheral blood leukocytes from humans with psychiatric disorders', pp. 174–8.
31 G. Rubinstein, 'Schizophrenia, Infection and Temperature. An Animal Model For Investigating Their Interrelationships', pp. 95–102.
32 R. F. Squires, 'How a poliovirus might cause schizophrenia: a commentary on Eagles' hypothesis', pp. 647–56.
33 J. O. Davis and H. S. Bracha, 'Famine and schizophrenia: first-trimester malnutrition or second-trimester beriberi', pp. 1–3.
34 H. W. Hoek et al., 'Schizoid personality disorder after prenatal exposure to famine', pp. 1637–9.
35 A. S. Brown et al., 'Neurobiological plausibility of prenatal nutritional dep-

rivation as a risk factor for schizophrenia', pp. 71–85.
36 E. Susser et al., 'Schizophrenia after prenatal famine. Further evidence', pp. 25–31.
37 R. S. Smith, 'The GI T-lymphocyte theory of schizophrenia: some new observations', pp. 27–30.
38 Brian Hyfryd, 'Neglect of the Body to the Detriment of the Patient: Management Notes', pp. 47–53.
39 James S. Howard, 'Requiem For Schizophrenia', pp. 148–55.
40 S. M. Ko, and T. C. Liu, 'Psychiatric syndromes in pernicious anaemia—a case report', pp. 92–94.
41 Breggin, op. cit., p. 122.
42 Mark Bowden, 'Study finds evidence for gene that may help cause schizophrenia,, p. 501.
43 Mark Bowden, 'Top human geneticists argue over ownership of schizophrenia research', p. 511.
44 K. C. Murphy et al., 'The molecular genetics of schizophrenia', pp. 147–57.
45 Peter McGuffin et al., 'Genetic basis of schizophrenia', pp. 678–83.
46 S. L. Varma, et al., 'Psychiatric morbidity in the first-degree relatives of schizophrenic patients', pp. 7–11.
47 P. J. Tienari and L. C. Wynne, 'Adoption studies of schizophrenia', pp. 233–37.
48 S. S. Kety et al., 'Mental illness in the biologic and adoptive families of adoptive individuals who have become schizophrenic: a preliminary report based on psychiatric interviews', pp. 147–65.
49 Donald W. Black et al., 'Schizophrenia, Schizophreniform Disorder, and Delusional (Paranoid) Disorders', p. 379.
50 Breggin, op. cit., pp. 118–121.
51 Jay Joseph, 'The Genetic Theory of Schizophrenia: a critical overview', pp. 119–45.
52 Ibid., p. 123.
53 Ibid., p. 126.
54 Ibid., pp. 126, 136–137.
55 Michael Owen and Peter McGuffin, 'The molecular genetics of schizophrenia: blind alleys, acts of faith, and difficult science', pp. 664–6.
56 Sigmund Freud, 'Psycho-analytic Notes on an Autobiographical Account of a Case of Paranoia (Dementia Paranoides)', *The Standard Edition of the Complete Psychological Works of Sigmund Freud*, pp. 3–82.
57 Black et al., op. cit., p. 380.
58 Jane Pearce, 'Harry Stack Sullivan: theory and practice', pp. 159–66.
59 Harry Stack Sullivan, *Schizophrenia as a Human Process*.
60 Harry Stack Sullivan, 'Erogenous Maturation', pp. 1–15.
61 Frieda Fromm-Reichman, 'Notes on the Development of Treatment of Schizophrenics by Psychoanalytic Psychotherapy', pp. 263–73.
62 Gordon Parker, 'Re-searching the schizophrenogenic mother', pp. 452–62.
63 Carol Eadie Hartwell, 'The schizophrenogenic mother concept in American

psychiatry', pp. 274–97.
64 Betty Friedan, *The Feminine Mystique*.
65 Stella Chess, 'The "blame the mother" ideology', pp. 95–107.
66 B. Ehrenreich, and D. English, *For Her Own Good*, p. 241.
67 Frank Simmers and Froma Walsh, 'The nature of the symbiotic bond between mother and schizophrenic', pp. 484–94.
68 Parker, *op.cit.*
69 Humphry Osmond, 'Dangerous psychosocial hypotheses', pp. 216–18.
70 Otto F. Wahl, 'Schizophrenogenic parenting in abnormal psychology textbooks', pp. 31–33.
71 Gregory Bateson et al., 'Towards a Theory of Schizophrenia'.
72 *Ibid.*, p. 15.
73 *Ibid.*, p. 18.
74 *Ibid.*, p. 8.
75 Bateson et al., *op. cit.*, p. 6
76 *Ibid.*, pp. 9, 10.
77 Susan L. Jones, 'The "damned if you do and damned if you don't" concept: The double bind as a tested theoretical formulation', pp. 162–9.
78 David M. Dush and Marvin Brodsky, 'Effects and implications of the experimental double bind', pp. 895–900.
79 Theodore Lidz et al., *Schizophrenia and the Family*, pp. 142–5.
80 *Ibid.*, p. 249.
81 Julian Leff, 'Social and Psychological Causes of the Acute Attack', p. 143.
82 Lidz et al., *op. cit.*, pp. 136–42, 264.
83 Leff, *op. cit.*, p. 143.
84 Theodore Lidz, 'Patients whose children became schizophrenic', pp. 408–11.
85 Leff, *op. cit.*, p. 144.
86 *Ibid.*, p. 145.
87 Deborah J. Lieber, 'Parental focus of attention in a videotape feedback task as a function of hypothesised risk for offspring schizophrenia', pp. 467–75.
88 N. M. Docherty, 'Communication deviance, attention, and schizotypy in parents of schizophrenic patients', pp. 750–56.
89 K. E. Wahlberg et al., 'Gene-environment interaction in vulnerability to schizophrenia: findings from the Finnish Adoptive Family Study of Schizophrenia', pp. 355–62.
90 Ian R. Falloon, 'Family stress and schizophrenia: Theory and practice', pp. 165–82.
91 William L. Cook et al., 'Expressed emotion and reciprocal affective relationships in families of disturbed adolescents', pp. 337–48.
92 Parker, *op. cit.*, pp. 452–62.
93 Froma W. Walsh, 'Concurrent grandparent death and birth of schizophrenic offspring: An intriguing finding', pp. 457–63.
94 Graziano Canton and Ida G. Fraccon, 'Life events and schizophrenia: A replication', pp. 211–16.
95 Hugh Freeman, 'Schizophrenia and city residence', pp. 39–50.

⁹⁶ D. Bhugra et al., 'Incidence and outcome of schizophrenia in whites, African-Caribbeans and Asians in London', pp. 791–98.
⁹⁷ Theodore R. Sarbin, 'Towards the Obsolescence of the Schizophrenia Hypothesis', p. 264.

Chapter Four

1. Anne Brown and Rebecca Weaver, 'Promising New Medications in Development'.
2. M. S. Humphreys et al., 'Dangerous Behaviour Preceding First Admission for Schizophrenia', pp. 501–5.
3. T. G. McGuire, 'Measuring the Economic Costs of Schizophrenia', pp. 375–88.
4. Richard Jed Wyatt et al., *An Economic Evaluation of Schizophrenia—1991*.
5. Ibid.
6. Loren R. Mosher, 'Are Psychiatrists Betraying Their Patients?', p. 40.
7. Ibid.
8. Ibid.
9. Stephen R. Marder and Richard C. Meibach, 'Risperidone in the treatment of schizophrenia', p. 825.
10. Editorial, *Science News*, Vol. 145, No. 25, 18 June 1994, p. 398.
11. Keith Hoeller, 'Psychiatric Drugs Harm Children'.
12. Ken Silverstein, 'Prozac.org: an influential mental health nonprofit finds its "grassroots" watered by pharmaceutical millions'.
13. Anne Deveson, 'Help for Families', p. 5.
14. SANE Australia, *Carers Handbook*, p. 26.
15. See for example, *SANE News*, Issue 9, Spring 1998, p. 8.
16. Silverstein, *op. cit.*
17. Dr Inge Southcott, 'Anguish over mental health Catch 22'.
18. Anne Deveson, 'Towards a better treatment of serious mental illness'.
19. Dr Kathleen Bocce, 'Mental health patients' families have few rights'.
20. Dr Robert Dixon, Letter to the editor.
21. Peter Macdonald, 'Mental Health Support and Counselling Services', *NSW Legislative Assembly Hansard*, 7 June 1995.
22. Ibid.
23. Dr. Refshauge, *Ibid.*
24. Inge Southcott, Letter to Peter Macdonald April 1994, quoted by Peter Macdonald in 'Mental Health Bill', *NSW Legislative Assembly Hansard*, 26 October 1995, p. 1.
25. Peter Macdonald, 'Mental Health Bill', *op. cit.*, p. 1.
26. Anne Deveson, *Tell Me I'm Here,* facing-cover page.
27. The Mental Health Act Implementation Monitoring Committee, *Report to the Honourable R. A. Phillips MP, Minister for Health on the NSW Mental Act 1990*, 'Preface', August 1992.
28. Ian W. Webster, Chairman of the Mental Health Act Implementation Monitoring Committee, Letter to the Hon. Ron Phillips MP, Minister for

Health, attached to *ibid.*
29   Human Rights and Equal Opportunity Commission, *Schizophrenia: occasional papers from the Human Rights Commissioner*, No. 1.
30   This was a judicial inquiry into psychiatric malpractice at a private hospital in Sydney called Chelmsford.
31   John Grigor, 'The Right To Treatment', in Human Rights and Equal Opportunity Commission, *op. cit.*, pp. 7–14.
32   Brian Burdekin, 'Human Rights Issues relating to Schizophrenia', in *Ibid.*, p. 2.
33   Anne Deveson, 'The Social Stigma of Schizophrenia as an Obstacle to the Exercise of Human Rights', in *Ibid.*, pp. 48–9.
34   *Mental Health Act 1990*, Section 9(1)(a), NSW Government Information Service, Reprinted as in force at 17 October 1994, p. 5.
35   *Ibid.*, Section 23(1), p. 10.
36   Mental Health Review Tribunal, *Annual Report*, 1993 p. 76, 1994 p. 74, 1995 p. 58.
37   *Ibid.*, 1994.
38   NSW Department of Health, *Caring for Health: proposals for reform—Mental Health Act 1990*, May 1996.
39   *Mental Health Legislation Amendment Bill 1997*, Schedule 1, 1.1 [1], p. 3.
40   United Nations, 'Principles for the Protection of Persons with Mental Illness and for the Improvement of Mental Health Care', in Australian Human Rights and Equal Opportunity Commission (eds.), *Human Rights and Mental Illness: report of the national inquiry into the human rights of people with mental illness.*
41   Fiona McDermott and Jan Carter, eds., *Commonwealth Department of Human Services and Health: issues for research, No. 4, mental disorders: prevention and human services research*, p. 3.
42   United Nations Commission on Human Rights, *op. cit.*, pp. 990–1.
43   Patricia B. Higgins, 'Clozapine and the treatment of schizophrenia', pp. 124–32.
44   John A. Robertson, 'Informed consent: a study of decisionmaking in psychiatry', p. 960.
45   V. Dharmananda, *Informed Consent to Medical Treatment: processes, practices and beliefs*, pp. 1–2.
46   The Nuremberg Code, reproduced in Carolyn Faulder, *Whose Body Is It? The Troubling Issue of Informed Consent*, p. 132.
47   Stephen Wear, *Informed Consent*, p. 135.
48   George J. Annas et al., *Informed Consent to Human Experimentation: the subject's dilemma*, p. 154.
49   H. Bursztajn et al., 'Parens patriae considerations in the commitment process', *Psychiatric Quarterly*, pp. 165–81.

Chapter Five

1   M. Goldwert, 'The Messiah-Complex in Schizophrenia', pp. 331–5.
2   Kenneth E. Lux, 'A Mystical-Occult Approach to Psychosis', p. 95.

3. Gillian Fulcher and Gary D. Bouma, 'Appendix A: the religious factor and modes of psychiatric treatment', pp. 221-31.
4. Gillian Fulcher and Gary D. Bouma, 'Appendix A: the religious factor and modes of psychiatric treatment', p. 226.
5. For a proposal to add this differential diagnosis to the *DSM* see, David Lukoff, 'The diagnosis of mystical experiences with psychotic features', pp. 155-82.
6. Joseph Campbell, 'Schizophrenia—the Inward Journey', in *Myths to Live By*, pp. 219-220.
7. F. C. Happold, *Mysticism*, p. 18.
8. Margaret Smith, 'The Nature and Meaning of Mysticism', in Richard Woods, (ed.), *Understanding Mysticism*, p. 19.
9. R. C. Zaehner, 'Mysticism Sacred and Profane', in Woods, *ibid.*, pp. 56-77.
10. Walter T. Stace, *The Teachings of the Mystics*, pp. 15-23.
11. E. G. Brown, 'A Year Among the Persians', quoted in Smith, *op. cit.*, p. 20.
12. Plato, *The Republic*, pp. 320-1.
13. *Ibid.*, p. 321.
14. Walter H. Principe, 'Mysticism: its meaning and varieties', in Harold Coward and Terence Penelhum, (eds.), *Mystics and Scholars*, p. 4.
15. Soren Kierkegaard, *The Last Years: journals 1853-55*, p. 132.
16. Warren Cohen, 'Kid looks like the mailman? Genetic labs boom as the nation wonders who's Daddy', pp. 62-3.
17. Alfred Lord Tennyson, in a letter to Mr. B. P. Blood, quoted in William James, *The Varieties of Religious Experience*, p. 370.
18. Louis Dupre, 'The Mystical Experience of the Self and Its Philosophical Significance', in Woods, *op. cit.*, p. 457.
19. *Ibid.*, p. 458.
20. Evelyn Underhill, 'The Essentials of Mysticism', in Woods, *op. cit.*, p. 38.
21. 'The Revelation of Jesus Christ', in Ernest Sutherland Bates, (ed.), *The Bible Designed To Be Read As Literature*, p. 1198.
22. Washington Irving, Life of Mohammed, Bell and Daldy, London 1869, quoted in Richard Maurice Bucke, *Cosmic Consciousness*, p. 126.
23. The Book of Exodus, in Bates, *op. cit.*, p. 82.
24. *Ibid.*, p. 83.
25. The Gospel according to John, in Bates, *op. cit.*, p. 1008.
26. The Gospel according to Mark, in Bates, *op. cit.*, p. 902.
27. George Fox, 'Journal', quoted in James, *op. cit.*, pp. 30-1.
28. James, *op. cit.*, p. 30.
29. Bucke, *op. cit.*, pp. 9-10.
30. Richard Maurice Bucke, *Proceedings and Transactions of the Royal Society of Canada*, Series II, Vol. 12, pp. 159-96,
31. Bucke, *Cosmic Consciousness*, p. 255.
32. *Ibid.*, p. 3.
33. Carole Angier, 'R. D. Laing: a divided self', p. 46.
34. R. D. Laing, *The Politics of Experience and The Bird of Paradise*, p. 112.

35 *Ibid.*, p. 97.
36 Gregory Bateson, (ed.), *Perceval's Narrative. A Patient's Account of his Psychosis*, p. xiii.
37 Laing, *op. cit.*, p. 103.
38 *Ibid.*, pp. 104–5.
39 *Ibid.*, p. 105.
40 *Ibid.*, p. 106
41 *Ibid.*, p. 107.
42 *Ibid.*, p. 117.
43 Peter Sedgwick, 'R. D. Laing: self, symptom and society', p. 41.
44 Ageha Bharati, 'Letter to Peter Sedgwick', November, 1971, reproduced in, in Robert Boyers and Robert Orrill, (eds.), *Laing and Anti-Psychiatry*, Penguin, Harmondsworth, 1972, *ibid.*, p. 46.
45 Leon Eisenberg, 'R. D. Laing: a biography, p. 939.
46 *Ibid.*
47 C. G. Jung, 'Schizophrenia', in *The Psychogenesis of Mental Disease*, p. 256.
48 C. G. Jung, 'The Psychology of Dementia Praecox', in Jung, *op. cit.*, pp. 1–153.
49 *Ibid.*, p. v.
50 *Ibid.*, p. 75.
51 *Ibid.*, p. 74.
52 C. G. Jung, 'The Content of the Psychoses', in Jung, *op. cit.*, pp. 153–78.
53 *Ibid.*, p. 158.
54 *Ibid.*, p. 159.
55 C. G. Jung, 'On the Problem of Psychogenesis', in Jung, *op. cit.*, p. 211.
56 C. G. Jung, 'Mental Disease and the Psyche', in Jung, *op. cit.*, p. 227.
57 C. G. Jung, 'On the Psychogenesis of Schizophrenia', in Jung, *op. cit.*, p. 234.
58 *Ibid.*, pp. 245, 246.
59 C. G. Jung, 'Recent Thoughts on Schizophrenia', in Jung, *op. cit.*, pp. 250–5.
60 *Ibid.*
61 *Ibid.*, pp. 254, 255.
62 C. G. Jung, 'Schizophrenia', in Jung, *op. cit.*, pp. 256–71.
63 *Ibid.*, p. 271.
64 John Weir Perry, *The Far Side of Madness*, p. 2.
65 *Ibid.*, p. 19.
66 *Ibid.*, p. 8.
67 *Ibid.*, p. 10.
68 John Weir Perry, interview with Michael O'Callaghan, reproduced in *Global Vision*, 1992–1995, accessed 14 September 1997, available on-line at http://www.ige.apc.org/glencree/dreamch2.html
69 *Ibid.*
70 John Weir Perry, *Trials of a Visionary Mind: Spiritual Emergency and the Renewal Process*, p. 58-9
71 *Ibid.*
72 Campbell, *op. cit.*, p. 201.

276 PUNISHING THE PATIENT

73 *Ibid.*, p. 202; Joseph Campbell, *The Hero With a Thousand Faces.*
74 Joseph Campbell, *The Masks of God* (4 volumes), Souvenir Press, London, 1973–1974.
75 Campbell, 'Schizophrenia—the Inward Journey', *op. cit.*, p. 202.
76 *Ibid.*, pp. 202–3.
77 *Ibid.*, p. 209.
78 John Weir Perry, *Roots of Renewal in Myth and Madness: the meaning of psychotic episodes.*
78 *Ibid.*, p. 195.
79 *Ibid.*
80 Perry, *Trials of a Visionary Mind, op. cit.*, p. 139.

Chapter Six

1 United Nations, 'International Covenant on Civil and Political Rights', pp. 32–3.
2 *Ibid.*, p. 25.
3 United Nations, 'Declaration on the Elimination of all Forms of Intolerance and of Discrimination Based on Religion or Belief', pp. 35–6.
4 John S. Mill, 'On Liberty', p. 135.
5 J. M. Robertson, *A History of Freethought*, p. 2.
6 Barrows Dunham, *The Heretics*, p. 2.
7 Karl Pearson, *The Ethic of Freethought*, p. 21.
8 United Nations Centre for Human Rights, *United Nations Action in the Field of Human Rights*, p. 110.
9 Margaret G. Wachenfeld, *The Human Rights of the Mentally Ill in Europe Under the European Convention on Human Rights*, p. 277.
10 Human Rights Committee, United Nations, CCPR/C/21/Rev.1/Add.4. p. 1, quoted in Human Rights and Equal Opportunity Commission, *Free to Believe? The Right to Freedom of Religion and Belief in Australia*, p. 21.
11 United Nations Centre for Human Rights, *op. cit.*, p. 110.
12 International Commission of Jurists, *Siracusa Principles on the Limitations and Derogation Provisions in the International Covenant on Civil and Political Rights.*
13 *Ibid.*, p. 6
14 *Ibid.*, p. 7.
15 *Ibid.*, p. 9
16 *Ibid.*
17 *Ibid.*, p. 8.
18 *Ibid.*, p. 765.
19 United Nations, 'International Covenant on Civil and Political Rights', Article 18.2, reproduced in Satish Chandra, (ed.), *op. cit.*, p. 32.
20 David Cohen and Michael McCubbin, 'The Political Economy of Tardive Dyskinesia: Asymmetries in Power and Responsibility', p. 472.
21 Norman L. Keltner et al., *Psychiatric Nursing*, p. 227.
22 Thomas Szasz, *Cruel Compassion: psychiatric control of society's*

unwanted, p. 167.
23   F. J. Ayds, 'The Early History of Modern Psychopharmacology', quoted in Keltner et al., *op. cit.*, p. 227.
24   Peter Breggin, 'Brain Damage, Dementia and Persistent Cognitive Dysfunction Associated With Neuroleptic Drugs: evidence, aetiology, implications', p. 445.
25   Peter Breggin and David Cohen, *Your Drug May Be Your Problem*, p. 77.
25   Keltner et al., *op. cit.*, p. 233.
26   Haldol Decanoate advertisement, *Archives of General Psychiatry*, August 1995.
27   J. N. Herrera, 'High Potency Neuroleptics and Violence in Schizophrenics', pp. 558–61.
28   Phillip Thomas, *The Dialectics of Schizophrenia*, pp. 111–12.
29   David Richman, 'Pursuing Psychiatric Pill Pushers', in Sherry Hirsch et al., (eds.), *Madness Network News Reader*, p. 113.
30   Seth Farber, *Madness, Heresy, and the Rumor of Angels*, p. 90.
31   *Ibid.*, p. 105.
32   United Nations, 'International Covenant on Economic, Social and Cultural Rights', Article 12 (1), reproduced in Satish Chandra, (ed.), *op. cit.*, p. 16.

Chapter Seven
1   Theodore R. Sarbin and James C. Mancuso, *Schizophrenia: medical diagnosis or moral verdict?*, p. 220.
2   Thomas Szasz, *The Manufacture of Madness: a comparative study of the inquisition and the mental health movement*.
3   Malleus Malificarum, quoted in Szasz, *The Manufacture of Madness*, p. 35.
4   *Ibid.*
5   See for example, Thomas Scheff, *Labelling Madness*.
6   American Psychiatric Association, *Diagnostic and Statistical Manual of Mental Disorders*, fourth edition, (DSM-IV), p. 274–277.
7   *Ibid.*, p. 285.
8   World Health Organisation, *The ICD-10 Classification of Mental Disorders and Behavioural Disorders: clinical descriptions and diagnostic guidelines*.
9   American Psychiatric Association, *op. cit.*, p. 765.
10 *Ibid.*
11 *Ibid.*, p. 767.
12 *Ibid.*, p. 275.
13 *Ibid.*, p. 276.
14 *Ibid.*
15 *Ibid.*
16 Thomas Szasz, 'Psychiatric diagnosis, psychiatric power and psychiatric abuse', pp. 135–8,
17 American Psychiatric Association, *op. cit.*, p. 764.
18 M. Spitze et al., 'Comprehension of metaphoric speech by healthy probands and schizophrenic patients: an experimental psychopathologic contribution

to concretism', pp. 282–92.
19. P. W. Corrigan et al., 'Situational familiarity and feature recognition in schizophrenia', pp. 153–61.
20. William Bradshaw, 'Evaluating Cognitive-Behavioural Treatment of Schizophrenia: four single-case studies', p. 419.
21. American Psychiatric Association, *op. cit.*, p. 276.
22. *Ibid.*, p. 764.
23. *Ibid.*, p. 278.
24. Paul Lysaker and Morris Bell, 'Work Performance Over Time for People With Schizophrenia', pp. 141–6.
25. Thomas Szasz, *Cruel Compassion: psychiatric control of society's unwanted*, p. 145.
26. Leonard Roy Frank, interview, in Seth Farber, p. 193.
27. Alan R. Beeber, 'Psychotherapy with Schizophrenics in Team Groups: a systems model', pp. 78–87.
28. Szasz, *The Manufacture of Madness*, p. 136.
29. *Ibid.*, pp. 127–8.
30. *Ibid.*, p. 316.
31. John Modrow, *How To Become A Schizophrenic: the case against biological psychiatry*, 1992.
32. *Ibid.*, p. 1.
33. *Ibid.*, p. 3.
34. Whistleblowers Australia, *Abuse of Medical Assessments to Dismiss Whistleblowers*.
35. Commonwealth Ombudsman, *AFP professional reporting & internal witnesses*, p. 53.
36. Louise Roy, *Psychiatry and the Suppression of Dissent*, unpublished report on the use of psychiatric labels to intimidate whistleblowers, December 1997.
37. Thomas Szasz, 'Psychiatric diagnosis, psychiatric power and psychiatric abuse', pp. 135–8,
38. Thomas Scheff, 'Schizophrenia as Ideology', in Scheff, (ed.), *Labelling Madness*, pp. 5–12.
39. Thomas Szasz, 'Idleness and Lawlessness in the Therapeutic State', p. 30–6.
40. *Ibid.*
41. *Ibid.*
42. Phillip D. Arben, 'Are Mental Illnesses Biological Diseases? Some Public Policy Implications', pp. 66–70.
43. Robert Spillane, professor in Management, Macquarie University, Sydney, reported in 'Mental illness myth: bosses', *Sunday Telegraph* (Sydney), 19 September 1999.
44. William Shakespeare, *King Lear*, Act II, Scene III.
45. American Psychiatric Association, *op. cit.*, p. 683.
46. *Ibid.*, pp. 472, 474.
47. John B. Murray, 'Munchausen Syndrome/Munchausen Syndrome by Proxy', pp. 343–53.

48   American Psychiatric Association, *op. cit.*, pp. 725-7.
49   *Ibid.*, p. 725.
50   B. E. Netter and D. J. Viglione Jr, 'An empirical study of malingering schizophrenia on the Rorschach', pp. 45-57.
51   R. Rogers et al., 'Feigning Schizophrenic Disorders on the MMPI-2: Detection of Coached Simulators, pp. 215-26.
52   David L. Rosenhan, 'On being Sane in Insane Places', pp. 250-8.
53   *Ibid*, p. 251.
54   Thomas J. Scheff, *Being Mentally Ill*, Aldine, New York, 1984, p. 190.
55   *Ibid.*
56   T. Millon, 'Reflections on Rosenhan's On being sane in insane places', pp. 456-61.
57   Stuart A. Kirk and Herb Kutchins, *The Selling of DSM: the rhetoric of science in psychiatry,* pp. 90-7.
58   R. L. Spitzer, 'On pseudoscience in science, logic in remission, and psychiatric diagnosis: a critique of Rosenhan's "On being sane in insane places", pp. 442-52.
59   Kirk and Kutchins, *op. cit.*, p. 93.
60   James T. Brown, 'Compensation neurosis rides again: a practitioner's guide to defending PTSD claims (post traumatic stress disorder)', pp. 467-82.
61   Maurice K. Temerlin, 'Suggestion Effects in Psychiatric Diagnosis', pp. 46-54.
62   *Ibid.*, p. 47.
63   *Ibid.*, pp. 47-8.
64   *Ibid.*, p. 48.
65   *Ibid.*, p. 52.
66   Janet Frame, *An Angel At My Table*, p. 78.
67   *Ibid.*, p. 79.
68   *Ibid.*, p. 108.

Chapter Eight

1   Michael S. Moore, 'Legal Conceptions of Mental Illness', in Baruch A. Brody and H. Tristram Engelhardt, Jr., (eds.), *Mental Illness: Law and Public Policy*, D. Reidel Publishing, Dordrecht/Boston, 1980, p. 27.
2   Jerome Neu, 'Minds on Trial', pp. 81-2.
3   Moore, *op. cit.*, p. 28.
4   *Ibid.*, p. 30.
5   William Glaberson, 'Killer Sues His Therapist and Wins $500,000', *New York Times,* 10 October, 1998, p. 1.
6   *Ibid.*
7   Thomas Szasz, letter to the Editor, *New York Times*, 14 October 1998.
8   Jeffrey A. Schaler, letter to the Editor, *New York Times,* 14 October 1998.
9   Mental Health Review Tribunal, *Annual Report* , 1996, pp. 37-57.
10   United Nations, 'International Covenant on Civil and Political Rights', Article 9, p. 29.
11   B. J. Carone et al., 'Posthospital Course and Outcome in Schizophrenia', pp.

247–53.
12. Peter Breggin and David Cohen, *Your Drug May Be Your Problem*, p. 78.
13. American Psychiatric Association, *Diagnostic and Statistical Manual of Mental Disorders* (DSM IV), fourth edition, p. 745.
14. United Nations, 'International Covenant on Civil and Political Rights', Article 7, p. 29.
15. United Nations, *Convention against Torture and Other Cruel, Inhuman or Degrading Treatment or Punishment*.
16. Elliot S. Valenstein, 'Historical Perspective', p. 15.
17. *Ibid.*
18. *Ibid.*, p. 17.
19. P. K. McCowan, 98th *Annual Report for 1937 of the Crichton Royal Institution*, Dumfries (Scotland). Quoted in L. C. Cook, 'Has fear any therapeutic significance in convulsion therapy?'
20. Marcus Schatner, 'Some observations in the treatment of dementia praecox with hypoglycemia: part 2, psychological implication', pp. 22–6.
21. Don Weitz, 'Cruel and Usual—A Human Rights Violation'.
22. Sylvia Plath, *The Bell Jar*, pp. 117–18.
23. Evelyn Crumpton et al., 'The role of fear in electroconvulsive treatment', pp. 29–33.
24. Deborah Dauphinais, *Medications for the treatment of schizophrenia: questions and answers*.
25. Darius Rejali, *Electric Torture: a global history of a torture technology*.
26. Neuropsychiatric Institute, *General Information*, Neuropsychiatric Institute (NPI), Prince Henry Hospital, Sydney, Australia, available on-line at http://acsusun.acsu.unsw.edu.au/~s8700122/npiphh.html/#NPS
27. F. A. Whitlock, 'Psychosurgery', in Erica M. Bates and Paul R. Wilson, (eds.), *Mental Disorder or Madness*, University of Queensland Press, St Lucia, 1979, p. 182.
28. Valenstein, *op. cit.*, p. 26.
29. *Ibid.*
30. Elliot S. Valenstein, 'Rationale and Surgical Procedures', Valenstein, (ed.), *op. cit.*, p. 69.
31. Valenstein, 'Historical Perspective', *op. cit.*, p. 27.
32. *Ibid.*, p. 26.
33. R. Anderson, 'Differences in the course of learning as measured by various memory tasks after amygdalectomy in man'.
34. P. MacDonald Tow, *Personality Changes Following Frontal Leucotomy*. Quoted in Breggin, in Valenstein, (ed.), *op. cit.*, p. 489.
35. Breggin, in Valenstein, (ed.), *op. cit.*, p. 489.
36. *Ibid.*
37. G. Johnson, 'The Biological Therapies' in Pierre J. V. Beumont and R. B. Hampshire (eds.), *Textbook of Psychiatry*, p. 330.
38. Harold I. Kaplan and Benjamin J. Sadock, *Synopsis of Psychiatry*, sixth edition, p. 816.

39 S. Tichurst, 'Dementia', in Robert Kosky et al., (eds.), *Mental Health and Illness: a textbook for students of health sciences*, pp. 269–70.
40 B. S. Gurian et al., 'Informed Consent for Neuroleptics with Elderly Patients in Two Settings', pp. 37–44.
41 Alison Motluk, 'Dementia drugs hasten mental decline', p. 9.
42 James W. Cooper, 'Drugs that cause falls in the nursing home', pp. 45–7.
43 Council on the Ageing (Australia), *Federal Budget Submission for 1995*, p. 9.
44 Human Rights and Equal Opportunity Commission, *Report of the National Inquiry into the Human Rights of People with Mental Illness*, p. 517.
45 *Ibid.* p. 245.
46 H. Molony, 'Mental retardation', in Beumont and Hampshire, (eds.), *op. cit.*, pp. 277–8.
47 Kaplan and Sadock, *op. cit.*, p. 799.
48 B. Bowers, 'Antipsychotics Evoke Youthful Concerns', p. 276.
49 *Ibid.*
50 Francis I. Dunne, 'Soviet and Western Psychology: a comprehensive study', p. 374.
51 Peter Breggin, *Toxic Psychiatry*, pp. 71–2.
52 Norman L. Keltner, 'Antipsychotic Drugs', in Norman Keltner et al., (eds.), pp. 230–1.
53 John Langone, 'A profession under stress; long ostracised by colleagues around the world, Soviet psychiatrists try to show that they are not instruments of oppression', pp. 94–6.
54 *Ibid.*
55 Victoria Pope, 'Mad Russians: victims of Soviet "punitive psychiatry" continue to pay a heavy price', pp. 38–43.
56 Keltner, *op. cit.*, pp. 230–1.
57 Thomas Szasz, 'Psychiatric Diagnosis, Psychiatric Power and Psychiatric Abuse', pp. 135–9.
58 Lawrence Stevens, *Psychiatric Drugs: cure or quackery?*
59 Heather Nolan, personal communication (letter to Richard Gosden), 26 February 1998.
60 *Ibid.*
61 *Ibid.*

Chapter Nine
1 A R. Yung et al., 'Monitoring and care of young people at incipient risk of psychosis', p. 300.
2 Tor K. Larsen and Stein Opjordsmoen, 'Early identification and treatment of schizophrenia: conceptual and ethical considerations', pp. 371–81.
3 Alison R. Yung and Patrick D. McGorry, 'The Prodromal Phase of First-Episode Psychosis: Past and Current Conceptualisations', pp. 353–70.
4 Chris Jackson and Max Birchwood, 'Early intervention in psychosis: Opportunities for secondary prevention', pp. 487–502.

5   Tor K. Larsen et al., 'First-Episode Schizophrenia: 1. Early Course Parameters', pp. 241–56.
6   Thomas H. McGlashan and Jan Olav Johannessen, 'Early Detection and Intervention With Schizophrenia: Rationale', pp. 209, 201, 212.
7   Jay W. Pettegrew et al., 'Alterations in Brain High-Energy Phosphate and Membrane Phospholid Metabolism in First-Episode, Drug-Naive Schizophrenics: A Pilot Study of the Dorsal Prefrontal Cortex by In Vivo Phosphorus 31 Nuclear Magnetic Resonance Spectroscopy', pp. 563-68.
8   Ian R. H. Falloon et al., 'Early Detection and Intervention for Initial Episodes of Schizophrenia', pp. 271–82.
9   Ibid., p. 279.
10 National Early Psychosis Project, *Australian clinical guidelines for early psychosis*, p. 11.
11 American Psychiatric Association, *Diagnostic and Statistical Manual of Mental Disorders, Third Edition — Revised, (DSM-III-R)*, pp. 194–5.
12 Yung et al., 'Monitoring and care of young people at incipient risk of psychosis', p. 289.
13 Ibid.
14 Ibid., p. 292.
15 Ibid., p. 293.
16 American Psychiatric Association, *Diagnostic and Statistical Manual of Mental Disorders, Fourth Edition, (DSM-IV)*, p. 768.
17 Patrick D. McGorry and Jane Edwards, *Early Psychosis Training Pack*, Module 1, p. 17, cited in table adapted from McGorry et al., 'The prevalence of prodromal features of schizophrenia in adolescence: a preliminary survey', *Acta Psychiatrica Scandanavica*, 92, 1995, pp. 241–9.
18 Yung et al., 'Monitoring and care of young people at incipient risk of psychosis', p. 299.
19 Ibid.
20 American Psychiatric Association, *op. cit.*, 1994, p. 643.
21 A. R. Yung, et al., 'Can we predict the onset of first-episode psychosis in a high-risk group?', p. 28.
22 Ibid., p. 26.
23 National Early Psychosis Project, *Australian Clinical Guidelines for Early Psychosis*, p. 13.
24 Ibid., p. 12.
25 Ibid., p. 19.
26 SANE Australia, *Something is not quite right*.
27 Ibid.
28 Ibid.
29 R. E. Kendell and W. Adams, 'Unexplained Fluctuations in the Risk for Schizophrenia By Month and Year of Birth', pp. 758–63.
30 C. E. Kim et al., 'Month of Birth and Schizophrenia in Korea. Sex, Family History and Handedness', pp. 829-31.
31 McGorry and Edwards, *Early Psychosis Training Pack*.

32   Gardiner-Caldwell Communications, *Influenza Bulletin*.
33   Daniel R. Weinberger, 'From neuropathology to neurodevelopment', pp. 552–8.
34   R. Livingston et al., 'Season of birth and neurodevelopmental disorders: summer birth is associated with dyslexia', pp. 612–16.
35   Anonymous, 'Young Adults Experiencing Psychosis Remain Undiagnosed', *Mental Health Net*, accessed August 1996, available on-line at, http:// www.cmhc.com/articles/young.htm
36   *Western Psychiatric Institute and Clinic (WPIC)*, accessed July 1998, available on-line at, http://brains2.wpic.pitt.edu/paces.html
37   Anonymous, 'Early Detection and Intervention in Schizophrenia: The Patient's Perspective', p. 4.
38   Early Psychosis Prevention and Intervention Centre, *PACE Background*.
39   National Early Psychosis Project, *Australian Clinical Guidelines for Early Psychosis*, p. 28.
40   Novartis (Sandoz Pharmaceuticals Corporation), Clozaril (clozapine) advertisement, *Archives of General Psychiatry*, Vol. 55, No. 1, January 1998, p. 8.
41   Janssen Pharmaceutica, Risperdal (risperidone) advertisement, *Psychiatric Services*, Vol. 49, No. 9, September 1998, p. 1124.
42   Eli Lilly and Company, Zyprexa (olanzapine) advertisement, *Psychiatric Services*, Vol 49, No. 3, March 1998, p. 310.
43   Zeneca Pharmaceuticals, Seroquel (quetiapine) advertisement, *Psychiatric Services*, Vol. 49, No. 3, March 1998, p. 284.
44   Risperdal (risperidone) advertisement, *op. cit.*
45   Seroquel (quetiapine) advertisement, *op. cit.*
46   Clozaril (clozapine) advertisement, *op. cit.*
47   J. K. Stanilla, J. de-Leon and G. M. Simpson, 'Clozapine withdrawal resulting in delirium with psychosis: a report of three cases', pp. 252–5.
48   American Psychiatric Association (DSM-IV), p, 273.
49   T. J. Crow, 'Sexual selection, Machiavellian intelligence, and the origins of psychosis', pp. 594–9.
50   McGorry and Edwards, *Early Psychosis Training Pack*, p. .9.
51   Yung et al., 'Monitoring and Care of Young People at Incipient Risk of Psychosis', p. 286.
52   *Report of the Royal Commission Into Deep Sleep Therapy*, Volume 2, pp. 48–58.
53   Peter Breggin, *Toxic Psychiatry*, p. 250.
54   John Marks, *The Search for the Manchurian Candidate*.
55   National Early Psychosis Project, *Australian Clinical Guidelines for Early Psychosis*, p. 13.
56   See for example, Alison R. Yung et al., 'Prediction of psychosis: A step towards indicated prevention of schizophrenia', *British Journal of Psychiatry*, pp. 14–20 and Richard Jed Wyatt et al., 'First-episode schizophrenia: Early intervention and medication discontinuation in the context of course and treatment', pp. 77–83.

57 D. E. Cameron, 'Early schizophrenia'. Quoted in Patrick McGorry, 'Preventive strategies in early psychosis', pp. 1–2.
58 Harry Stack Sullivan, 'Discussion', in D. Ewen Cameron, 'Early schizophrenia', p. 579.
59 Peter Breggin and David Cohen, *Your Drug May Be Your Problem*, p. 189.

Conclusion
1 American Psychiatric Association, *Diagnostic and Statistical Manual of Mental Disorders*, Fourth edition, p. 283.

Bibliography

American Psychiatric Association, *Diagnostic and Statistical Manual of Mental Disorders, Third Edition—Revised, (DSM-III-R)*, American Psychiatric Association, Washington, 1987.
——, *Diagnostic and Statistical Manual of Mental Disorders (DSM IV)*, Fourth Edition, American Psychiatric Association, Washington, 1994.
Anderson, R., 'Differences in the course of learning as measured by various memory tasks after amygdalectomy in man', in E. Hitchcock, L. Laitinen and K. Vaernet (eds.), *Psychosurgery*, Charles C. Thomas, Springfield Ill., 1972.
Andreasen, Nancy C., Laura Flashman, Michael Flaum, Stephan Arndt, Victor Swayze II, Daniel S. O'Leary, James C. Ehrhardt and William T. C. Yuh, 'Regional brain abnormalities in schizophrenia measured with magnetic resonance imaging', *JAMA, Journal of the American Medical Association*, Vol. 272, No. 22, 14 December 1994, pp. 1763–70.
Angier, Carole, 'R. D. Laing: A Divided Self', *New Statesman*, Vol. 25, No. 4294, 26 July 1996, p. 46.
Annas, George J., Leonard H. Glantz, and Barbara F. Katz, *Informed Consent to Human Experimentation: the subject's dilemma*, Ballinger Publishing Company, Cambridge, Mass., 1977.
Arben, Phillip D., 'Are Mental Illnesses Biological Diseases? Some Public Policy Implications', *Health & Social Work*, Vol. 21, No. 1, February 1996, pp. 66–70.
'Atypical treatments for schizophrenia', *Lancet*, Vol. 339, No. 8788, 1 February 1992, pp. 276–8.
Bates, Ernest Sutherland (ed.), *The Bible Designed To Be Read As Literature*, William Heinemann, London, 1920.
Bateson, Gregory, Don D. Jackson, Jay Haley, and John Weakland, 'Towards a Theory of Schizophrenia', *Behavioral Science*, Vol. 1, No. 4, October 1956, reproduced in Milton M. Berger, *Beyond the Double Bind*, Brunner/Maze, New York, 1978, pp. 3–27.
Bateson, Gregory, *Perceval's Narrative. A Patient's Account of his*

Psychosis, Stanford University Press, Stanford, 1961.
Beeber, Alan R., 'Psychotherapy with Schizophrenics in Team Groups: a systems model', *American Journal of Psychotherapy,* Vol. 45, No. 1, 1991, pp. 78–87.
Berrios, German E., *The History of Mental Symptoms,* Cambridge University Press, Cambridge, 1996.
Berrios, German and Roy Porter (eds.), *A History of Clinical Psychiatry: the origin and history of psychiatric disorders,* New York University Press, New York, 1996.
Beumont, Pierre J. and R. B. Hampshire (eds.), *Textbook of Psychiatry,* Blackwell, Melbourne, 1989.
Bhugra, Dinesh (ed.), *Psychiatry and Religion: context, consensus and controversies,* Routledge, London, 1996.
Bhugra, D., J. Leff, R. Mallett, G. Der, B. Corridan and S. Rudge, 'Incidence and outcome of schizophrenia in whites, African-Caribbeans and Asians in London', *Psychological Medicine,* Vol. 27, No. 4, July 1997, pp. 791–8.
Black, Donald W., William R. Yates and Nancy C. Andreasen, 'Schizophrenia, Schizophreniform Disorder, and Delusional (Paranoid) Disorders', in John A. Talbott, Robert E. Hales and Stuart C. Yudofsky (eds.), *Textbook of Psychiatry,* American Psychiatric Press, Washington, 1988, pp. 357–402.
Bleuler, Eugen, *Dementia Praecox or The Group of Schizophrenias,* translated by Joseph Zinkin International Universities Press, New York, 1950.
Bocce, Kathleen, 'Mental health patients' families have few rights', Letters to the Editor, *Sydney Morning Herald,* 2 June 1995.
Bowden, Mark, 'Study finds evidence for gene that may help cause schizophrenia', *Knight-Ridder/Tribune News Service,* 1 May 1995, p. 501.
——, 'Top human geneticists argue over ownership of schizophrenia research', *Knight-Ridder/Tribune News Service,* 11 May 1995, p. 511.
Bower, Bruce, 'Schizophrenia: genetic clues and caveats', *Science News,* Vol. 134, No. 20, 12 Nov. 1988, p. 308.
——, 'Brain Anatomy Yields Schizophrenia Clues', *Science News,* Vol. 137, No. 12, 24 March 1990, p. 182.
——, 'Antipsychotics Evoke Youthful Concerns', *Science News,* Vol. 140, No. 18, 2 November 1991, p. 276.
Bradshaw, William, 'Evaluating Cognitive-Behavioural Treatment of Schizophrenia: four single-case studies', *Research on Social Work*

Practice, Vol. 7, No. 4, October 1997, p. 419.
Breggin, Peter, 'Brain Damage, Dementia and Persistent Cognitive Dysfunction Associated With Neuroleptic Drugs: evidence, aetiology, implications', *Journal of Mind and Behaviour*, Vol. 11, Nos. 3 and 4, summer and autumn 1990, pp. 425–63.
——, *Toxic Psychiatry*, Fontana, London, 1993.
Breggin, Peter and Cohen, David, *Your Drug May Be Your Problem*, Perseus Books, Reading, Massachusetts, 1999.
Brown, A. S., E. S. Susser, P. D. Butler, R. Richardson-Andrews, C. A. Kaufmann and J. M. Gorman, 'Neurobiological plausibility of prenatal nutritional deprivation as a risk factor for schizophrenia', *Journal of Nervous and Mental Disorders*, Vol. 184, No. 2, February 1996, pp. 71–85.
Brown, Anne and Weaver, Rebecca, 'Promising New Medications in Development', *NARSAD Research Newsletter*, summer 1998 available on-line at http://www.nami.org/medicat/9809meds.htm
Brown, James T., 'Compensation neurosis rides again: a practitioner's guide to defending PTSD claims', *Defence Counsel Journal*, Vol. 63, No. 4, 1996, pp. 467–82.
Browne, Anthony, Health Editor, 'Doctors could soon prescribe behaviour-controlling chemicals to pre-teens against their parents' wishes', *The Observer*, 27 February, 2000.
Bucke, Richard Maurice, *Cosmic Consciousness*, E. P. Dutton, New York, 1969.
Burdekin, Brian, Federal Human Rights Commissioner, opening address to Sydney hearings, National Inquiry into Human Rights and Mental Illness, 17 June 1991.
Bursztajn, H., T. G. Gutheil, R. M. Hamm, A. Brodsky and M. J. Mills, 'Parens patriae considerations in the commitment process', *Psychiatric Quarterly*, Fall 1988, Vol. 59, No. 3, pp. 165–81.
Cameron, D. E., 'Early schizophrenia', *American Journal of Psychiatry*, Vol. 95, 1938, pp. 567–78.
Campbell, Joseph, *The Hero With a Thousand Faces*, Princeton University Press, Princeton N.J., 1968.
——, 'Schizophrenia—the Inward Journey', in Joseph Campbell, *Myths To Live By*, Condor Books, New York, 1970.
——, *The Masks of God*, (4 volumes), Souvenir Press, London, 1973–74.
Canton, Graziano and Ida G. Fraccon, 'Life events and schizophrenia: a replication', *Acta Psychiatrica Scandinavica*, Vol. 71, No. 3, March 1985, pp. 211–16.

Chapman, Loren J. and Jean P. Chapman, *Disordered Thought in Schizophrenia*, Prentice-Hall, Englewood Cliffs, New Jersey, 1973.

Chess, Stella, 'The "blame the mother" ideology', *International Journal of Mental Health*, Vol. 11, Nos. 1–2, 1982, pp. 95–107.

Clayer, John R., Alexander C. McFarlane, Clara L. Bookless, Tracy Air, Graham Wright and Andrew S. Czechowicz, 'Prevalence of psychiatric disorders in rural South Australia', *The Medical Journal of Australia*, Vol. 163, 7 August 1995, pp. 124–8.

Coggiano, M. A., R. C. Alexander, D. G. Kirch, R. J. Wyatt and H. Kulaga, 'The Continued Search for Evidence of Retroviral Infection in Schizophrenic Patients', *Schizophrenia Research*, Vol. 5, No. 3, 1991, pp. 243–7.

Cohen, David and Michael McCubbin, 'The Political Economy of Tardive Dyskinesia: Asymmetries in Power and Responsibility', *Journal of Mind and Behaviour*, Vol. 11, Nos. 3 and 4, summer and autumn 1990, pp. 465–88.

Cohen, David, *Soviet Psychiatry: politics and mental health in the USSR today*, Paladin, London, 1989.

Cohen, Warren, 'Kid looks like the mailman? Genetic labs boom as the nation wonders who's Daddy', *US News and World Report*, Vol. 122, No. 3, 27 Jan. 1997, pp. 62–63.

Commonwealth Ombudsman, *AFP professional reporting & internal witnesses*, Australian Commonwealth Government, Canberra, November 1997.

Cook, William L., Angus M. Strachan, Michael J. Goldstein and David J. Miklowitz, 'Expressed emotion and reciprocal affective relationships in families of disturbed adolescents', *Family Process*, Vol. 28, No. 3, September 1989, pp. 337–48.

Cooper, James W., 'Drugs that cause falls in the nursing home', *Nursing Homes*, Vol. 42, No. 4, May 1993, pp. 45–7.

Corrigan, P. W., R. Silverman, J. Stephenson, J. Nugent-Hirschbeck, and B. J. Buican, 'Situational familiarity and feature recognition in schizophrenia', *Schizophrenia Bulletin*, Vol. 22, No. 1, 1996, pp. 153–61.

Council on the Ageing (Australia), *Federal Budget Submission for 1995*, Melbourne, December 1994.

Coward, Harold and Terence Penelhum (eds.), *Mystics and Scholars*, Wilfrid Laurier University Press, Waterloo, Ont., 1977.

Crow, T. J., 'Sexual selection, Machiavellian intelligence, and the origins of psychosis', *Lancet*, 342, 1993, 594–9.

Crumpton, Evelyn, Norman Q. Brill, Samuel Eiduson and Edward Geller,

'The role of fear in electroconvulsive treatment', *Journal of Nervous and Mental Disorders*, Vol. 136, 1963, pp. 29–33.

Dauphinais, Deborah, *Medications for the treatment of schizophrenia: questions and answers*, Pamphlet produced by U.S. Department of Health and Human Services, Washington, 1992.

Davis, J. O. and H. S. Bracha, 'Famine and schizophrenia: first-trimester malnutrition or second-trimester beriberi', *Biological Psychiatry*, Vol. 40, No. 1, 1 July 1996, pp. 1–3.

Davis, L. J., 'Diagnostic and Statistical Manual of Mental Disorders, 4th ed.', *Harper's Magazine*, Vol. 294, No. 1761, 1997, p. 61.

Deveson, Anne, 'The Social Stigma of Schizophrenia as an Obstacle to the Exercise of Human Rights', in Human Rights and Equal Opportunity Commission, *Schizophrenia: occasional papers from the Human Rights Commissioner*, No. 1, Human Rights and Equal Opportunity Commission, Sydney, December 1989, pp. 44–9.

——, *Tell Me I'm Here*, Penguin, Ringwood, 1991.

——, 'Towards a better treatment of serious mental illness', *Sydney Morning Herald*, 31 May 1995.

——, 'Help for Families', *SANE News*, Issue 8, Winter 1998.

Dharmananda, V., *Informed Consent to Medical Treatment: processes, practices and beliefs*, Law Reform Commission of Western Australia, Perth, 1992.

Dixon, Robert, Letter to the Editor, *Sydney Morning Herald*, 2 June 1995.

Docherty, N. M., 'Communication deviance, attention, and schizotypy in parents of schizophrenic patients', *Journal of Nervous and Mental Disease*, Vol. 181, No. 12, December 1993, pp. 750–6.

Double, Duncan, *Antipsychiatry*, available on-line at http://ourworld.compuserve.com/homepages/Duncan_Double/

Double, D. B. 'Understanding Schizophrenia', Letter to Editor, *British Medical Journal*, 24 August 1992 available on-line at http://www.uea.ac.uk/~wp276/schizo.htm.

Dunne, Francis I., 'Soviet and Western Psychology: a comprehensive study', *British Medical Journal*, Vol. 305, No. 6849, 8 August 1992, p. 374.

Dush, David M. and Marvin Brodsky, 'Effects and implications of the experimental double bind', *Psychological Reports*, Vol. 48, No. 3, June 1981, pp. 895–900.

'Early Detection and Intervention in Schizophrenia: the patient's perspective', *Schizophrenia Review*, Vol. 6, No. 1, January 1998, p. 4.

Early Psychosis Prevention and Intervention Centre, *PACE Background*, Early Psychosis Prevention and Intervention Centre, accessed July

1998, available on-line at http://brains2.wpic.pitt.edu/paces.html.

Editorial, *Science News,* Vol. 145, No. 25, 18 June 1994, p. 398.

Ehrenreich, B. and D. English, *For Her Own Good,* Doubleday, New York, 1987.

Eisenberg, Leon, 'R. D. Laing: a biography', *Lancet,* Vol. 344, No. 8927, 1 October 1994, p. 939.

Eli Lilly and Company, Zyprexa (olanzapine) advertisement, *Psychiatric Services,* Vol. 49, No. 3, March 1998, p. 310.

Engel, George L., 'The Need for a New Medical Model: a challenge for biomedicine', *Science,* Vol. 196, No. 4286, 8 April 1977.

Falloon, Ian R., 'Family stress and schizophrenia: theory and practice', *Psychiatric Clinics of North America,* Vol. 9, No. 1, March 1986, pp. 165–82.

Falloon, Ian R. H., Robert R. Kyd, John H. Coverdale and Tannis M. Laidlaw, 'Early Detection and Intervention for Initial Episodes of Schizophrenia', *Schizophrenia Bulletin,* Vol. 22, No. 2, 1996, pp. 271–82.

Farber, Seth, *Madness, Heresy, and the Rumor of Angels: the revolt against the mental health system,* Open Court, Chicago, 1993.

Faulder, Carolyn, *Whose Body Is It? The Troubling Issue of Informed Consent,* Virago Press, London, 1985.

Farber, Seth, *Madness, Heresy, and the Rumor of Angels: the revolt against the mental health system,* Open Court, Chicago, 1993.

Frame, Janet, *An Angel At My Table,* Vintage, Auckland, 1984.

Freud, Sigmund, *The Standard Edition of the Complete Psychological Works of Sigmund Freud,* Hogarth Press, London, 1958.

Fromm-Reichman, Frieda, 'Notes on the Development of Treatment of Schizophrenics by Psychoanalytic Psychotherapy', *Psychiatry,* Vol. 11, 1948, pp. 263–73.

Fulcher, Gillian and Gary D. Bouma, 'Appendix A: the religious factor and modes of psychiatric treatment', in Gary D. Bouma, *The Research Process,* Oxford University Press, Oxford, 1996, pp. 221–31.

Fulford, K. W. M., 'Religion and Psychiatry: extending the limits of tolerance', in Dinesh Bhugra (ed.), *Psychiatry and Religion: context, consensus and controversies,* Routledge, London, 1996, pp. 5–22.

Fulford, K. W. M., A. Y. U. Smirnov and E. Snow, 'Concepts of Disease and the Abuse of Psychiatry in the USSR', *British Journal of Psychiatry,* Vol. 162, 1993, pp. 801–10.

Gabbard, G. O., 'Mind and brain in psychiatric treatment', *Bulletin of the Menninger Clinic,* Vol. 58, No. 4, 1994, pp. 427–46.

Gardiner-Caldwell Communications, *Influenza Bulletin*, accessed July 1998, available on-line at http://www.eswi.com/bull/5/home.htm.

Glaberson, William, 'Killer Sues His Therapist and Wins $500,000', *New York Times,* 10 October 1998, p. 1.

Goldwert, M., 'The Messiah-Complex in Schizophrenia', *Psychological Reports*, Vol. 73, No. 1, 1993, pp. 331–5.

Halpern, A. L., 'Current Dilemmas in the Aftermath of the US Delegation's Inspection of the Soviet Psychiatric Hospitals', Paper presented at the Emerging Issues For The 1990s In Psychiatry, Psychology And Law, *Proceedings of the 10th Annual Congress of the Australian and New Zealand Association of Psychiatry, Psychology and Law*, Melbourne, 1989.

Happold, F. C., *Mysticism,* Penguin, Harmondsworth, 1963.

Hartwell, Carol Eadie, 'The schizophrenogenic mother concept in American psychiatry', *Psychiatry Interpersonal and Biological Processes*, Vol. 59, No. 3, August 1996, pp. 274–97.

Herrera, J. N., John J. Sramek, Jerome F. Costa, Swati Roy, Chris W. Heh and Bich N. Nguyen, 'High Potency Neuroleptics and Violence in Schizophrenics', *Journal of Nervous and Mental Disorders*, Vol. 176, No. 9, 1988, pp. 558–61.

Hietala, Jarmo, Erkka Syvalahti, Klaus Vuorio, Viljo Rakkolainen, Jorgen Bergman, Merja Haaparanta, Olof Solin, Mikko Kuoppamaki, Olli Kirvela, Ulla Ruotsalainen and Raimo K. R. Salokangas, 'Presynaptic dopamine function in striatum of neuroleptic-naive schizophrenic patients', *Lancet,* 28 October 1995, Vol. 346, No. 8983, pp. 1130–2.

Higgins, Patricia B., 'Clozapine and the treatment of schizophrenia', *Health & Social Work,* Vol. 20, No. 2, 1995, pp. 124–32.

Hirsch, Sherry, Joe Adams, Leonard Frank, Wade Hudson, and David Richman (eds.), *Madness Network News Reader,* Glide, San Francisco, 1974.

Hoek, H. W., E. Susser, K. A. Buck, H. Lumey, S. P. Lin and J. M. Gorman, 'Schizoid personality disorder after prenatal exposure to famine', *American Journal of Psychiatry,* Vol. 153, No. 12, December 1996, pp. 1637–9.

Hoeller, Keith, 'Psychiatric Drugs Harm Children', *Seattle Post-Intelligencer,* April 1997.

Howard, James S., 'Requiem For Schizophrenia', *Integrative Physiological & Behavioral Science,* Vol. 31, No. 2, April-June 1996, pp. 148–55.

Human Rights and Equal Opportunity Commission, *Schizophrenia:*

Occasional papers from the Human Rights Commissioner, No. 1, Human Rights and Equal Opportunity Commission, Sydney, December 1989.

——, *Human Rights and Mental Illness: report of the national inquiry into the human rights of people with mental illness*, Australian Government Publishing Service, Canberra, 1993.

——, *Free to Believe? The Right to Freedom of Religion and Belief in Australia*, Human Rights and Equal Opportunity Commission, Sydney, 1997.

——, *Article 18: freedom of religion and belief*, Human Rights and Equal Opportunity Commission, Sydney, July 1998.

Humphreys, M. S., E. C. Johnstone, J. F. MacMillan and P. J. Taylor, 'Dangerous Behaviour Preceding First Admission for Schizophrenia', *British Journal of Psychiatry*, Vol. 161, 1992, pp. 501–5.

Hyfryd, Brian, 'Neglect of the Body to the Detriment of the Patient: management notes', *Journal of Nutritional & Environmental Medicine*, Vol. 7, No. 1, March 1997, pp. 47–53.

International Commission of Jurists, *Siracusa Principles on the Limitations and Derogation Provisions in the International Covenant on Civil and Political Rights*, American Association for the International Commission of Jurists, Washington, 1985.

Jackson, Chris and Max Birchwood, 'Early intervention in psychosis: opportunities for secondary prevention', *British Journal of Clinical Psychology*, Vol. 35, No. 4, November 1996, pp. 487–502.

James, William, *The Varieties of Religious Experience*, Fontana, London, 1960.

Janssen Pharmaceutica, Risperdal (risperidone) advertisement, *Psychiatric Services*, Vol. 49, No. 9, September 1998, p. 1124.

Jones, Susan L., 'The "damned if you do and damned if you don't" concept: The double bind as a tested theoretical formulation', *Perspectives in Psychiatric Care*, Vol. 15, No. 4, 1977, pp. 162–9.

Joseph, Jay, 'The Genetic Theory of Schizophrenia: a critical overview', *Ethical Human Sciences and Services*, Vol. 1, No. 2, 1999, pp. 119–45.

Jung, C. G., *The Psychogenesis of Mental Disease*, R. F. C. Hull (trans.), Routledge and Kegan Paul, London, 1960.

Kaplan, Harold I., and Benjamin J. Sadock, *Synopsis of Psychiatry: behavioural sciences, clinical psychology*, Sixth Edition, Williams and Wilkins, Baltimore, 1991.

Keltner, Norman L., Lee Hilyard Schwecke and Carol E. Bstrom (eds.),

Psychiatric Nursing, Mosby, St Louis, 1995.

Kendell, R. E. and W. Adams, 'Unexplained Fluctuations in the Risk for Schizophrenia By Month and Year of Birth', *British Journal of Psychiatry,* Vol. 158, 1991, pp. 758–63.

Kety, S. S., D. Rosenthal, P. H. Wender et al., 'Mental illness in the biologic and adoptive families of adoptive individuals who have become schizophrenic: a preliminary report based on psychiatric interviews', in R. Fieve, D. Rosenthal and H. Brill (eds.), *Genetic Research in Psychiatry,* John Hopkins University Press, Baltimore, 1975, pp. 147–65.

Khouri, Philippe, 'Continuum versus dichotomy in theories of schizophrenia', *Schizophrenia Bulletin,* Vol. 3, No. 2, 1977, pp. 262–7.

Kierkegaard, Soren, *The Last Years: journals 1853–55,* Fontana, London, 1965.

Kirk, Stuart A. and Herb Kutchins, *The Selling of DSM: the rhetoric of science in psychiatr,* Aldine De Gruyter, New York, 1992.

Kleinman, Arthur and Alex Cohen, 'Psychiatry's Global Challenge', *Scientific American,* March 1997.

Klerman, G. L., 'The Advantages of DSM III', *American Journal of Psychiatry,* No. 141, 1984.

Ko, S. M. and T. C. Liu, 'Psychiatric syndromes in pernicious anaemia— a case report', *Singapore Medical Journal,* Vol. 33, No. 1, February 1992, pp. 92–4.

Kraepelin, E., *Lectures on Clinical Psychiatry* Bailliere, Tindall and Cox, London, 1906.

Kubota, Yo, 'The Institutional Response', in C. G. Weeramantry (ed.), *Human Rights and Scientific and Technological Development,* United Nations University Press, Tokyo, 1990.

Laing, R. D., *The divided self: an existential study in sanity and madness,* Penguin, Harmondsworth, 1965.

——, *The Politics of Experience and The Bird of Paradise,* Penguin, Harmondsworth, 1967.

Langone, John, 'A profession under stress; long ostracised by colleagues around the world, Soviet psychiatrists try to show that they are not instruments of oppression', *Time,* Vol. 133, No. 15, 10 April 1989, pp. 94–6.

Larsen, Tor K., Thomas McGlashan, and Lars Conrad Moe, 'First-Episode Schizophrenia: 1. Early Course Parameters', *Schizophrenia Bulletin,* Vol. 22, No. 2, 1996, pp. 241–56.

Larsen, Tor K. and Stein Opjordsmoen, 'Early identification and treatment of schizophrenia: conceptual and ethical considerations',

Psychiatry: Interpersonal and Biological Processes, Vol. 59, No. 4, 1996, pp. 371–81.

Leff, Julian, 'Social and Psychological Causes of the Acute Attack', in J. K. Wing (ed.), Schizophrenia: Towards a New Synthesis, Academic Press, London, 1978.

Leifer, Ronald, 'The Medical Model as the Ideology of the Therapeutic State', Journal of Mind and Behavior, Vol. 11, Nos. 3 and 4, 1990, pp. 247–58.

Lewis, Philip E. T. and Koshy, Paul, 'Youth employment, unemployment and school participation', Australian Journal of Education, April 1999, Vol 43, p. 42.

Lidz, Theodore, 'Patients whose children became schizophrenic', Journal of Nervous and Mental Disease, Vol. 172, No. 7, July 1984, pp. 408–11.

Lidz, Theodore, Stephen Fleck and Alice R. Cornelison, Schizophrenia and the Family, International Universities Press, New York, 1965.

Lieber, Deborah J., 'Parental focus of attention in a videotape feedback task as a function of hypothesised risk for offspring schizophrenia', Family Process, Vol. 16, No. 4, December 1977, pp. 467–75.

Lifton, Robert Jay, The Nazi Doctors: medical killing and the psychology of genocide, Basic Books, New York, 1986.

Livingston, R., B. S. Adams and H. S. Bracha, 'Season of birth and neurodevelopmental disorders: summer birth is associated with dyslexia', Journal of the American Academy of Child and Adolescent Psychiatry, Vol. 32, No. 3, May 1993, pp. 612–16.

Lukoff, David, 'The diagnosis of mystical experiences with psychotic features', Journal of Transpersonal Psychology, Vol. 17, No. 2, 1985, pp. 155–82.

Lux, Kenneth E., 'A Mystical-Occult Approach to Psychosis', in Peter A. Magaro, The Construction of Madness, Pergamon Press, Oxford, 1976.

Lysaker, P. and M. Bell, 'Work Rehabilitation and Improvements in Insight in Schizophrenia', Journal of Nervous and Mental Disease, Vol. 183, No. 2, 1995, pp. 103–6.

Macdonald, Peter, 'Mental Health Support and Counselling Services', Legislative Assembly , 7 June 1995, Hansard 51st Parliament 1995-1998.

——, 'Mental Health Amendment Bill', Legislative Assembly, 26 October 1995, Hansard 51st Parliament 1995-1998.

Marder, Stephen R. and Richard C. Meibach, 'Risperidone in the treatment of schizophrenia', American Journal of Psychiatry, Vol. 151, No.

6, 1994, p. 825.

Marks, John, *The Search for the Manchurian Candidate*, W. W. Norton and Company, New York, 1979.

McCowan, P. K. 98th *Annual Report for 1937 of the Crichton Royal Institution*, Dumfries (Scotland). Quoted in L. C. Cook, 'Has fear any therapeutic significance in convulsion therapy?', *Journal of Mental Science*, Vol. 86, No. 484, 1940.

McDermott, Fiona and Jan Carter (eds.), *Commonwealth Department of Human Services and Health: issues for research, No. 4, mental disorders: prevention and human services research*, Australian Government Publishing Service, Canberra, 1995.

McGlashan, Thomas H. and Jan Olav Johannessen, 'Early Detection and Intervention With Schizophrenia: rationale', *Schizophrenia Bulletin*, Vol. 22, No. 2, 1996, pp. 201–22.

McGorry, Patrick D. and Jane Edwards, *Early Psychosis Training Pack*, Gardiner-Caldwell Communications, Macclesfield, Cheshire, 1997.

McGuffin, Peter, Michael J. Owen and Anne E. Farmer, 'Genetic basis of schizophrenia', *Lancet*, Vol. 346, No. 8976, 9 September 1995, pp. 678–83.

McGuire, T. G., 'Measuring the Economic Costs of Schizophrenia', *Schizophrenia Bulletin*, Vol. 17, No. 3, 1991, pp. 375–88.

McKenna, Kathleen, Charles T. Gordon, Marge Lenane, Debra Kaysen, Kimberly Fahey and Judith L. Rapoport, 'Looking for childhood-onset schizophrenia: the first 71 cases screened', *Journal of the American Academy of Child and Adolescent Psychiatry*, Vol. 33, No. 5, 1994, pp. 636–45.

McNeil Pharmaceutical, Haldol Decanoate advertisement, *Archives of General Psychiatry*, August 1995.

Mental Health Act Implementation Monitoring Committee, *Report to the Honourable R. A. Phillips MP, Minister for Health on the NSW Mental Act 1990*, August 1992.

Mental Health Review Tribunal, *Annual Report, 1992*, NSW Government, Sydney.

——, *Annual Report, 1993*, NSW Government, Sydney.

——, *Annual Report, 1994*, NSW Government, Sydney.

——, *Annual Report, 1995*, NSW Government, Sydney.

——, *Annual Report, 1996*, NSW Government, Sydney.

——, *Annual Report, 1997*, NSW Government, Sydney.

——, *Executive Summary for period January 1994 to June 1995*, NSW Government, 1995.

'Mental illness myth: bosses', *Sunday Telegraph* (Sydney), 19 September 1999.
Messite, Jacqueline and Steven D. Stellman, 'Accuracy of death certificate completion: the need for formalized physician training', *JAMA, Journal of the American Medical Association*, Vol. 275, No. 10, 1996, pp. 794–7.
Mill, John S., 'On Liberty', in Mary Warnock (ed.), *Mill: Utilitarianism and Other Writings*, World Publishing, New York, 1962.
Millon, T., 'Reflections on Rosenhan's "On being sane in insane places"', *Journal of Abnormal Psychology*, Vol. 81, 1975, pp. 456–61.
Modrow, John, *How to Become a Schizophrenic: the case against biological psychiatry*, Apollyon Press, Seattle, 1992.
Moore, Michael S., 'Legal Conceptions of Mental Illness', in Baruch A. Brody and H. Tristram Engelhardt, Jr. (eds.), *Mental Illness: law and public policy*, D. Reidel Publishing, Dordrecht/Boston, 1980.
Mosher, Loren R., 'Are Psychiatrists Betraying Their Patients?', *Psychology Today*, Vol. 32, Issue 5, September 1999, p. 40.
Motluk, Alison, 'Dementia drugs hasten mental decline', *New Scientist*, Vol. 153, No. 2067, 1 Feb. 1997, p. 9.
Murphy, K. C., A. G. Cardno and P. McGuffin, 'The molecular genetics of schizophrenia', *Journal of Molecular Neuroscience*, Vol. 7, No. 2, 1996, pp. 147–57.
Murray, John B., 'Munchausen Syndrome/Munchausen Syndrome by Proxy', *Journal of Psychology*, Vol. 131, No. 3, 1997, pp. 343–53.
National Early Psychosis Project, Australian Commonwealth Government, available on-line at http://yarra.vicnet.net.au/eppic/nepp.html.
——, *Australian Clinical Guidelines for Early Psychosis*, Australian Commonwealth Government, National Early Psychosis Project, Melbourne, 1998.
Netter, B. E. and D. J. Viglione Jr, 'An empirical study of malingering schizophrenia on the Rorschach', *Journal of Personal Assessment*, Vol. 62, No. 1, 1994, pp. 45–57.
Neu, Jerome, 'Minds on Trial', in Baruch A. Brody and H. Tristram Engelhardt, Jr. (eds.), *Mental Illness: law and public policy*, D. Reidel Publishing, Dordrecht/Boston, 1980.
Neuropsychiatric Institute, *General Information*, Neuropsychiatric Institute (NPI), Prince Henry Hospital, Sydney, Australia, available on-line at
http://acsusun.acsu.unsw.edu.au/~s8700122/ npiphh.html/#NPS.

New South Wales Parliament, *NSW Mental Health Act 1990, Reprinted as in force at 17 October* NSW Government Information Service, Sydney, 1994.

——, *Mental Health Legislation Amendment Bill 1997*, NSW Government Information Service, Sydney, 1997.

Nolan, Heather, Former patient, Personal Communication (letter to Richard Gosden), 26 February 1998.

Novartis (Sandoz Pharmaceuticals Corporation), Clozaril (clozapine) advertisement, *Archives of General Psychiatry*, Vol. 55, No. 1, January 1998, p. 8.

NSW Health, 'Mental Health Legislation Amendment Bill 1996', in Centre for Mental Health (eds.), *Caring for Health: Proposals for Reform—Mental Health Act 1990*, NSW Health, Sydney, 1996.

O'Callaghan, Michael, *Global Vision, 1992–1995*, accessed 14 September 1997, available on-line at http://www.ige.apc.org/glencree/dreamch2.html.

'Olanzapine For Schizophrenia', *Medical Letter on Drugs & Therapeutics*, Vol. 38, No. 992, 17 January 1997, pp. 5–7.

O'Reilly, R. L., 'Viruses and Schizophrenia', *Australian & New Zealand Journal of Psychiatry*, Vol. 28, No. 2, 1994, pp. 222–8.

Osmond, Humphry, 'Dangerous psychosocial hypotheses', *Journal of Orthomolecular Psychiatry*, Vol. 11, No. 3, 1982, pp. 216–18.

Owen, Michael and Peter McGuffin, 'The molecular genetics of schizophrenia: blind alleys, acts of faith, and difficult science', *British Medical Journal*, Vol. 305, No. 6855, 19 September 1992, pp. 664–6.

Parker, Gordon, 'Re-searching the schizophrenogenic mother', *Journal of Nervous and Mental Disease*, Vol. 170, No. 8, August 1982, pp. 452–62.

Pathe, Michele T., and Paul E. Mullen, 'The Dangerousness of the DSM-III-R', *Journal of Law and Medicine*, Vol. 1, July 1993.

Pearce, Jane, 'Harry Stack Sullivan: theory and practice', *Managed Environment Systems*, Vol. 14, No. 4, July 1984, pp. 159–66.

Pearson, Karl, *The Ethic of Freethought*, T. Fisher Unwin, London, 1888.

Perry, John Weir, *The Far Side of Madness*, Prentice-Hall, Englewood Cliffs, New Jersey, 1974.

——, *Roots of Renewal in Myth and Madness: the meaning of psychotic episodes*, Jossey-Bass, San Francisco, 1976.

——, *Trials of the Visionary Mind: spiritual emergency and the renewal process*, State University of New York Press, Albany, 1999.

Pettegrew, Jay W., Matcheri S. Keshavan, Kanagasabai Panchalingam,

Sandra Strychor, David B. Kaplan, Marjorie G. Tretta, and Maureen Allen, 'Alterations in Brain High-Energy Phosphate and Membrane Phospholid Metabolism in First-Episode, Drug-Naive Schizophrenics: A Pilot Study of the Dorsal Prefrontal Cortex by In Vivo Phosphorus 31 Nuclear Magnetic Resonance Spectroscopy', *Archives of General Psychiatry,* Vol. 48, June 1991, pp. 563–8.

Pierrakos, John C., 'Psychiatric Implications of Energy Fields in Man and Nature', in Stanley R. Dean (ed.), *Psychiatry and Mysticism,* Nelson Hall, Chicago, 1975, pp. 145–151.

Plath, Sylvia, *The Bell Jar,* Bantam, New York, 1972.

Plato, *The Republic,* Desmond Lee (trans.), Penguin, London, 1955.

Pope, Victoria, 'Mad Russians: victims of Soviet "punitive psychiatry" continue to pay a heavy price', *US News & World Report,* 16 December 1996, pp. 38–43.

Rejali, Darius, *Electric Torture: A Global History of a Torture Technology,* February 1999, available on-line at http://humanities.uchicago.edu/cis/torture/abstract/dariusrejali.html.

Report of the Royal Commission Into Deep Sleep Therapy, Justice J. P. Slattery, Royal Commissioner, New South Wales Government, Sydney, 1990.

Reuter Information Service, *Drugmakers look for home-runs with schizophrenia drugs,* Chicago, Nando.net, 1996, available on-line at http://somerset.nando.net/newsroom/ntn/health/032496/health3_14068.html.

Reznek, Lawrie, *The Nature of Disease,* Routledge and Kegan Paul, London and New York, 1987.

Richard Woods (ed.), *Understanding Mysticism,* The Athlone Press, London, 1981.

Richman, David, 'Pursuing Psychiatric Pill Pushers', in Sherry Hirsch, Joe Adams, Leonard Frank, Wade Hudson, and David Richman (eds.), *Madness Network News Reader,* Glide, San Francisco, 1974.

Richt, J. A., R. C. Alexander, S. Herzog, D. C. Hooper, R. Kean, S. Spitsin, K. Bechter, R. Schuttler, H. Feldmann, A. Heiske, Z. F. Fu, B. Dietzschold, R. Rott and H. Koprowski, 'Failure to detect Borna disease virus infection in peripheral blood leukocytes from humans with psychiatric disorders', *Journal of Neurovirology,* Vol. 3, No. 2, 3 April 1997, pp. 174–8.

Robertson, J. M., *A History of Freethought,* Watts and Co., London, 1936.

Robertson, John A., 'Informed consent: a study of decisionmaking in psychiatry', *Science,* Vol. 226, 23 November 1984, p. 960.

Rogers, R., R. M. Bagby, D. Chakraborty, 'Feigning Schizophrenic Disorders on the MMPI-2: Detection of Coached Simulators', *Journal of Personality Assessment,* Vol. 60, No. 2, 1993, pp. 215–26.

Rosenhan, David L., 'On Being Sane in Insane Places', *Science,* Vol. 179, 19 January 1973, pp. 250–8.

Roy, Leena and Suby Roy, 'Does the theory of logical types inform a theory of communication?', *Journal of Genetic Psychology,* Vol. 148, No. 4, December 1987, pp. 519–25

Roy, Louise, *Psychiatry and the Suppression of Dissent,* unpublished report on the use of psychiatric labels to intimidate whistleblowers, December 1997.

Royal College of Psychiatrists, 'Stereotypical attitudes towards Christian names and gender may influence diagnosis', Press release, Annual Conference, July 2000.

Rubinstein, G., 'Schizophrenia, Infection and Temperature. An Animal Model for Investigating their Interrelationships', *Schizophrenia Research,* Vol. 10, No. 2, 1993, pp. 95–102.

Russell, Andrew T., 'The Clinical Presentation of Childhood-Onset Schizophrenia', *Schizophrenia Bulletin,* Vol. 20, No. 4, 1994, pp. 631–46.

Sandyk, R., S. R. Kay and A. E. Merriam, 'Atrophy of the Cerebellar Vermis: Relevance to the Symptoms of Schizophrenia', *International Journal of Neuroscience,* Vol. 57, Nos. 3 and 4, 1991, pp. 205–212.

SANE Australia, *Carers Handbook,* SANE Australia, Melbourne, 1996.

——, *Something is not quite right,* pamphlet produced by SANE Australia, Melbourne, 1998.

Sarbin, Theodore R., 'Towards the Obsolescence of the Schizophrenia Hypothesis', *Journal of Mind and Behaviour,* Vol. 11, Nos. 3 and 4, 1990, pp. 259–83.

Sarbin, Theodore R. and James C. Mancuso, *Schizophrenia: medical diagnosis or moral verdict?,* Pergamon Press, New York, 1980.

Schaler, Jeffrey A., Letter to the Editor, *New York Times,* 14 October 1998.

Schatner, Marcus, 'Some observations in the treatment of dementia praecox with hypoglycemia: part 2, psychological implication', *Psychiatric Quarterly,* Vol. 12, No. 1, 1938, pp. 22–6.

Scheff, Thomas (ed.), *Labelling Madness,* Prentice-Hall, Englewood Cliffs, N.J., 1975.

——, *Being Mentally Ill,* Aldine, New York, 1984.

Schizophrenia Information Centre, 'Schizophrenia: the early signs', *Schizophrenia Information Centre Bulletin*, NSW Association For Mental Health, Gladesville.

Sedgwick, Peter, 'R. D. Laing: self, symptom and society', in Robert Boyers and Robert Orrill (eds.), *Laing and Anti-Psychiatry*, Penguin, Harmondsworth, 1972.

Shakespeare, William, 'King Lear', in W. J. Craig (ed.), *Shakespeare Complete Works*, Oxford University Press, London, 1969, pp. 908–42.

Shaw, C., 'The World Psychiatric Association and Soviet Psychiatry', in Robert Van Voren (ed.), *Soviet Psychiatric Abuse in the Gorbachev Era*, International Association on the Political Use of Psychiatry, Amsterdam, 1992.

Shiovitz, T. M., T. L. Welke, P. D. Tigel, R. Anand, R. D. Hartman, J. J. Sramek, N. M. Kurtz and N. R. Cutler, 'Cholinergic rebound and rapid onset psychosis following abrupt clozapine withdrawal', *Schizophrenia Bulletin*, Vol. 22, No. 4, 1996, pp. 591–5.

Silverton, Leigh and S. Mednick, 'Class drift and schizophrenia', *Acta Psychiatrica Scandinavica*, Vol. 70, No. 4, October 1984, pp. 304–9.

Silverstein, Ken, 'Prozac.org: an influential mental health nonprofit finds its "grassroots" watered by pharmaceutical millions', *Mother Jones*, November/December 1999, available on-line at http://www.motherjones.com/mother_jones/ND99/nami.html.

Simmers, Frank and Froma Walsh, 'The nature of the symbiotic bond between mother and schizophrenic', *American Journal of Orthopsychiatry*, Vol. 47, No. 3, July 1977, pp. 484–94.

Smith, R. S., 'The GI T-lymphocyte theory of schizophrenia: some new observations', *Medical Hypotheses*, Vol. 37, No. 1, January 1992, pp. 27–30.

Southcott, Inge, 'Anguish over mental health Catch 22', Letters to the Editor, *Sydney Morning Herald*, 26 May 1995.

——, letter to Peter Macdonald, in Peter Macdonald, 'Mental Health Support and Counselling Services', Legislative Assembly, 26 October 1995, *Hansard 51st Parliament 1995-1998*.

Spitze, M., M. Lukas, S. Maier and L. Hermle, 'Comprehension of metaphoric speech by healthy probands and schizophrenic patients: An experimental psychopathologic contribution to concretism', *Nervenarzt*, Vol. 65, No. 5, May 1994, pp. 282–92.

Spitzer, R. L., 'On pseudoscience in science, logic in remission, and psychiatric diagnosis: a critique of Rosenhan's "On being sane in insane places" ', *Journal of Abnormal Psychology,* Vol. 84, 1975, pp. 442–52.

Squires, R. F., 'How a poliovirus might cause schizophrenia: a commentary on Eagles' hypothesis', *Neurochemical Research,* Vol. 22, No. 5, May 1997, pp. 647–56.

Stace, Walter T., *The Teachings of the Mystics,* Mentor, New York, 1960.

Stanilla, J. K., J. de-Leon and G. M. Simpson, 'Clozapine withdrawal resulting in delirium with psychosis: a report of three cases', *Journal of Clinical Psychiatry,* Vol. 58, No. 6, June 1997, pp. 252–5.

Stevens, Lawrence, *Psychiatric Drugs: cure or quackery?,* accessed March 1998, available on-line at http://www.cjnetworks.com/~cgrandy/stevens/psychiatric_drugs.html.

Sullivan, Harry Stack, 'Erogenous Maturation', *Psychoanalytical Review,* Vol. 61, 1926, pp. 1–15.

——, 'Discussion', in D. Ewen Cameron, 'Early schizophrenia', *American Journal of Psychiatry,* 95, 1938, pp. 578–80.

——, *Schizophrenia as a Human Process,* W. W. Norton and Company, New York, 1962.

Susser, E., R. Neugebauer, H. W. Hoek, A. S. Brown, S. Lin, D. Labovitz and J. M. Gorman, 'Schizophrenia after prenatal famine. Further evidence', *Archives of General Psychiatry,* Vol. 53, No. 1, January 1996, pp. 25–31.

Szasz, Thomas S. (ed.), *The Age of Madness,* Routledge and Kegan Paul, London, 1973.

——, *The Manufacture of Madness: a comparative study of the inquisition and the mental health movement,* Paladin, St Albans, 1973.

——, *The Myth of Mental Illness,* revised edition, Harper and Row, New York, 1974.

——, *Law, Liberty, and Psychiatry: an inquiry into the social uses of mental health practices,* Routledge and Kegan Paul, London, 1974.

——, *Schizophrenia: the sacred symbol of psychiatry,* Syracuse University Press, Syracuse, New York, 1976.

——, *Psychiatric Slavery,* The Free Press, New York, 1977.

——, 'Diagnoses are not diseases', *Lancet,* Vol. 338, No. 8782, 21 December 1991, pp. 1574–7.

——, 'Psychiatric Diagnosis, Psychiatric Power and Psychiatric Abuse', *Journal of Medical Ethics,* Vol. 20, No. 3, September 1994, pp. 135–9.

——, *Cruel Compassion: psychiatric control of society's unwanted,* John Wiley and Sons, New York, 1994.

——, 'Idleness and Lawlessness in the Therapeutic State', *Society,* Vol. 32,

No. 4, 1995, pp. 30–6.
——, 'The Case Against Psychiatric Coercion', *Independent Review*, Vol. I, No. 4, spring 1997, pp. 1086–653.
——, Letter to the Editor, *New York Times*, 14 October 1998.
Temerlin, Maurice K., 'Suggestion Effects in Psychiatric Diagnosis', in Thomas Scheff, *Labelling Madness*, Prentice-Hall, Englewood Cliffs, N.J., 1975, pp. 46–54.
Tennyson, Alfred Lord, letter to Mr. B. P. Blood, quoted in William James, *The Varieties of Religious Experience*, Fontana, London, 1960.
Thomas, Phillip, *The Dialectics of Schizophrenia*, Free Association Books, London, 1997.
Tichurst, S., 'Dementia', in Robert Kosky, Hadi Salimi Eshkevari and Vaughan Carr (eds.), *Mental Health and Illness: a textbook for students of health sciences*, Butterworth-Heinemann, Sydney, 1991.
Tienari, P. J. and L. C. Wynne, 'Adoption studies of schizophrenia', *Annals of Medicine*, Vol. 26, No. 4, August 1994, pp. 233–7.
Torrey, E. Fuller, 'A Viral-Anatomical Explanation of Schizophrenia', *Schizophrenia Bulletin*, Vol. 17, No. 1, 1991, pp. 15–18.
Treffert, Darold A., 'Balancing Legal Realities: The Courts, the Legislature and Public Psychiatry', in C. Christian Beels and Leona L. Bachrach (eds), *Survival Strategies for Public Psychiatry*, Jossey-Bass Inc., San Francisco, 1989.
United Nations, *Convention against Torture and Other Cruel, Inhuman or Degrading Treatment or Punishment*, G. A. res. 39/46, annex, 39 U. N. GAOR Supp. (No. 51) at 197, U. N. Doc. A/39/51 (1984), entered into force 26 June 1987, available on-line at http://www.umn.edu/humanarts/instree/h2catoc.htm.
——, 'International Covenant on Economic, Social and Cultural Rights', in Satish Chandra (ed.), *International Documents on Human Rights*, Mittal Publications, New Delhi, 1990, pp. 11–23.
——, 'International Covenant on Civil and Political Rights' in Satish Chandra (ed.), *International Documents on Human Rights*, Mittal Publications, New Delhi, 1990, pp. 24–52.
——, 'Principles for the Protection of Persons with Mental Illness and for the Improvement of Mental Health Care', in Australian Human Rights and Equal Opportunity Commission, *Human Rights and Mental Illness: report of the national inquiry into the human rights of people with mental illness*, Australian Government Publishing Service, Canberra, 1993, pp. 989–1005.
——, 'Declaration on the Elimination of all Forms of Intolerance and of

Discrimination Based on Religion or Belief', UN Resolution 36/55, 25 November 1981, reproduced in Human Rights and Equal Opportunity Commission, *Free to Believe? The Right to Freedom of Religion and Belief in Australia*, Human Rights and Equal Opportunity Commission, Sydney, 1997, pp. 35–6.

United Nations Centre for Human Rights, *United Nations Action in the Field of Human Rights*, United Nations, Geneva, 1994.

Valenstein, Elliot S. (ed.), *The Psychosurgery Debate*, W. H. Freeman, San Francisco, 1980.

Van Drimmelen-Krabbe, Jenny J., T. Bedirhan Ustun, David H. Thompson, Andre L'Hours, John Orley and Norman Sartorius, 'Homosexuality in the International Classification of Diseases: a clarification', *JAMA, Journal of the American Medical Association*, Vol. 272, No. 21, 1994, p. 1660.

Varma, S. L., A. M. Zain and S. Singh, 'Psychiatric morbidity in the first-degree relatives of schizophrenic patients', *American Journal of Medical Genetics*, Vol. 74, No. 1, 21 February 1997, pp. 7–11.

Volkmar, Fred R., 'Childhood and adolescent psychosis: a review of the past 10 years', *Journal of the American Academy of Child and Adolescent Psychiatry*, Vol. 35, No. 7, 1996, pp. 843–52.

Wachenfeld, Margaret G., *The Human Rights of the Mentally Ill in Europe Under the European Convention on Human Rights*, Nordic Journal of International Law and The Danish Center For Human Rights, Copenhagen, 1992.

Wahl, Otto F., 'Schizophrenogenic parenting in abnormal psychology textbooks', *Teaching of Psychology*, Vol. 16, No. 1, February 1989, pp. 31–3.

Wahlberg, K. E., L. C. Wynne, H. Oja, P. Keskitalo, L. Pykalainen, I. Lahti, J. Moring, M. Naarala, A. Sorri, M. Seitamaa, K. Laksy, J. Kolassa and P. Tienari, 'Gene-environment interaction in vulnerability to schizophrenia: findings from the Finnish adoptive family study of schizophrenia', *American Journal of Psychiatry*, Vol. 154, No. 3, March 1997, pp. 355–62.

Walsh, Froma W., 'Concurrent grandparent death and birth of schizophrenic offspring: an intriguing finding', *Family Process*, Vol. 17, No. 4, December 1978, pp. 457–63.

Warner, Richard, *Recovery From Schizophrenia*, Routledge & Kegan Paul, London, 1985.

Warnock, Mary (ed.), *Mill: utilitarianism and other writings*, World Publishing, New York, 1962.

Wear, Stephen, *Informed Consent,* Kluwer Academic Publishers, Dordrecht, 1993.

Weatherall, M., 'An end to the search for new drugs', *Nature,* Vol. 296, 1 April 1982.

Weinberger, Daniel R., 'From neuropathology to neurodevelopment: schizophrenia, part 2', *Lancet,* Vol. 346, No. 8974, 26 August 1995, pp. 552–8.

Weitz, Don, 'Cruel and Unusual—A Human Rights Violation', unpublished article, posted on, *Support Coalition SCI list* (internet discussion list), 4 December 1998.

Western Psychiatric Institute and Clinic (WPIC), accessed July 1998, available on-line at http://brains2.wpic.pitt.edu/paces.html.

Whistleblowers Australia, *Abuse of Medical Assessments to Dismiss Whistleblowers,* 1998, available on-line at, http://www.uow.edu.au/arts/sts/bmartin/dissent/documents/psychiatry.html

Whitlock, F. A., 'Psychosurgery', in Erica M. Bates and Paul R. Wilson (eds.), *Mental Disorder or Madness,* University of Queensland Press, St Lucia, 1979, pp. 181–201.

Wiesel, F. A., 'Neuroleptic Treatment of Patients with Schizophrenia. Mechanisms of Action and Clinical Significance', *British Journal of Psychiatry,* No. 23, 1994, pp. 65–70.

Williams, Gareth and Jennie Popay, 'Lay Knowledge and the Privilege of Experience', in J. Gabe, D. Kelleher, and G. Williams (eds.), *Challenging Medicine,* Routledge, London, 1994.

Wing, J. K., 'Psychiatry in the Soviet Union', *British Medical Journal,* 9 March 1974.

Wold, P. N. and S. Soled, 'The family history of mental illness and welfare dependence', *Journal of Clinical Psychiatry,* Vol. 39, No. 4, April 1978, pp. 328–31.

Wolf, Moisey, Solomon Wolf and William Harwell Wilson, 'Clozapine Treatment in Russia: A Review of Clinical Research', *Psychiatric Services,* Vol. 46, No. 3, March 1995.

Woods, Richard (ed.), *Understanding Mysticism,* The Athlone Press, London, 1981.

World Health Organisation, *The ICD-10 Classification of Mental Disorders and Behavioural Disorders: clinical descriptions and diagnostic guidelines,* World Health Organisation, Geneva, 1992.

Wright, Robert, 'The Biology of Violence', *New Yorker,* March 1 1995, pp. 68–77.

Wyatt, Richard Jed, Ioline Henter, Megan C. Leary and B. A. Edward Taylor, *An Economic Evaluation of Schizophrenia—1991*, Neuroscience Research Center, Neuropsychiatry Branch, National Institute of Mental Health.

'Young Adults Experiencing Psychosis Remain Undiagnosed', *Mental Health Net*, accessed August 1996, available on-line at http://www.cmhc.com/articles/young.htm.

Yung, Alison R., Patrick D. McGorry, Colleen A. McFarlane, Henry J. Jackson, George C. Patton and Arun Rakkar, 'Monitoring and Care of Young People at Incipient Risk of Psychosis', *Schizophrenia Bulletin*, Vol. 22, No. 2, 1996, pp. 283–304.

Yung, Alison R. and Patrick D. McGorry, 'The Prodromal Phase of First-Episode Psychosis: Past and Current Conceptualisations', *Schizophrenia Bulletin*, Vol. 22, No. 2, 1996, pp. 353–70.

Yung, Alison R. and Patrick D. McGorry, 'Is pre-psychotic intervention realistic in schizophrenia and related disorder?', *Australian and New Zealand Journal of Psychiatry*, No. 31, 1997, pp. 799–805.

Yung, Alison R. et al., 'Prediction of psychosis: a step towards indicated prevention of schizophrenia', *British Journal of Psychiatry*, Vol. 172, Supplement, June 1998, pp. 14–20.

Yung, Alison R., Lisa J. Phillips, Patrick D. McGorry, Mats A. Halgren, Colleen A. McFarlane, Henry J. Jackson, Shona Francey and George C. Patton, 'Can we predict the onset of first-episode psychosis in a high-risk group?', *International Clinical Psychopharmacology*, Vol. 13 (suppl.1), 1998, pp. s23–s30.

Zeneca Pharmaceuticals, Seroquel (quetiapine) advertisement, *Psychiatric Services*, Vol. 49, No. 3, March 1998, p. 284.

Index

Abbott Laboratories 95
action, consequences of 154
admission principles 104
adolescent thinking 228 *see also*
 magical thinking
adolescents 7, 11, 65, 217, 226, 229, 231, 243, 244
 and neuroleptics 217 ff.
adoption studies 72–3 *see also*
 theories: environmental; Kety study
adult identity 185–6 *see also* Szasz, Thomas
'affectation' 136–7 *see also* Jung, Carl
akathisia, neuroleptic-induced 204
alienation 11 *see also* social alienation
alienists 129
alogia 175–6, 178
 defined 175–6
alternative meaning 257–8 *see also*
 life meaning; quest for meaning
Alzheimer 34
Alzheimer's disease 65
American Law Institute 199
American Psychiatric Association (APA) 10, 40–1, 92 *see also*
 pharmaceutical: industry
American psychiatric profession 10, 59
 and commitment to scientific medicine 10
Amnesty International 20, 212
amygdalotomy 214
anti-depressants 8
antisocial behaviour 15
anti-psychiatry movement 130 ff. *see also* Weitz, Don
Antisocial Personality Disorder 11
approaches

biopsychosocial 89
 medical/psychiatric 9
 mystical 130 ff.
 psychoanalytical 54
archetypes 138–9 *see also* Jung, Carl; 142; Perry, John Weir; 146; Campbell, Joseph
Article 1 154 *see also* United Nations Declaration on the Elimination of all Forms of Intolerance and of Discrimination Based on Religion or Belief
Article 2 153
 and mentally ill 153 *see also*
 International Covenant on Civil and Political Rights
Article 7 204 ff.
Article 9 218
Article 12 21, 164
Article 18 152 ff., 164, 256
 uncertainty in 157–8 *see also*
 International Covenant on Civil and Political Rights
AstraZeneca 237, 238 *see also* Zeneca
at-risk people 225, 228, 231, 241, 243
Australia, research 226–31
Australian Clinical Guidelines for Early Psychosis 226, 231–2, 234, 241, 244, 245 *see also*
 Schizophrenia Australia Foundation: Checklist 2
Australian Council on the Ageing 216
Australian Human Rights and Equal Opportunity Commission 15–17, 100, 256 *see also* rights, human
 on early diagnosis and treatment 15–16

autism 35, 46
avolition 177–9 *see also* symptoms: negative

Bacon, Francis 129
Baillarger, Jules 31
Bateson, Gregory 81-3, 85, 130–1 *see also* theories: double bind; theories: family
behaviour *see also* problems: of behaviour
    disorders 11
    setting 174
belief 151
    in 'real' schizophrenics 250
        definition of 256
        holding of 157
        manifestation of 157–9
beliefs 3, 234
    culturally unacceptable 159, 171
    false 158, 170–1
    cultural 167, 170
    ordinarily accepted 159
    popularity of 48
    unusual 3
The Bell Jar 210–11

biomedical treatments 92 *see also* drugs; treatment: drugs
biopsychiatrists 222
The Bird of Paradise 133
births and incidence 66
Blake, William 129
Bleuler, Eugen 33-7, 136, 138, 167
brain 207, 215 *see also* drugs: neuroleptic; Jung, Carl
    abnormalities 64–5, 75
    architecture 32, 63, 254
    atrophy 216,
    blocking higher thinking centres 159–61
    chemistry 5, 13, 215, 240, 254
    damage 216, 225
    disease 137, 166, 253, 258
    dopamine neurotransmitter system 160
    dysfunction 136, 139, 182
    -mapping 211
    toxin in 138–9
Breggin, Peter 59, 69, 72, 214, 247
Bristol-Myers Squibb 95
British empiricism 32
British Journal of Psychiatry 245
Bucke, Richard Maurice 127–9, 146
Buckingham Project 225
Buddhism 119
Burdekin, Brian 24 ff., 100
Burdekin Inquiry 24–6
    and 'consumers' 26
business community 186

Cameron, D. Ewen 245–6
Campaign to Extend Involuntary Treatment in New South Wales (NSW) 97–102
Campbell, Joseph 115, 145–9, 258
cardiazol 209
catatonia 35, 42, 45, 212
catatonic behaviour 170, 173
    defined 173
catatonic-like behaviour states as a side effect of drug treatment 161
Catatonic Type *see* schizophrenia: sub-types
central nervous system 65, 67
cerebral syphilis 33, 66
character traits 12
Chelmsford Royal Commission 100
'chemical lobotomy' 160 *see also* drugs: neuroleptic
'chemical straitjacket' 215
children 7, 11, 13, 109
    'hyperactive' 8
    and neuroleptics 217
chlorpromazine 159–163 *see also* drugs: antipsychotic; drugs: neuroleptic; Thorazine
Christian Church 116
Christianity 115
CIA 245
civil liberties 3, 11, 18, 19, 25, 26, 91, 96, 102, 202, 251
civilisation
    earliest 142, 146 *see also* Perry,

John Weir
    outcome of *see* Jung, Carl
class *see* social class; social status
classification systems 3, 52 *see also*
    Diagnostic and Statistical Manual of
    Mental Disorders; International
    Classification of Diseases
    biological 52
    botanical 52
client 251 *see also* relatives; State
clinical guidelines *see* Australian
    Clinical Guidelines for Early
    Psychosis; symptoms; Schizophrenia
    Australia Foundation
clinical
    psychologists 12, 91, 92
    social workers 12, 91, 106–7
    trials 109
clozapine (Clozaril) 58-60, 218, 238
    see also drugs: neuroleptic: 'atypical'
coercion *see* psychiatry; rights of the
    individual to freedom from
Cohen, David 247
Columbia University 93
Columbia Psychiatry Institute 93
community counselling orders (CCOs)
    203
    in NSW 19
community treatment orders (CTOs)
    203, 215
    in NSW 19
community-based catchment system
    225
community views 9, 10
components, biological and
    environmental *see* approaches:
    biopsychosocial
'concrete' *see* alogia
concreteness 175–7
    in patients 175–6
    in diagnosticians 175–6
conduct disorder 15, 217 *see also*
    adolescents; children
    defined by *DSM-IV* 15
    and neuroleptics and lack of
        therapeutic rationale 217
conferences, organisation of 237 *see*
    also drug: companies
confidentiality 23, 103
conscience 153 ff. *see also* freedom
    collective 212
consciousness, 138, 142, 146, 149,
    160, 209 *see also* Bucke, Richard
    Maurice; mentally ill person; Perry,
    John Weir
    altered states 3, 117, 122, 158
    levels 127–8, 148, 149
    normal human 119, 127
consensus-building *see* medical model
consent *see also* informed consent;
    State
    presumed (to treatment) 109
    proxy 10
    parens patriae 109–10
    treatment 23
    withholding 104
consumer support groups *see* interest
    groups
consumerism 249, 257
'consumers' 4, 26, 91, 94 *see also*
    Burdekin inquiry; interest groups
    primary (patients) 94
    secondary (usually relatives) 94,
        97, 102
controversy 3 *see also* schizophrenia:
    theories of cause
    over classification system 3
    over diagnosis 3
    over treatments 3
Convention against Torture and
    Other Cruel, Inhuman or Degrading
    Treatment or Punishment 206
Cosmic Consciousness 127 *see also*
    Bucke, Richard Maurice
Crichton, Alexander 30
criminal
    justice system 91; 250
    liability 20
    offences 203, 207 *see also* rights:
        of misfits
cultural
    -outsider-schizophrenic 168–71,
        185
    acceptance 170, 179

bias 174
change 79–80, 144
culturally
 based prejudices 152
 defined boundaries 169
Curling, T.B. 51
cyclical mood disorders 33

danger 157 *see also* physical
 dangerousness; harm
dangerous 151, 158, 249
 drugs 4 *see also* physical
 dangerousness; harm
Dante 129
delusion, shared collective 167
Delusional Disorder 47–8
 sub-types 47
 grandiose 200
delusions 3, 38–9, 41–2, 44, 45, 46,
 47, 48, 114, 139, 152, 158, 159,
 170, 175, 179, 216, 220, 250, 255
 types 42, 170
dementia 216, 218, 260
'dementia praecox' 33, 36, 136–7
 as the foundation for the modern
 description of schizophrenia 34,
 136
Dementia Praecox 34
democratic societies 25, 220–1, 257
 see also psychiatric: abuse
developed countries *see* drugs: market
 expansion: in developed countries
developing countries *see* drugs:
 market expansion: in developing
 countries
developmental disorder 46
Deveson, Anne 97, 99–100
deviance 16, 47, 181, 229
 medical containment 7
 'medicalisation' of 13, 20, 111
 in developing countries 20
 mental 175
 and personality types 10, 32
 group 86
 in the language of parents and
 patients 86 *see also* informed
 consent; consent: presumed

deviants 166
diagnosis, 10, 41, 170, 221, 240
 despite no medical problems 4
 and drug treatment 4 *see also*
 drugs: treatment; treatment
 early 15–16
 international 10
 uncertainty 25, 48, 172, 194
 false 165
 false positive 25, 228, 241
 misuse 221
 paradox 244
 and solitary individuals 115
 subjective nature of 25, 47, 62, 74
diagnosing by suggestion 192
diagnostic
 agreement 12
 criteria 4, 40–1, 44, 74, 169 ff.,
 175–84, 228, 249, 259
 decisions 114
 indicator 174
 manuals see *DSM-II*; *DSM-III*;
 DSM-III-R; *DSM-IV*; *Malleus
 Maleficarum*
 methods 253
 techniques 9
 tools 3 *see also* Australian Clinical
 Guidelines for Early Psychosis;
 Diagnostic and Statistical Manual
 of Mental Disorders;
 International Classification of
 Diseases
 Soviet 220 *see also DSM-II*; *DSM-
 III*; *DSM-III-R*; *DSM-IV*
*Diagnostic and Statistical Manual of
 Mental Disorders* 10–13
 and Australian psychiatrists 10–12
 see also DSM-II; *DSM-III*; *DSM-
 III-R*; *DSM-IV*
Diehl, Scott 70–1
disease *see also* schizophrenia
 categories 187
 criteria 51–2
 drug-induced 238
 and human values 52
 meanings of 48–9
 model 252 *see also* psychiatrists

organic 138
and relatives 94, 109, 183, 251–2
diseased minds 9, 166, 252
disordered thinking 3
disordered thoughts *see* thought disorder
disorders *see also* behaviour; cyclical moods; *DSM-IV*
   medical, symptoms that overlap with schizophrenia 260
   and work 11
disorganised
   behaviour 174
   speech 170, 172, 174
   thinking 42, 45
Disorganised Type *see* schizophrenia: sub-types
disruptive behaviour 91
distortions of thinking and perception 41–2
disturbances of association and affectivity 35, 138 *see also* Bleuler
doctor/patient relationship 4
dopamine *see* brain; drugs: neuroleptic
dopamine hypothesis *see* theories: 'dopamine' *see also* brain
drug
   companies 4, 96–7, 99
   influence of 234, 237, 247, 250, 262 *see also* pharmaceutical: companies
   disorders 4
   therapy *see* treatment: drug
drug-free residential facility 261–2 *see also* Perry, John Weir
drug treatment 53, 98, 260
   forced 4, 5, 164 *see also* drugs; treatment: forced
drug 4, 7, 13, 18, 54, 55, 89, 110
   anti-psychotic 159, 161, 212, 216 *see also* drugs: neuroleptic; chlorpromazine
   captive market 19
   company profits 19
   conventional 61
   generics 60–1

   long-acting 19
   as management not cure 4
   mind-altering 163 *see also* treatment: side effects; drugs: neuroleptic
   neuroleptic 15, 55–60, 61, 62, 64, 69, 92, 93, 107, 150, 159–64, 197, 204, 214–23, 236, 254
     'atypical' 58, 60, 93–4, 234, 236, 237, 239, 246
      and expansion of market 223
     as chemical restraint 216–17
     complaints by involuntary patients 107
     and injurious falls in nursing homes 216
     intoxication 254
     lack of therapeutic rationale 217–18
     long-acting 215
     market expansion 20, 236
      in developed countries 20
      in developing countries 20
     market in the United States 219, 220
     as prophylactic treatment 237–40
     as punishment and torture 218–23
     as rape 221
     and right to liberty 214–218 *see also* right to liberty
     side effects 4, 56–9, 62, 160, 204, 217, 222
      and dangerous behaviour 57
      and suicide 204
   and side effects 4, 222
   and sudden death 238 *see also* disease: drug-induced; drugs: neuroleptic
   as treatment 4, 114
   United States' market 19–20
   withdrawal and psychotic reaction 240
DSM *see also* Diagnostic and Statistical Manual of Mental Disorders

and empowerment of medical
  practitioners 11
DSM-II 72 see also Diagnostic and
  Statistical Manual of Mental
  Disorders
DSM-III 10, 190 see also Diagnostic
  and Statistical Manual of Mental
  Disorders
DSM-III-R 226, 227, 228
DSM-IV 10, 11, 15, 16, 40–1, 44, 46,
  47, 56, 114, 158, 170–9, 187–9,
  194, 205, 219–20, 225, 227, 229,
  242, 260 see also Diagnostic and
  Statistical Manual of Mental
  Disorders
  and essential features 41
due process 106
Dufor, Jean Francois 30
duration of untreated psychosis
  (DUP) 224–5

early detection 225
early intervention in psychosis 226,
  237 see also Early Psychosis
  Prevention and Intervention Centre
early psychosis 224–47, 248
  concept 244 see also symptoms;
    treatment
Early Psychosis Prevention and
  Intervention Centre (EPPIC) 226,
  228, 237, 242–3, 245
Early Psychosis Training Pack 235,
  236, 244 see also Australian Clinical
  Guidelines for Early Psychosis
ECT 210–12, 222, 245 see also 'fear
  therapy'
ego 141–3
elderly people 109, 216 see also
  nursing homes
electroconvulsive therapy 114, 208
  see also ECT
Eli Lilly 60, 95, 137
emotional rapport 137 see also Jung,
  Carl
employers and personality types 11
Enlightenment 38
Ennis, Bruce 25

Esquirol, Jean Etienne 31
ethical
  burdens 240
  questions 229
  responsibility 238
ethics 107, 108–9, 190, 249–50, 255
  see also scientific research
eugenics policies 72
European Christian tradition 155,
  and heretics 155, 167 see also
    Christianity
exclusion of other conditions 45–6
experience see also mystical
  schizophrenic 139
  'split' see Laing, R.D.
experts, judgement of 251
extrapyramidal side effects (EPSEs)
  57–9 see also drugs: neuroleptics:
  side effects
Ey, Henri 32

Factitious Disorder 187, 188, 194 see
  also Munchausen Syndrome
family 180, 183, 213, 220, 234
  groups 182
  history 232
  propensities 69–71 see also
    theories: genetic
  types
    skewed and schismatic 84–5 see
      also theories: family stress;
      Lidz, Theodore
fantasy, impulses of 35
Food and Drug Administration 59
'fear therapy' 208, 210, 221 see also
  ECT
Flynn, Laurie 96 see also interest
  groups
forced psychiatric intervention 6, 7
  see also treatment: forced
Fox, George 126
fragmentation between thought and
  feeling see Bleuler
Frame, Janet 195–6
Frank, Leonard Roy 25, 179–80
freedom of thought and belief 5, 152
  ff. see also right: to freedom of

thought and belief; conscience
Freeman, Walter 213
Freud, Sigmund 39, 76-8, 136, 195
Freudian
  psychoanalytic techniques 76
  training 143
Fromm-Reichman, Frieda 79
frontal-lobe dysfunction 63
functionality test 49–50

Gardiner-Caldwell Communications 235 *see also* pharmaceutical
Gautama the Buddha 129
general paresis 66
general practitioners 8
genetic component 66, 86 *see also* theories: genetic
global culture of the market place 26
Greek philosophers 116
Group of Schizophrenias see Dementia Praecox

Haldol 217, 218, 220 *see also* haloperidol
haloperidol 94, 161–2
hallucinations 3, 29–32, 35, 39, 41, 42, 44–5, 46, 49, 76, 123, 125, 139, 152, 161, 170, 171, 175, 216, 219, 250, 255 *see also* symptoms; psychotic, as a side effect of drug treatment; diagnostic manuals; voices
  auditory 42, 66, 84, 171
  defined *see DSM-IV*
  normal 31–2
harm 15, 50–1, 97, 154–5, 164, 203 *see also* disease; physical dangerousness
  from early diagnosis and treatment 15
  and the exercise of human rights 20
  to a person's social identity 102
  'serious' vs. 'serious physical' 102
Hartley, David 30
heretics 167 *see also* European Christian tradition

Hobbes, Thomas 29
homelessness 16
homosexuality 49–50
hostel settings 216
How to Become a Schizophrenic 182 *see also* Modrow, John
human behaviour and internal and external controls 114
human identity 10
Human Rights *see* rights, human
human rights bodies *see* UN Commission on Human Rights; Burdekin Inquiry
Human Rights Commission 26
human rights organisations 255–7 *see also* Australian Human Rights and Equal Opportunity Commission; Burdekin inquiry; Human Rights Committee of the United Nations; rights, human; UN Commission on Human Rights
Human Rights Committee of the United Nations 156
Huntington's Chorea 69
hypotheses
  brain-atrophy 63–4
hypothetical mental patient 158–9

ICI 96
Idleness and Lawlessness in the Therapeutic State 185
inability to work 179
incarceration 5, 19, 21, 25, 91, 96, 158–9, 190, 195, 204, 221
incarcerated people 215
identical twins 64 *see also* twins
identity
  adult 186
  vs. self-identity *see* self-identity
impairment in communication 173
individual autonomy 107 *see also* informed consent
infection therapies
infectious organisms *see* theories: biological
influenza-vaccination programme 236
informed consent 3–4, 23, 104,

107–1, 216 *see also* rights; consent: presumed
  moral, ethical and legal considerations 107–8
  paradoxes 109
  treatment without 3–4
  withholding 104
inner revelation 260
Inquiry into Human Rights and Mental Illness 217
Inquisitors 167
insanity
  defence 292
  as defined
    in Britain 199
    by the American Law Institute 199
  plea 197–203
insight 110, 197, 207, 257
  'lack of' 110, 220
instincts 138–9 *see also* Jung, Carl
Institute of Psychiatry of the USSR Academy of Medical Sciences 219
insulin coma 208
interest groups 90 ff.
  and medical model 90 ff., 103
  pharmaceutical industry 92
    funding of consumer support groups 94–7, 102
    funding of scientific research 92–4
  psychiatric researchers
  relatives 94–6 *see also* relatives
International Classification of Diseases (ICD-10) 10, 16–17, 40–1, 44, 46, 114, 170 *see also* unemployment
  description of schizophrenia 27
International Covenant on Civil and Political Rights (ICCPR) 152 ff., 203, 205–6, 218, 256
International Covenant on Economic, Social and Cultural Rights (ICESCR) 21, 164 *see also* rights, human
international law 5, 108, 152
international lobbying campaign 4
intolerance 38, 143, 166, 250

involuntary
  admissions 203
  commitment 18, 24, 96, 97, 98, 102, 195 *see also* Frame, Janet
  detention 23
  and the UN *see* United Nations
  hospitalisation 158, 203, 204
  participants 177
  patients 4, 9, 18–19, 21, 23, 104–5, 210, 215 *see also* drugs: captive market; drugs: neuroleptic
  as mystical voyagers 133
  numbers in NSW 19
  proportion 104–5
  treatment 19, 91, 255, 257

James, William 126–7
Janssen Cilag 96, 235, 237
Jesus 125, 129
John the Baptist 125
John of Ephesus 124
Joseph, Jay 72
Jung, Carl 34, 130, 135–40, 142–3
Jungian *see* Jung, Carl; theories
justice 5, 7
  system, and precautionary control measures 201–2

Keltner, Norman 71
Kendler, Kenneth 70–1
Kety, Seymour 71
Kety study 72–3
King Lear 186–7
Kirk and Kutchins 190
Kraepelin, Emile 33–4, 37, 136, 167
  see also theories: associationist
  fragmentation between thought and feeling 34
  and 'fundamental symptoms' 35
  'split mind' 34

'labelling' 169, 181, 185, 230 *see also* schizophrenic role: scripting of laboratory tests 3, 12, 15, 25, 47
  absence of 28, 159, 195
Laing, R.D. 37, 130–5, 148, 150, 258
Largactil 220 *see also* Thorazine

law 198 *see also* international law; legal devices; legislation; rights, human
lay beliefs *see* community views
learning disorders 11
legal devices 19, 257
  redress 257
  system 198
legislation 4, 7–8, 19, 23, 91, 95, 96, 103, 106, 157, 159, 206, 215 *see also* Campaign to Extend Involuntary Treatment in NSW; NSW Mental Health Act
Leifer, Ronald 9
libertarian philosophy 185 *see also* Szasz, Thomas
liberty 202 *see also* right to liberty
libido 76
Lidz, Theodore 84–6 *see also* theories: family stress
life meaning 157–9 *see also* quest for meaning
lobotomy operations 213
Locke, John 29-30, 32-3
London Health Sciences Centre, Ontario 236

Macdonald, Peter Dr 1, 98, 99, 101–2
madness 207
  simulation of 186–7
magical thinking 227, 228, 229, 242, 247 *see also* adolescents
  and rates 228, 243
Magnetic resonance imaging (MRI) 64
'Malingering' 187–8, 194 *see also* DSM-IV
Malleus Maleficarum see medieval witches
manic depression 65
The Manufacture of Madness 181 *see also* scapegoat; Szasz, Thomas
marital relationships 84–5 *see also* theories: family environment
Marks, John 245
masturbation 174–5

maternal over-protection 79 *see also* theories: family environment; Fromm-Reichman, Frieda
McNeil Pharmaceuticals 219
McGorry, Patrick Dr 245–6
medical model 28ff., 38, 40, 48, 53, 90, 92, 93, 95, 103, 107, 110, 135, 139, 241
  authoritarian imposition 201 *see also* justice: system
  confusion in 89
  consensus-building 110–11, 252–3
  critics of 165 ff., 201
  damage to 241
  deficiencies 28
  fashions in 90, 134
  flaws in 165
  key words 20
  lack of scientific evidence 28, 252, 258
  logic of denial 110
  origins of 28
  paradoxes in 104
  quality of findings 93
  researchers and public relations 235, 236
  subjective diagnoses 3, 28, 253
  types 53, 139
  unproven assumptions 252
  vs. human communication 36
medical problems 5
medicalisation 38 *see also* deviance
medical/psychiatric approach 9
  and determinism 9
medication, efficacy of 54
  forced 200
  neuroleptic 201, 227 *see also* drugs
medieval witches 181
  and analogy with modern schizophrenics 167–8
Mellaril 217
mental disease 12, 17, 22, 27, 111, 114, 149–50, 166, 197, 250, 253, 255 *see also* Bleuler; Jung, Carl; Kraepelin
  concept preceding schizophrenia 29, 136

matching symptoms with specific 33
pre-twentieth century concepts in England, France and Italy 29–30
and science 22, 255
weakness of concept 194
mental disorder 3, 5, 16, 44, 47, 175, 191, 246
  defined by *DSM-IV* 26
  spectrum 47
mental health 114, 155, 164
  care costs 13, 262
  law 1
  legislation 199, 200, 207
  model 262
  preventive programmes 15
  professional irresponsibility 201
  professionals 4, 127, 179
    literature 179
    predisposition to label mystics with mental illness 127
NSW Mental Health Act 1983 99
NSW Mental Health Act 1990 99
NSW Mental Health Amendment Bill 1995 98, 100
mental health industry 92
  expansion of 12, 18, 102
  services 91
  costs 91
'mental illness' 10, 166, 199 *see also Diagnostic and Statistical Manual of Mental Disorders*
mental illness 3, 5, 6, 9, 10, 17, 25, 38, 110, 112, 127, 130, 218, 241, 244, 256 *see also* mental health: professionals
  'alleged' 24–5 *see also* schizophrenia: alleged
  determination of 103, 172–3
  indications of 6
  manifestations of 256
  as metaphor 166
  United Nations Principles for the Protection of Persons ... 22 ff.
mental patients, chronic 185
mental pathology 9
mentally ill 188
  sterilisation of 72
mentally ill person
  and freedoms 153
  assumption of unconsciousness 106–7, 109
mentally retarded people 217
methodology 190 *see also* Rosenhan, David
Michéa, Claude 31
middle-class values 6
Mill, John Stuart 154 ff.
mind
  concept of 75, 166
  disease of 258
mind/brain dichotomy 89
minds
  diagnosticians' 173
  patients' 173, 215
M'Naghten, Daniel 198–9
mobile treatment teams 19, 215
modern industrial societies 149, 151–2
Modrow, John 182
Mohammed 124–5, 129
mood 41, 42, 45
moral model 9
  and free choice 9
mortality, knowledge of, and anxiety about 119–21, 146, 149, 154
Moses 125
mother/child bonding *see* theories: family environment; Fromm-Reichman, Frieda
Mother Jones 95
movement disorders 160, 254–5 *see also* chlorpromazine; drugs: neuroleptic
mystical
  considerations 138
  emergencies 165
  experience 5, 115–19, 124–130 ff., 135–6, 139, 140, 149, 151, 153 *see also* spiritual/mystical emergency
    attaining 121–2
    meaning 135, 149
    and meditation 122, 133–4

and modern life 149
and soundness of mind 127
and transcendence 122-3, 130
practice 142
mysticism 116 ff., 142, 165
definitions 116-17
and psychiatry 127
mystics 115-16, 123-4 *see also* Fox, George; Jesus; John the Baptist; John of Ephesus; Laing, R.D.; Mohammed; Moses; struggle for social status and power
and academic analysts 123
and religious movements 115
myth-of-mental-illness school 165 ff., 185-6, 188 *see also* Szasz, Thomas
mythology 145 ff. *see also* Campbell, Joseph
Munchausen Syndrome 187 *see also* Factitious Disorder

National Alliance for the Mentally Ill (NAMI) *see also* consumer interest groups
and the medical model 95
National Early Psychosis Project (NEPP) 226
National Institute of Mental Health 14, 72, 91, 92, 140
National Mental Health Association 237
National Mental Health Strategy 14
Nature 70
nature/nurture 53
Nazi Germany 182 *see also* psychiatric: abuse; psychiatric: profession
neuroleptic *see* drugs
New Testament 125
non-democratic political systems 257
non-medical models 111, 112 ff.
non-medical people as front-line diagnosticians 234 *see also* Schizophrenia Foundation Australia: Checklist 2
Normal 257, 259
normal

behaviour 250
boundary with schizophrenic symptoms 248
doctor/patient contractual arrangements 4
Novartis 95, 237
NSW Mental Health Act 1-2, 18, 24, 97, 101
and involuntary commitment 24, 101-2
NSW Mental Health Review Tribunal 18-19
nursing homes 216

'occupational dysfunction' 17, 110 *see also* social/occupational dysfunction
Oedipus complex 78
olanzapine (Zyprexa) 60, 61 *see also* drugs: neuroleptic: 'atypical'
outpatients, commitment of 19, 20, 215
in NSW 19, 101
by relatives and friends 101
in the United States 19, 215

'paleological thinking' 38
Paranoid Type *see* schizophrenia: subtypes; schizophrenia: and paranoia
parental role models 71-2, 84 *see also* Lidz, Theodore; theories: family stress
Parkinsonism 217
Parkinson's disease 55, 56
paternity, uncertainty about 120-1
pathology, evolving definition of 167
patient access to information 104
patients *see also* involuntary: patients
listening to 140
as not understood 173
pseudo- 189-90
unwilling 4
as witty 36
patients' rights 100 *see also* rights, human; rights: of voluntary patients
patterns of speech 43 *see also* disorganised thinking

pellagra 68
People Against Coercive Treatment (PACT) 209
Perry, John Weir 140–50, 255, 258, 261
Personal Assistance and Crisis Evaluation (PACE) 226, 228–30, 237, 241, 243
Personality Changes Following Frontal Leucotomy 214
personality disorders 11, 18, 246 *see also* Antisocial Personality Disorder
pharmaceutical
   companies 92, 93, 109, 237, 241
     grants 92
     and clinical trials 109
     by name: Abbott Laboratories 95; AstraZeneca 237, 238; Bristol-Myers Squibb 95; Eli Lilly 95, 237; ICI 96; Janssen Cilag 96, 235, 237; McNeil Pharmaceuticals 219; Novartis 95, 237; Pfizer 95, 234, 236; Sandoz 96; SmithKline Beecham 235; Solvay Pharma 235; Wyeth-Ayerst 95; Zeneca 236 *see also* drug: companies
   industry 92, 249
   market 19–20
   marketing 235
   profits 61
   research 60 *see also* interest groups
phenomenology 139–40 *see also* Jung, Carl
Phillpot, William 67
physical dangerousness 24, 91, 97–8, 101, 204
   and sports 204
placebo 94
Plath, Sylvia 210
Plato 117, 141
play-acting, medicalisation of 188
Plyushch, Leonid 219
poets 129
political, economic or social status and diagnosis 24

The Politics of Experience 133
power 146, 154
   moral 137
   psychiatric 220
   relationships 137 *see also* Jung, Carl
precautionary measure 203, 223 *see also* justice: system
pre-psychosis researchers 242 *see also* early psychosis
pre-psychotic *see* early psychosis; schizophrenia: extending the definition
preventive medicine 14, 224, 241, 245, 259 *see also* drugs: neuroleptic: 'atypical': expansion of the market
   government-sponsored 245
'primary process' thinking 39, 76
problem of living 4 *see also* problems
problem, mental 5
problem of the mind 5
problem of social adjustment 5
problems
   of behaviour 8, 105–6
   of character 7, 9
   of discipline 7
   of intelligence 7
   of living 4, 110
   of morals 7
procedural safeguards 104
'prodrome' 240 *see also* psychosis: definition: extension of
Program for Assessment and Care in Early Schizophrenia (PACES) 236
psychiatric
   abuse 20–1, 165, 219, 220–2
   belief 197
   critics 165 ff.
   diagnoses 189, 190 *see also* diagnosis
   injustice 221
   interception 248–9
   journals 93
   literature 171, 175, 225, 238, 240
   malpractices 100
   misuse of power 259
   myth 187

in Nazi Germany 20
practice 156–7
survivors 179, 209 see also Weitz, Don
theories 134 see also theories; World Psychiatric Assocation's Committee to Review the Abuse of Psychiatry
psychiatric research 37, 55, 89, 138–9, 226, 247
  anomalous nature 247
  in Australia 226
  tendency to literal 36
  and methodological problems 74, 80, 94
  and dangerousness 204
  and drug: companies 247 see also conferences
psychiatrists see also psychiatric profession: training
  American 12
  beliefs of compilers of DSM-IV 170–1
  British 52
    and Christian names of patients 52
    competence 113
  and disease model 251
  dissident 111, 168, 219
  European 59
  Melbourne 113–14
    and religion 113
  Russian 59
  scientific identity 133
  Soviet 218, 219, 220, 221
  vulnerability to 'prestige suggestion' 193
psychoanalysis 141
psychoanalytic approaches 54
psychological distress 115
  origin 138
psychologists see clinical: psychologists
psychology 191
psychotherapy 52, 143 see also talking therapy
psychiatric profession 52, 56, 80, 92, 151, 249
  biomedically oriented elements 262
  factions 53
  knowledge 254
  knowledge-deficit 112, 168
  in Nazi Germany 20
    and 'medical killing' 20
  and religious affiliation 114
  in the Soviet Union 21, 24–5, 27
  training 112, 113, 150
  in the United States 190
  in the West 21, 220
psychiatry see also International Classification of Diseases
  classification system 3, 12, 33
  as 'degradation ceremonial' 132
  expansion of 7, 26
  Kraepelinian 133
  mainstream 3
  in the Soviet Union 21–2, 24, 26, 221, 249–50
  Soviet 218
  in Western democracies 250
psychiatry and coercion 18–19, 21, 23, 27, 47, 103, 105, 153, 159, 179–80, 197 ff., 207, 209, 234, 256, 257 see also mysticism
psychosurgery 208, 212
  in Britain 212–13
  and change in intellectual functions 213–14
  in the United States 212–13
psychosis 5–6, 11, 16, 40, 41, 47, 56, 60, 68–9, 73, 75, 106, 138, 140, 144, 148, 165, 194, 228–9, 238, 242, 255, 258, 259
  approaching 228
  concept, flaws in 242
  and definitions 41, 230, 242
    extension of 226, 227, 241
    lack of precise 230
  drug-induced 240
  increasing the incidence 239
  lack of treatment and onset 231
  lifetime prevalence 242
  rates compared with pre-psychotic 242–4

and risk factors 14, 232, 234, 235
  threshold 230, 242
  transition to full 228, 229–30,
    240, 241
psychotic
  diagnosed as 3 see also psychosis
  disorders 3 see also schizophrenia:
    as most serious sub-type of
    episode 33 see also Laing, R.D.
'public health' 157
'public morals' 157
'public order' 157
'public safety' 157
punishment 5, 206 ff. see also rights:
  to protection against torture; torture

Quaker religion 126
quest for meaning 257–8
quetiapine (Seroquel) 236, 238 see
  also drugs: neuroleptic: atypical

race 14
racial groups 152
  identity see also theories: social
    stress
rationality 38, 44
  continuum 44
'rebirthing experience' 134 see also
  Laing, R.D.
receptive aphasia 42
Reformation 155
Refshauge, Dr Andrew 98
relationship between an individual
  and a professional expert 108
relatives 4, 40, 41, 91, 105–6, 109,
  227, 232, 234, 251, 255 see also
  theories: family stress; theories:
  family environment; theories: social
religion 155 ff. see also Christianity;
  client; European Christian tradition;
  religious beliefs
religious
  beliefs 48, 112–13, 151
  phenomena 139
  rights of minorities 155 see also
    psychiatrists
Residual Type see schizophrenia: sub-
types
right to act 155
right to manifest a belief 157
rights
  and democratic societies 20–1,
    24–5, 257
  economic, social, cultural 21
  to freedom of thought and belief
    152–6
  to freedom of thought, conscience
    and religion 153
  'Fundamental Freedoms and Basic
    Rights' 103
  to liberty 5, 24, 203, 214–18
  and medical containment 7
  and Nazi atrocities 20
  political see rights, human
  to protection against torture, cruel,
    inhuman or degrading treatment
    24, 215
  various 103
  of voluntary patients 23
rights, human 4, 5, 15, 20, 25, 90 ff.,
  100, 103–4, 151–3, 164, 197 ff.,
  202–3, 255 see also informed
  consent; Inquiry into Human Rights
  and Mental Illness; 'the right to
  treatment'; 'right to refuse
  treatment'; rights of the individual
  to avoid coercion and
  discrimination; right to liberty;
  activists 152
  advocates 26
  areas of protection 103
  duplicity in interpretation of 110
  and freedoms of others 1157
  harm to the exercise of 20
  law 205, 251
  of misfits 250 see also criminal:
    justice system
  'right to informed consent' 104
  supporting the medical model 103
    see also United Nations Principles
    for the Protection of Persons
  violation of 5, 20, 21, 151
  watchdog groups 15, 255–6
'right to refuse treatment' 107, 111

see also informed consent
'right to treatment' 4, 5, 18, 20, 23, 100, 103, 104–7, 110, 164
   paradoxes 107, 164
risk factors 16
risperidone (Risperdal) 93–4, 237 *see also* drugs: neuroleptic: 'atypical'
Ritalin 8
   in the United Kingdom 8
   in the United States 8
role-player, schizophrenic as 169, 184–96
Rosenhan, David 189-91
Rousseallian humanism 130
Royal College of Psychiatrists 52, 65

sales promotion 93 *see also* scientific research 93
Sandoz 96
SANE Australia *see* Schizophrenia Australia Foundation
Sarbin, Theodore 89
Sartre, Jean Paul 130
scapegoat schizophrenic 169, 180–4, 185; *see also The Manufacture of Madness*; Szasz, Thomas
Schaler, Jeffrey 201
Scheff, Thomas 190
'schizophrenia' 166
schizophrenia
   as adaptive behaviour 37–8
   alleged 153, 158, 164
   costs 91–2
   culturally determined 173
   diagnosed 152, 194, 197, 200
   diagnosis 170, 249–50, 253, 257
      and assumed incapacity for rational decisions 109
      in children, mean age 13
   as disease 28, 33, 49, 52, 110, 115, 139, 223
   disintegration of ideas in 136 *see also* Jung, Carl; theories: Jungian
   extending the definition 224
   ICD-10's description of 17
   identifying factors 17
   incidence 225
   invention of 169
   'latent' 73
   and mental illness 202–3
   as mind playing tricks on itself 195
   as most serious sub-type of psychotic disorders 3
   and mystical practices 113–14
   mystical problem associated with 149–50
   as myth 242 *see also* myth-of-mental illness
   as mythological mystical journey *see* Campbell, Joseph
   and paranoia 75 *see also* Paranoid Type
   and polio 66–7
   and political dissidents 22, 27, 218, 220, 249 *see also* psychiatry: Soviet
   as problems of living *see* problems: of living
   prodromal 227, 229, 239, 241, 243 *see also* psychosis: definitions: extension of
   psychogenesis 136–6 *see also* Jung, Carl
   rates 20, 22
   research industry 92
   risk factors 236
   simulated 189–191 *see also* symptoms: simulated
   'sluggish' 22, 25, 72, 219, 220
   as spiritual/mystical emergency *see* spiritual/mystical emergency
   as split mind *see* Bleuler
   sub-types 46, 220
   theories of cause 4, 9, 34, 53, 60, 89, 255
      biological 53–4, 65, 133, 135–7
      environmental 71–2, 74, 135
      in past experience and present environment 53–4
   types 197 *see also* mental disorder
Schizophrenia Australia Foundation 95, 99, 100, 232
   Checklist 2 232–4
   and drug: companies 99, 232

and medical model 95 *see also* interest groups
Schizophrenia Fellowship 99, 101
'schizophrenia gene' 69–71 *see also* theories: genetic
Schizophrenia Information Centre 13
schizophrenic concerns 144 *see also* Perry, John Weir
schizophrenics
    as parasites 185 *see also* Szasz, Thomas
    'real' 250–1, 258, 261–2
    as 'seers' 144, 151 *see also* Perry, John Weir
schizophrenic role, scripting of 169
'schizophrenogenic mother' 78–80, 81, 87 *see also* theories: family environment; Fromm-Reichman, Frieda
schizotypal personality disorder 227, 228
    symptoms of 228 *see also* DSM-IV
Schreber, Daniel Paul 76
science 32, 108
    and Nazi war criminals 108 *see also* mental disease: and science
Science 190
scientific
    evidence 252–3 *see also* medical model
    knowledge 167
    research 62, 92–3, 167
        into biological theories 62–3, 65
        ethics 62, 190
        method 138
        and artefacts of neuroleptic medication 62, 64–5, 254
        and sales promotion 93
        and side effects of drug treatment 62, 254 *see also* interest groups: pharmaceutical industry
The Search for the Manchurian Candidate 245
Second International Conference on Early Psychosis 237
'secondary process' thinking 39

sedation as management technique 217
self-appraisal 11
self-consciousness 120 *see also* consciousness
self-control 38
self-identity 21, 117, 122, 142, 149
self-protection 154
sense perceptions *see* consciousness: levels
severe depression 211
sex-link 74
sexual
    abuse 204
    dysfunction 11
Shakespeare, William 129
shamanism 116
Sharan, S. N. 85–6
Shellharbour Hospital 221
Sharpe, Douglas 210
shock therapy 207
shock treatment 210
Shrink Resistant: the struggle against psychiatry in Canada 209
sick role 185
'simple' schizophrenia 17 *see also* schizophrenia: sub-types
Siracusa Principles 156–7
SmithKline Beecham 235
Snezhnevsky, Andrei 219 *see also* schizophrenia: 'sluggish'
social alienation 5, 111 *see also* alienation
social
    class 88, 136–7, 147
    control 14, 17, 91, 215, 234, 249–50, 257
    exclusion 104
    functioning, as a key determinant 172
    nuisance 220
    and occupational dysfunction *see* social/occupational dysfunction
    problem
        serious 168 *see also* scapegoat; cultural outsider; role-player
    problems 184, 250, 259

relationships, difficulties in 165
status 136, 179, 244
workers *see* clinical: social workers
socially alienated class 203 *see also* social alienation
socially unacceptable 11
social/occupational dysfunction 3, 4, 5, 16, 17, 110, 170, 172–3, 178, 248, 250
as diagnostic tool 3 *see also* adolescents
societal views *see* community views
socio-economic status 16, 73
sociology 191
Socrates 117
Solvay Pharma 235
somatic therapy 113–14
SOS programme 237
Southcott, Inge Dr 97–9
spiritual aspect 257
spiritual/mystical emergency 4, 5, 110–11, 112 ff., 130, 135, 144–9, 164, 165, 166, 168, 255, 258–9, 261–2 *see also* Campbell, Joseph
Spitzer, Robert 190 *see also DSM-III*
State, the 91, 110, 251–2
Stevens, Lawrence 221
stream-of-consciousness 36
stress 78, 87 *see also* theories: family stress; theories: social stress; symptoms; Jung, Carl
struggle for social status and power 121
and mystics 121
sub-coma insulin 210
substance abuse 11
substance-related disorders 4 *see also* treatment: advocates of drug
sub-types 16, 46
suicide 101–2
and neuroleptic medication 205
and statistical evidence 101
supposedly high rate 204
Sullivan, Harry Stack 77–8, 246–7 *see also* theories: family environment
superstition 155
support groups 4, 18, 90ff

surveys
Australia 8, 10, 226–7
New Zealand 8
United States 8
suspiciousness 244–5
and irony 244–5
symptoms 4, 36, 46, 65, 91, 92, 113–14, 131, 135, 136, 138, 139, 140–1, 166, 204, 219–20, 241, 248, 253 *see also* catatonic behaviour; delusions; disorganised speech; disorganised thinking; *DSM-IV*; drugs: side effects; drugs: neuroleptic: side effects; hallucinations; schizotypal personality disorder; voices
accessory 35 *see also* Bleuler
active phase 45–6
acute 212 *see also* ECT
clinical guidelines (Australia) 231–2, 234, 235, 237
and compilers of 235
cultural bias 174
definition of 27
disease interpretation 252
duration 45
fundamental 35
as manufactured 130 *see also* Szasz, Thomas
as manufactured artefacts 165 ff., 180
'negative' 3, 43–5, 170, 175–80, 220
non-deteriorating 34
as pathology 92
'positive' 3, 43, 63, 170, 175, 200
pre-psychotic 225
lack of consensus 226, 245, 248
see also schizophrenia
primary 138, 158
'prodromal' 224, 226, 227, 228, 229, 231 *see also* early psychosis; schizophrenia: extending the definition
psychotic, as a side effect of drug treatment 161
schizoid 133 *see also* Laing, R.D.

schizotypal 231
secondary 138
simulated 169, 188–91
of stress 139
words used 177
Substance-related disorders 261
Szasz, Thomas 16, 130, 168, 179, 181, 185-6, 201-2, 220

talking therapists 54
talking therapy 53–4, 75, 89, 91, 113 *see also* psychotherapy
  varieties 76
  and personal responsibility 114
tardive dyskinesia *see* drugs: neuroleptic: and side effects
Temerlin, Maurice 191–4
Tennyson, Alfred Lord 121–2
theories 53, 90
  associationist 32
  biochemical 55, 138
  biological 62, 69, 75, 133, 135, 136–7
  biology vs. experience 53–4
  developmental 76–8
  'dopamine' 55–6, 217, 218
  double bind 81–4
  enlarged ventricles 64–5
  environmental 71–2, 74, 75
  evolutionary 140–9 *see also* Perry, John Weir; Campbell, Joseph
  faculty 32
  family environment 78–9
  family stress 84–8
  genetic 69–75
  Jungian 135–40, 148
  link with influenza 236
  mystical 130–5, 149–50 *see also* Campbell, Joseph
  nutritional 67–9
  psychogenesis 137–8 *see also* Jung, Carl
  regression 38–40
  rise and fall 89, 90
  'season of birth' 232, 235, 236
  social stress 88
  unconfirmed 235
  viral 66–7
therapies, proliferation of 89 *see also* biomedical treatments; 'fear therapy'; infection; insulin coma; psychosocial; psychotherapy; shock; talking therapies
thinking processes, effects on *see* treatment: effects on
Thorazine 162, 163, 220 *see also* chlorpromazine
thought disorder 32, 35, 36, 75
  early theories 32
Time 219, 220
torture 204–5, 212
Tow, P. MacDonald 214
tranquillisers major 159 *see also* drugs: neuroleptic
treatment 3, 9, 18
  adverse reactions to 241 *see also* drugs
  advocates of drug 20
  claims to prevent psychosis and lack of evidence 230–1
  coercion 159 ff.
  cruel 204–14, 222
  as dehumanising and depersonalising 222
  drug 53, 89, 92
    dangerous 89
    forced 4, 164, 169, 197, 203, 221, 249, 257 *see also* involuntary
  drugs
    as punishment and torture 214–18
  effects on thinking processes 160 ff.
  first choice 215
  forced 2, 3, 4, 5, 96, 98, 102, 110, 152, 156, 197, 209–10, 221
  humane 104
  involuntary *see* forced (above)
  medical
    as experimental 206
    more sophisticated 208
    rationale for 206
    as torture 207

methods of 53–4
neuroleptic 160–2 *see also* drugs:
  neuroleptic
and psychiatrists' beliefs 197
and torture, difference 212 *see also* ECT
and psychiatrists' religious
  affiliations 113–14
pre-psychosis programme 225,
  234, 242
pre-psychosis 242
  literature 242 *see also*
    psychiatric: literature
in pre-psychotic state 230
torture 212, 218–23
unnecessary 230
views on 53
without drugs 255
without normal evidence for
  mental illness 241
treatment-as-animals 38
treatment decisions 114 *see also*
  psychiatrists: and religion 114
troublesome citizens 27
truth 5, 7, 255
twins 73–5 *see also* adoption studies;
  Kety study; theories: genetic

unconscious 142, 148
Undifferentiated Type *see*
  schizophrenia: sub-types
unemployment 16, 17–18, 88, 179
  in Australia 17
  and ICD-10's description of
    schizophrenia 17
  levels 27 *see also* social class
United Nations (UN) 5, 103
  Centre for Human Rights 155
  Commission on Human Rights
    22–3, 155
  Declaration on the Elimination of
    all Forms of Intolerance and of
    Discrimination Based on Religion
    or Belief 154
  General Assembly 23, 108
  and international psychiatric
    practice 22

  and international standards 108
  Principles for the Protection of
    Persons with Mental Illness and
    for the Improvement of Mental
    Health Care 23 ff., 103–5
    and more coercion 23
    paradoxes 104
    and involuntary detention 23–4
Universal Declaration of Human
  Rights 153
unrequited love as a pathological
  symptom 47
United States' policy analysts 186

The Varieties of Religious Experience
  127–8 *see also* James, William
violation *see* rights, human
visionary states 148
visions 123
Vitamin B12 deficiency *see* theories:
  nutritional
voices 3, 42, 45, 123, 171–2, 175,
  189, 250 *see also* hallucinations
voluntary patients 4, 9, 91, 104
  and rights *see* rights *see also*
    informed consent

watchdog groups *see* Australian
  Human Rights and Equal
  Opportunity Commission; rights,
  human: watchdog
Watts, James 213
Weitz, Don 209
welfare burden 186
  dependency *see* social class
Western Psychiatric Institute and
  Clinic (WPIC) 236
whistleblower 183–4 *see also*
  scapegoat
Whistleblowers Australia 184
Williamson, Wendell 200
'word salad' *see* receptive aphasia
workplaces 183 *see also* scapegoat
World Health Organisation (WHO)
  10, 40
World Psychiatric Association (WPA)
  22, 218, 219

expulsion of the Soviet
  professional organisation 22
and international standards 22, 24,
  25, 104
World Psychiatric Association's
  Committee to Review the Abuse of
  Psychiatry 184
Wyeth-Ayerst 95

ziprasidone (Zeldox) 234 *see also*
  pharmaceutical: companies: by
  name; drugs: neuroleptic: atypical;
  Australian Human Rights and Equal
  Opportunity Commission
Zeneca 236 *see also* AstraZeneca